Series Editor

Prof. Dr. Michael J. Parnham
PLIVA
Research Institute
Prilaz baruna Filipovica 25
10000 Zagreb
Croatia

Cytokines in Severe Sepsis and Septic Shock

Heinz Redl
Günther Schlag[†]

Editors

Birkhäuser Verlag
Basel · Boston · Berlin

Editors

Prof. Dr. Heinz Redl
Prof. Dr. Günther Schlag†
Ludwig Boltzmann Institute for
Experimental and Clinical Traumatology
Donaueschingenstrasse 13
A-1200 Vienna

Austria

A CIP catalogue record for this book is available from the Library of Congress, Washington D.C., USA

Deutsche Bibliothek Cataloging-in-Publication Data

Cytokines in severe sepsis and septic shock / ed. by H. Redl, G. Schlag... - Basel ; Boston ;
Berlin : Birkhäuser, 1999
    (Progress in inflammation research)
    ISBN 3-7643-5877-7 (Basel...)
    ISBN 0-8176-5877-7 (Boston)

© 1999 Birkhäuser Verlag, P.O. Box 133, CH-4010 Basel, Switzerland
Printed on acid-free paper produced from chlorine-free pulp. TCF ∞
Cover design: Markus Etterich, Basel
Printed in Germany
ISBN 3-7643-5877-7
ISBN 0-8176-5877-7

9 8 7 6 5 4 3 2 1

Contents

List of contributors

Edward Abraham, Division of Pulmonary Sciences and Critical Care Medicine, Box C272, University of Colorado Health Sciences Center, 4200 E. Ninth Avenue, Denver, Colorado 80262, USA; e-mail: edward.abraham@uchsc.edu

Alfred Ayala, Center for Surgical Research, Rhode Island Hospital, Middle House II, 593 Eddy Street, Providence, RI 02903, USA; e-mail: Aayala@RIHOSP.edu

Soheyl Bahrami, Ludwig Boltzmann Institute for Experimental and Clinical Traumatology, Donaueschingenstr. 13, A-1200 Vienna, Austria

Michael Bergmann, Chirurgische Forschungslaboratorien, Universitätsklinik für Chirurgie/Akh, N. Währinger Gürtel 18–20, A-1090 Wien, Austria

Maarten G. Bouma, Department of Surgery, Maastricht University (Fac. II), P.O. Box 616, NL-6200 MD Maastricht, The Netherlands

Wim A. Buurman, Department of Surgery, Maastricht University (Fac. II), P.O. Box 616, NL-6200 MD Maastricht, The Netherlands;
e-mail: w.buurman@ah.unimaas.nl

Jean-Marc Cavaillon, Unité d'Immuno-Allergie, Institut Pasteur, 28 rue Dr. Roux, F-75724 Paris cedex 15, France; e-mail: jmcavail@pasteur.fr

Irshad H. Chaudry, Center for Surgical Research, Rhode Island Hospital, Middle House II, 593 Eddy Street, Providence, RI 02903, USA;
e-mail: IChaudry@lifespan.org

David Creery, Eaton North 9-234, Toronto Hospital, General Division, 200 Elizabeth Street, Toronto, Ontario, Canada, M5G 2C4

Regina Flach, Klinische Forschergruppe "Schock und Multiorganversagen" der DFG, Zentrum für Chirurgie, Universitätsklinikum Essen, Hufelandstr. 55, D-45122 Essen, Germany

Sergio Grinstein, Division of Cell Biology, The Hospital for Sick Children, 555 University Avenue, Toronto, Ontario M5G 1X8, Canada

C. Erik Hack, Central Laboratory of the Netherlands Red Cross Blood Transfusion Service, Plesmanlaan 125, NL-1066 CX Amsterdam, The Netherlands

David J. Hackam, Department of Surgery, The Toronto Hospital, 200 Elizabeth Street EN9-232, Toronto, Ontario M5G 2C4, Canada, and Division of Cell Biology, The Hospital for Sick Children, 555 University Avenue, Toronto, Ontario M5G 1X8, Canada; e-mail: dhackam@torhosp.toronto.on.ca

Thomas Hirsch, Klinische Forschergruppe "Schock und Multiorganversagen" der DFG, Zentrum für Chirurgie, Universitätsklinikum Essen, Hufelandstr. 55, D-45122 Essen, Germany

Bernhard Holzmann, Department of Surgery, Klinikum rechts der Isar, Technical University of Munich, Ismaninger Str. 22, D-81675 Munich, Germany; e-mail: holzmann@nt1.chir.med.tu-muenchen.de

Hartmut Jaeschke, Pharmacia & Upjohn, Inc., Kalamazoo, MI, USA

John C. Marshall Eaton North 9-234, Toronto Hospital, General Division, 200 Elizabeth Street, Toronto, Ontario, Canada, M5G2C4; e-mail: jmarshall@torhosp.toronto.on.ca

Brigitte Neumann, Department of Surgery, Klinikum rechts der Isar, Technical University of Munich, Ismaninger Str. 22, D-81675 Munich, Germany; e-mail: Brigitte.Neumann@lrz.tum.de

Steven M. Opal, Infectious Disease Division, Memorial Hospital of Rhode Island, 111 Brewster Sreet, Pawtucket, RI 02860, USA; e-mail: Steven_Opal@brown.edu

Michael A. Rogy, University of Vienna, AKH Wien, Department of Surgery, Währingergürtel 18-20, A-1090 Wien, Austria; e-mail: Michael.Rogy@akh-wien.ac.at

Erich Roth, Chirurgische Forschungslaboratorien, Universitätsklinik für Chirurgie/ Akh, Währinger Gürtel 18-20, A-1090 Wien, Austria; e-mail: E.Roth@akh-wien.ac.at

Ori D. Rotstein, Department of Surgery, The Toronto Hospital, 200 Elizabeth Street EN9-232, Toronto, Ontario M5G 2C4, Canada; e-mail: orotstein@torhosp.toronto.on.ca

F. Ulrich Schade, Klinische Forschergruppe "Schock und Multiorganversagen" der DFG, Zentrum für Chirurgie, Universitätsklinikum Essen, Hufelandstr. 55, D-45122 Essen, Germany; e-mail: shock@uni-essen.de

Ralph R. Schumann, Universitätsklinikum Charité, Medizinische Fakultät der Humboldt-Universität zu Berlin, Institut für Mikrobiologie und Hygiene, Dorotheenstr. 96–98, D-10117 Berlin, Germany

Scott I. Simon, Section of Leukocyte Biology, Children's Nutrition Research Center, 1100 Bates, Room 6014, Houston, Texas 77030-2600, USA

C. Wayne Smith, Section of Leukocyte Biology, Children's Nutrition Research Center, 1100 Bates, Room 6014, Houston, Texas 77030-2600, USA

Wolfgang Strohmaier, Ludwig Boltzmann Institute for Experimental and Clinical Traumatology, Donaueschingenstrasse 13, A-1200 Wien, Austria

Frank Stüber, Klinik und Poliklinik für Anästhesiologie und spezielle Intensivmedizin, Friedrich-Wilhelms-Universität Bonn, Siegmund-Freud-Str. 25, D-53105 Bonn, Germany; e-mail: umc80e@ibm.rhrz.uni-bonn.de

Franz Tatzber, Institute for Biochemistry, Schubertstrasse 1, A-8010 Graz, Austria

Christoph Thiemermann, The William Harvey Research Institute, St. Bartholomew's and the Royal London School of Medicine and Dentistry, Charterhouse Square, London EC1M 6BQ, UK; e-mail: c.thiemermann@mds.qmw.ac.uk

Ping Wang, Center for Surgical Research, Rhode Island Hospital, Middle House II, 593 Eddy Street, Providence, RI 02903, USA

Timothy D. Warner, The William Harvey Research Institute, St. Bartholomew's and the Royal London School of Medicine and Dentistry, Charterhouse Square, London EC1M 6BQ, UK

R. William G. Watson, Surgical Professorial Unit, Mater Hospital, University College Dublin, 47 Eccles Street, Dublin 7, Ireland; e-mail:research@profsurg.iol.ie

Peter Zabel, Forschungszentrum Borstel, Zentrum für Medizin und Biowissenschaften, Parkallee 35, D-23845 Borstel, Germany

René Zellweger, Department of Trauma Surgery, University of Zurich, CH-8091 Zürich, Switzerland

Preface and introduction

Heinz Redl and Günther Schlag[+]

Ludwig Boltzmann Institute for Experimental and Clinical Traumatology, Vienna, Austria

The word "sepsis" derives from the Greek meaning decay or rottenness. Traditionally this term has been used to describe the process of infection accompanied by the host's systemic inflammatory response. Based on that understanding, previous clinical studies have been designed to include only patients with positive blood cultures [1, 2]. However, the frequent occurrence of a septic response without the demonstration of microorganisms in the circulation has led to a new definition and understanding of sepsis, mainly as the systemic response of the host to an often undetectable microbiological or non-microbiological process [3].

The general consensus is that cytokines are central to the inflammatory response, particularly in sepsis. It is now known that not only Gram-negative but also Gram-positive, viral, and fungal infections initiate the complex cascades of cytokine release. Probably the most important aspect of bacterial action is the release of toxic bacterial products. In particular endotoxin from Gram-negative bacteria (see chapter by Schade) and super antigens (see chapter by Neumann and Holzmann), as well as pore-forming toxins [4] from Gram-positive bacteria, induce cytokine formation. The importance of this cytokine release is evident from both diagnostic and therapeutic (mostly experimental) studies, and the action of cytokines may be the key to our understanding of the pathophysiology of the sepsis syndrome.

Therefore we set out to put together 20 chapters to deal with the different aspects of cytokine induction, monitoring, cytokine actions and therapeutic opportunities in this complicated network (Fig. 1). We were most fortunate that world experts were willing to contribute to this endeavor despite their normal workload, and we would like to take this opportunity to thank all of them.

Most of the cytokines are not produced, at least not detectably under baseline normal conditions, but are induced during infection/gut translocation by bacteria/bacterial products, as described in the first two chapters by Schade and Holzmann. From the recognition/binding of bacterial products there are several intermediate steps – the signal transduction cascade – that lead to transcription of the specific mRNAs (as described by Rotstein). Both the transcription and many posttranscriptional events are dependent on multiple factors such as sex, age and nutrition-

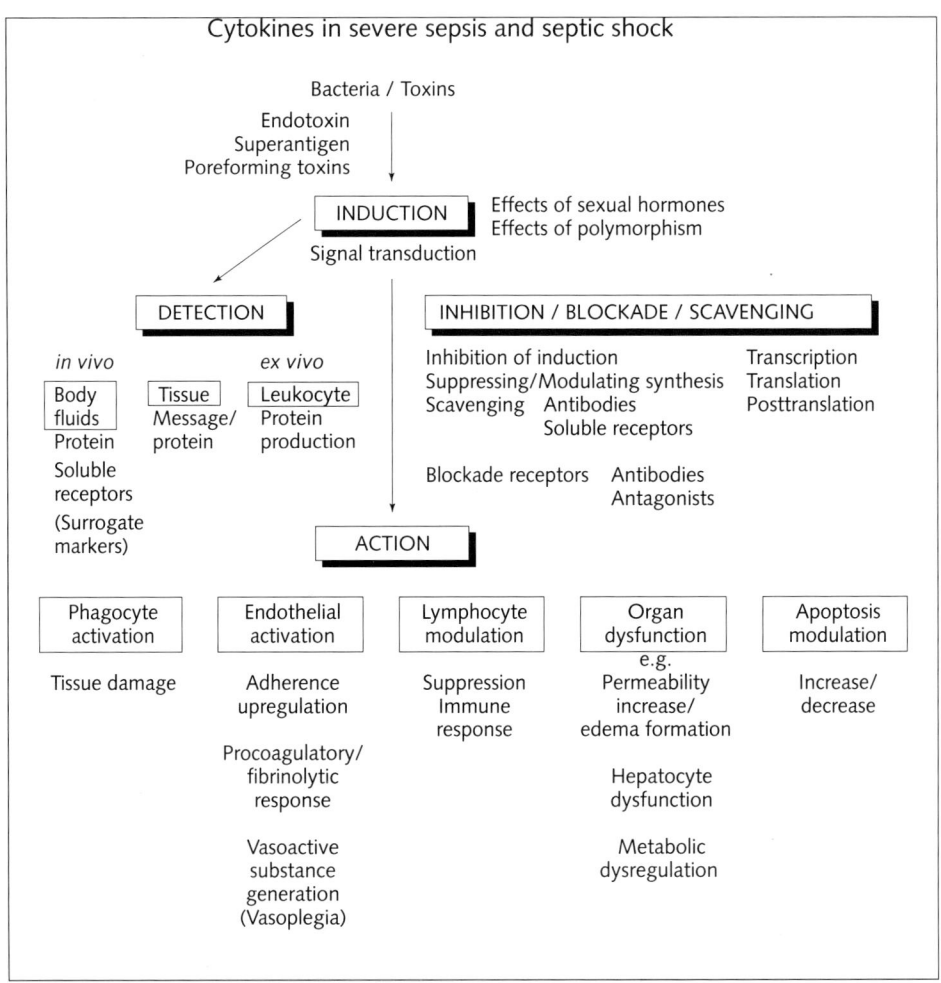

Figure 1
Schematic representation of the topics covered in this book.

al status, as well as genetic predisposition in term of polymorphisms. These aspects are combined in the section predisposing factors and discussed by Zellweger and Chaudry and by Stüber.

One important aspect in the understanding of the cytokine network in sepsis is the ability to detect and measure the cytokines (as discussed by Cavaillon), which is a difficult task due to their local production and action, low levels, and short half-life. The short half-life in plasma is due partly to binding to receptors, including the soluble circulating cytokine receptors, which not only neutralize cytokines but are diagnostic tools in themselves (as discussed by Buurman). An approach to avoid the difficulties associated with cytokine monitoring is the use of so-called surrogate markers for sepsis monitoring, of which the macrophage activation marker neopterin [5] and procalcitonin [6] are the best known (see chapter by Strohmaier).

Cytokines act in an autocrine, paracrine and hormonal fashion, and a few selected actions of cytokines are discussed in the third section. One of the cytokine-induced events is the production of vasoactive mediators, such as nitric oxide (NO) formation from inducible NO synthase (iNOS) [7, 8], which can lead ultimately to vasoplegia or the counteracting cytokine-dependent production of endothelin [9] (discussed in the chapter by Thiemermann). Many studies of NOS inhibition have been performed, with partly contradictory results; the discrepancies are mainly related to type, dose, and time of inhibitor application (for recent review see [10]). With an appropriate study design, non-selective inhibitors are also beneficial, even in non-human primates [11]; on the other hand, new interesting approaches with so-called selective iNOS inhibitors have been tried [12]. The vasoregulatory activities are endothelial-related, similar to adherence molecule upregulation (see chapter by Smith) and many procoagulatory and fibrinolytic events induced by cytokines. The important procoagulatory action of cytokines and fibrinolysis are thoroughly discussed by Hack.

A very recent aspect of the action of cytokines is their influence on apoptosis, with increasing or suppressing effects depending on the cytokine. This is discussed with respect to neutrophils in the chapter by Watson. A completely different action of cytokines is the redirection of metabolism, an important long-term aspect, as described by Roth.

Whenever something is supposed to be a key actor in inducing sepsis and organ failure, countermeasures are proposed. However, sepsis reactions take place within the complicated network of a partly overactivated and partly oversuppressed local and systemic inflammatory response [13], so it is often difficult to identify the good guys and the bad guys. Despite this lack of knowledge and the limited or even nonexistent monitoring possibilities, enormous resources have been put into therapeutic studies (see chapters by Opal and Abraham).

There are several potential levels and time windows for interference in the sepsis process (Fig. 1), and chapters were solicited dealing with the different possible levels of interference. The conceptually less difficult therapeutic intervention is scavenging the inducers, e.g. endotoxin, as described by Opal, because there is little to no interference with the body's immune system. One particularly promising tool is bactericidal permeability-increasing protein, with excellent efficacy in gut translocation [14] and in sepsis in non-human primates [15], and meningococcemia patients [16]. If the inducers cannot be fought as a first line of defense, there is still the possibility of attenuating the host's cytokine response while interfering at the transcriptional or posttranscriptional level of cytokine production, as outlined in the chapter by Zabel and Bahrami, with the potential benefit of reducing, but not eliminating, cytokine production. The neutralization of potentially (teleologically) useful cytokines, an inherent problem of therapeutic strategies with anti-cytokine anti-bodies, soluble receptor constructs or cytokine receptor blockers, is discussed by Abraham. That a blockade to cytokines is not the only useful therapeutic approach in sepsis is outlined in the chapter by Chaudry, where different possibilities of immunomodulation are described. Finally, there is a chapter on potential future applications of gene therapy to modulate the sepsis response, especially with anti-inflammatory cytokines (Rogy). However, there are several hurdles to be overcome before the technique can be used in patients.

So far there has been only meagre success of clinical trials in sepsis patients (as discussed in the final section by Marshall). According to Knaus, approximately 7500 patients have been enrolled in 22 multicenter phase II/III clinical trials of immunotherapy [17].

Lack of success has been attributed in part to the following:

- inactive or inadequate drugs (e.g. HA-1A against LPS, sTNF receptor 75 kDa against TNF)
- heterogeneous patient populations (case mix)
- imprecise inclusion criteria, e.g. SIRS or sepsis criteria [1]
- using only outcome as a measure of efficacy; this may be insufficient (small signal to noise ratio), since improved organ function may not always translate into improved survival
- difficult timing of pharmacological intervention (when and for how long?)

Furthermore, some investigators claim that preclinical trials with inappropriate models would lead to suboptimal clinical protocols. Therefore, the two last chapters by Marshall deal with the problems of preclinical models (as also discussed in [18]), the clinical set-up and possible improvements in sepsis trials.

Improvements could include

- increase in homogeneity of patients enrolled, by conducting medium-sized instead of large clinical trials, but only with patients exhibiting similar underlying disease
- risk classification with scoring systems, e.g. by Pilz [19] or calculated risk stratification [20, 21]
- selection of only moderately severe cases with a high likelihood of improvement upon therapeutic intervention.

A further crucial issue is monitoring of the inflammatory/immunological status. This can be done by measuring circulating mediators, e.g. cytokines (see chapter by Cavaillon for possibilities and limitations) or surrogate markers as discussed by Strohmaier. Furthermore, the status of circulating cells, e.g. monocytes for levels of HLA-DR expression [22], can be used.

Criteria for inclusion/exclusion of patients could be based on these diagnoses. On the other hand, an evaluation based on the microcirculatory assessment of patient status (regional perfusion), e.g. tonometry (pHi) [23] and muscle pO_2 [24], should be considered.

We sincerely hope that this collection of contributions by outstanding scientists will boost the understanding of the role of cytokines in the development and consequences of sepsis and thus help to achieve improvements in diagnosis and treatment.

Acknowledgments

We would like to dedicate this book to the partners and families of the contributors as some slight compensation for the reduced attention from the authors and editors. We also want to thank M. Serres and C. Wilfing for their excellent support in putting this book together, as well as M. Großauer for preparing this article.

References

1   Bone RC, Fisher CJ Jr., Clemmer TP, Slotman GJ, Metz CA,Balk RA (1987) A controlled clinical trial of high-dose methylprednisolone in the treatment of severe sepsis and septic shock. *N Engl J Med* 317: 653–658

2   Sprung CL, Caralis PV, Marcial EH, Pierce M, Gelbard MA, Long WM, Duncan RC, Rendler MD, Karpf M (1984) The effect of high dose corticosteroids in patients with septic shock: a prospective, controlled study. *N Engl J Med* 311: 1137–1143

3   Goris RJ, te Boekhorst TP, Nuytinck JK, Gimbrere JS (1985) Multiple-organ failure. Generalized autodestructive inflammation? *Arch Surg* 120: 1109–1115

4   Bhakdi S, Tranum-Jensen J (1991) Alpha toxin of Staphylococcus aureus. *Microbiol Rev* 55: 733–751

5   Strohmaier W, Redl H, Schlag G, Inthorn D (1987) D-erythro-neopterin plasma levels in intensive care patients with and without septic complications. *Crit Care Med* 15: 757–760

6   Assicot M, Gendrel D, Carsin H, Raymond J, Guilbaud J, Bohuon C (1993) High serum procalcitonin concentration in patients with sepsis and infection. *Lancet* 341: 515–518

7   Kilbourn RG, Szabo C,Traber DL (1997) Beneficial versus detrimental effects of nitric oxide synthase inhibitors in circulatory shock: lessons learned from experimental and clinical studies. *Shock* 7: 235–246

8   Kilbourn R, Griffith O (1992) Overproduction of nitric oxide in cytokine-mediated and septic shock. *J Natl Cancer Inst* 84: 827–831

9   Redl H, Schlag G, Bahrami S, Kargl R, Hartter W, Woloszczuk W, Davies J (1994) Big-endothelin release in baboon bacteria is partially TNF dependent. *J Lab Clin Med* 124: 796–801

10   Schlag G, Redl H (eds) (1998) *Sixth Wiggers Bernard Conference: Shock, Sepsis, and Organ Failure – Nitric Oxide Synthase Inhibition.* Springer-Verlag, Heidelberg, Berlin

11   Schlag G, Redl H, Gasser H, Davies J, Rees D, Grover R (1997) Delayed treatment with the NO-synthase inhibitor 546C88 in a baboon model of septic shock. *Am J Respir Crit Care Med* 155: A263

12   Bahrami S, Strohmaier W, Gasser H, Peichl G, Fürst W, Fitzal F, Werner ER, Schlag G

(1997) 2,4-Diamino-5,6,7,8-tetrahydro-6-(1-erythro-1,2-dihydroxypropyl) pteridine (4-ABH4) reduces nitric oxide formation and improves survival rate in experimental endotoxin shock. *Shock* 8 (Suppl.): 54

13 Yao YM, Redl H, Bahrami S, Schlag G (1998) The inflammatory basis of trauma/shock-associated multiple organ failure. *Inflamm Res* 47: 201–210

14 Yao YM, Bahrami S, Leichtfried G, Redl H, Schlag G (1995) Pathogenesis of hemorrhage-induced bacteria-endotoxin translocation in rats: effects of recombinant bactericidal-increasing protein (rBPI21). *Ann Surg* 221: 398–405

15 Schlag G, Redl H, Davies J, Scannon PJ (1997) The protective effect of bactericidal permeability increasing protein (rBPI21) is more related to its anti-bactericidal than anti-endotoxin properties in baboon sepsis. *Shock* 8 (Suppl.): 20

16 Giroir BP, Quint PA, Barton P, Kirsch EA, Kitchen L, Goldstein B, Nelson BJ, Wedel NI, Carroll SF, Scannon PJ (1997) Preliminary evaluation of recombinant amino terminal fragment of human bactericidal permeability increasing protein in children with severe meningococcal sepsis. *Lancet* 350: 1439–1443

17 Knaus WA (1996) Scrutinizing sepsis: cells, cytokines, computer, and clinical sense. *Second Annual: Sepsis/SIRS: Reducing mortality to patients & suppliers, February 12–13, 1996.* Washington, DC: 1

18 Redl H, Schlag G, Bahrami S, Yao YM (1996) Animal models as the basis of pharmacologic interventions in trauma and sepsis. *World J Surg* 20: 487–492

19 Pilz G, Fateh-Moghadam S, Viell B, Bujdoso O, Döring G, Marget W, Neumann R, Werdan K (1993) Supplemental immunoglobulin therapy in sepsis and septic shock – comparison of mortality under treatment with polyvalent i.v. immunoglobulin versus placebo: protocol of a multicenter, randomized, prospective, double-blind trial. *Theor Surg* 8: 61–83

20 Knaus WA, Sun X, Hakim RB, Wagner DP (1994) Evaluation of definitions for adult respiratory distress syndrome. *Am J Respir Crit Care Med* 150: 311–317

21 Fisher CJ Jr., Dhainaut JF, Opal SM, Pribble JP, Balk RA, Slotman GJ, Iberti TJ, Rackow EC, Shapiro MJ, Greenman RL et al (1994) Recombinant human interleukin 1 receptor antagonist in the treatment of patients with sepsis syndrome. Results from a randomized, double-blind, placebo-controlled trial. Phase III rhIL-1ra Sepsis Syndrome Study Group. *JAMA* 271: 1836–1843

22 Volk HD, Reinke P, Falck P, Staffa G, Briedigkeit H, vonBaehr R (1989) Diagnostic value of an immune monitoring program for the clinical management of immunosuppressed patients with septic complications. *Clin Transplant* 3: 246–252

23 Gutierrez G, Palizas F, Doglio G, Wainsztein N, Gallesio A, Pacin J, Dubin A, Schiavi E, Jorge M, Pusajo J et al (1992) Gastric intramucosal pH as a therapeutic index of tissue oxygenation in critically ill patients. *Lancet* 339: 195–199

24 Boekstegers P, Weidenhöfer S, Zell R, Holler E, Kapsner T, Redl H, Schlag G, Kaul M, Kempeni J, Werdan K (1994) Changes in skeletal muscle PO2 after administration of anti-TNF alpha-antibody in patients with severe sepsis: comparison to interleukin-6 serum levels, APACHE II, and Elebute scores. *Shock* 1: 246–253

Induction

Endotoxin as an inducer of cytokines

F. Ulrich Schade[1], Regina Flach[1], Thomas Hirsch[1] and Ralph R. Schumann[2]

[1]Klinische Forschergruppe "Schock und Multiorganversagen" der DFG, Zentrum für Chirurgie, Universitätsklinikum Essen, Hufelandstr. 55, D-45122 Essen, Germany; [2]Universitätsklinikum Charité, Medizinische Fakultät der Humboldt-Universität zu Berlin, Institut für Mikrobiologie und Hygiene, Dorotheenstr. 96–98, D-10117 Berlin, Germany

Endotoxins were suspected of being related to the pathophysiology of Gram-negative bacterial infections since the time when R. Pfeiffer and E. Centanni independently found that different species of these microorganisms contained a heat stable pyrogenic material. This was termed endotoxin based on its tight association with the microorganisms. Intensive studies, in particular during the last two decades, have established the detailed chemical structure of the endotoxins in most of the clinically-relevant microbes (reviewed in [1]). The finding that application of highly purified endotoxins to experimental animals and humans induces major signs of bacteriosis, such as fever, hemodynamic disorders, shock, and many others (reviewed in [2]) gave reason to suspect endotoxin as being a major component in the pathogenesis of sepsis. Bacterial components, including endotoxins, have been administered to patients for almost one hundred years as a treatment for malignancies [3] and as an experimental model for the acute inflammatory response with similarities to the initial response of humans to bacterial sepsis.

Effects of endotoxin on humans

The intravenous application of 2–4 ng/kg endotoxin to human volunteers causes a monophasic rise in core temperature which is accompanied by chills and rigors within one hour after endotoxin administration [4]. The peak core temperature rises to 38.5°–40°C and symptoms of nausea, headache and myalgia reach a maximum within 2 h [5]. Studies performed in humans have shown that pyrogenic doses of endotoxin evoke a hyperdynamic cardiovascular response. Furthermore, it was found in healthy volunteers that endotoxin altered pulmonary function with a fall in PaO_2 and $PaCO_2$ and widening of the alveolar-arterial oxygen gradient [6]. Bronchoalveolar lavage indicated an increase in the permeability to small molecules, while changes in the permeability to larger molecules were minimal [6].

As a consequence of the application of low doses of endotoxin (2–4 ng/kg), the coagulation system and the fibrinolytic system are activated, which is gradually inhibited by increasing levels of plasminogen activator inhibitor 1 within 2–3 h [5, 7]. The plasma contact system is activated, resulting in the formation of bradykinin which causes vasodilatation and increased transcapillary flux [8].

Several findings suggest that neutrophils are activated as a consequence of endotoxin administration. The content of neutrophil elastase is increased in the circulation 2–3 h after endotoxin [7], cell surface C3-receptors are upregulated by 3 h post endotoxin [9] and neutrophils were found to be primed for enhanced superoxide production *ex vivo* [10] as a result of endogenous mediator production caused by endotoxin. Alveolar macrophages obtained from normal humans after endotoxin were found to exhibit a similar pattern of priming [11].

Two cases have been reported in which high doses of endotoxin were applied to humans. A 14 year old boy received 100 ml of packed erythrocytes contaminated with endotoxin from *Pseudomonas fluorescens* (40000 EU/ml) and developed a life-threatening septic shock [12]. In a suicide attempt, a laboratory worker injected 1 mg purified *Salmonella minnesota* lipopolysaccharide (LPS) i.v. [13]. Both patients survived.

The above data show that small doses of endotoxin induce sepsis-like symptoms in humans, leading to the formation of major inflammatory mediators, and in higher amounts may cause life-threatening circulatory and multiple-organ failure.

Endotoxins in septic shock

While it has been suggested for a long time that endotoxins play a major role in human sepsis shock, quantitative studies of LPS in the plasma of septic patients were not possible until the introduction of the Limulus amoebocyte lysate (LAL) assay [14]. It was first reported by Levin et al. that the clinical severity of sepsis caused by Gram-negative bacteria was correlated with positive Limulus determinations in plasma. This finding was confirmed by others [15, 16]. In particular in systemic meningococcal disease, circulating levels of LPS have been correlated quantitatively to the activation of mediator systems, especially TNFα, involved in the pathogenesis of septic shock and revealed a dose-dependent association of plasma endotoxin levels with mortality [17]. In these patients levels of endotoxin correlated with disease severity. Plasma levels of 800ng/l or higher predicted the development of persistent septic shock, impaired renal function, ARDS, and massive coagulopathy.

Therefore, in systemic meningococcal disease a clear relationship seems to exist between endotoxemia, as determined by Limulus assay in the plasma, and Gram-negative bacteremia. However, in patients of diverse pathogenicity, including Gram-positive bacteremia, this correlation is much less than clear. Danner et al. examined

100 patients with septic shock and found that in 43% of these, plasma specimens were positive in a sensitive chromogenic Limulus assay [18]. In patients with positive blood cultures, endotoxemia was associated with high mortality. Interestingly, only 26% of the endotoxemic patients had documented Gram-negative bacteremia, on the other hand, 14% of endotoxin-negative patients grew Gram-negative organisms from their blood culture. Further, circulating endotoxin was found in some patients with isolated Gram-positive bacteremia or Candida septicemia. Therefore, a positive Limulus test did not predict the presence of Gram-negative sepsis or the absence of Gram-positive or fungal sepsis.

Recently a multicenter study was carried out to examine the use of a chromogenic LAL blood assay in a population of 346 patients with sepsis syndrome in eight clinical centers in the USA. [19]. No correlation was found between a positive LAL result and Gram-negative bacteremia or Gram-negative infection. Furthermore, no association was found between endotoxemia and mortality in patients with positive blood cultures, as was reported by Danner et al. [18]. Therefore, the predictive value of endotoxin determination in sepsis patients seems to be limited. One major reason for this discrepancy may be that "the microbiology of the 'sepsis syndrome' population varies widely from center to center and is influenced by treatment modalities and therapies for the sepsis syndrome that change over time", as stated in [19].

From this data it is suggested that endotoxin is an important mediator of septic shock although bacterial products other than endotoxin, and host-related factors, may be important contributors to toxicity and mortality in Gram-negative septic shock. This supports efforts to develop antiendotoxin therapies for treating patients with this disease. Such efforts include the use of crossreacting antibodies against endotoxin (reviewed in [68]). Future therapies may evolve from the knowledge of the interactions of endotoxins with mammalian cells.

Endotoxin recognition and host regulation of LPS activity

LPS in the circulation of the host will be bound to a certain degree by "high density lipoprotein" (HDL), which attenuates its effects both [20–22] *in vitro* and *in vivo*. Apolipoproteins and "low density lipoprotein" (LDL) have also been shown to bind LPS, inhibit its cell-stimulatory potential [23, 24], and LDL-receptor knock-out mice were protected against endotoxic shock [25]. Several humoral factors have been described exhibiting the ability to bind LPS: the cationic proteins (CAP) 18, 37, and P15A/P15B, a 28 kDa mannose binding protein, albumin, transferrin, lactoferrin, hemoglobin, and lysozyme (reviewed in [26]). It has, however, not been shown as to whether binding of these molecules to endotoxin is specific or modulates the activity of LPS.

The cellular LPS receptor CD14 and the "missing link"

There is much evidence that the massive activation of cells by LPS is regulated by an LPS receptor complex. Work of several groups indicates that part of an LPS receptor is represented by the cell surface molecule CD14 [27–29]. Cellular CD14 can bind LPS, which initiates cell activation, and blocking of this interaction prevents most of the cellular effects of endotoxin. Since CD14 lacks a transmembrane domain, an as yet undefined co-receptor that initiates signaling subsequent to the binding of LPS to CD14 has been supposed.

The CD14 molecule is a 53kDa glycoprotein found on the cell surface of numerous cell types [30]. Furthermore, two soluble forms of the protein exist and can be found in high concentrations in human serum [31]. These molecules are also involved in LPS-recognition, one apparently being directly secreted, while a second, slightly smaller soluble form of CD14, can be found in normal serum most likely due to shedding of the surface receptor. Soluble CD14 can mediate the binding of LPS to cells that don't express cellular CD14, such as endothelial and other cells [32, 33].

Anti-CD14 antibodies exhibited a protective effect in a vertebrate animal model of sepsis [34]. Transgenic mice overexpressing CD14 were more sensitive to LPS and the CD 14 "knock out" (CD14$^{-/-}$) mouse exhibited a significantly reduced susceptibility to experimental sepsis induced by LPS or bacteria [35, 36]. On the other hand, soluble CD14 (sCD14) was recently shown to protect against LPS effects [37].

Lipopolysaccharide binding protein (LBP): potential dual function

As well as sCD14, LPS binding protein (LBP) seems to be essential for recognition and binding of LPS. LBP is an acute phase protein of the liver and is synthesized in hepatocytes as a glycosylated 58 kDa protein [38]. It is constitutively secreted into the blood stream, but synthesis can be greatly enhanced during the acute phase response (30-fold in humans) [39]. This rise in LBP level is caused by transcriptional activation of the LBP gene involving acute phase-typical transcription factors and is mediated by IL-1 and IL-6 [40,41]. LBP binds to the Lipid A portion of LPS and the binding site has recently been identified by mutagenesis experiments [42]. More recently, LBP has been found to also bind to certain phospholipids, thus relating its structural homology to other lipid binding proteins, such as phospholipid transfer protein (PLTP) [43, 44]. By analysis of their genes and genomic organization it was found that LBP belongs to a family of lipid binding proteins including bactericidal permeability increasing protein (BPI), and cholesterol ester transfer protein (CETP) [45–48].

LPS-induced TNF production and TNF mRNA expression in rabbit peritoneal macrophages are enhanced when LPS is complexed to low-dose LBP, most likely due to monomerization of LPS complexes and presentation to the CD14 receptor [49, 50]. Macrophages, furthermore, detect and bind LPS faster and easier when it is complexed with LBP, so LBP acts as an opsonin for Gram-negative bacteria [51]. In initial animal studies, a protective effect of anti-LBP antibodies was observed [52].

Acute phase concentrations of LBP, as we have shown recently, can block LPS effects *in vitro* and protect mice from an otherwise lethal infection [53]. *In vitro*, LPS fails to induce cytokine production in the murine macrophage cell line RAW 264.7 when high concentrations of LBP are present. Low concentrations of LBP, corresponding to constitutive mouse LBP levels, enhance TNFα production of RAW 264.7 cells induced by subthreshhold levels of LPS. In line with this, an i.p. injection of high concentrations of LBP blocked the *in vivo* cytokine production induced by LPS, prevented liver injury, and significantly reduced the lethality of an LPS or bacteria injection in mice. The *ex vivo* LPS responsiveness of blood from LBP "knock out" (LBP$^{-/-}$) mice for cytokine production was diminished, and these mice also survived an otherwise lethal LPS-shock in a D-galactosamine model. LBP$^{-/-}$ mice, however, were more susceptible to the lethal consequences of infection than normal mice [54, 55]. Here, apparently, LBP also exhibits a protective role as the lack of LBP in the LBP$^{-/-}$ mouse leads to a more severe outcome.

The ability of LPS to induce numerous responses in the host including the massive release of cytokines by defense cells is, therefore, modulated by certain LPS-recognizing host proteins. The host reaction to the release of small quantities of endotoxin clearly depends on serum factors and receptors found on responsive cells which may serve two goals: enhancement of cell stimulation for initiation of a broad innate immune response; and binding, removal, and thus detoxification of LPS. These may be of potential therapeutic use.

Endotoxin tolerance

In numerous studies it has been shown that pretreatment with a low amount of endotoxin 1–4 days before a challenge with endotoxin will afford substantial protection to experimental animals and humans (reviewed in [56, 57]). This phenomenon was termed endotoxin tolerance and its molecular background has so far not been completely elucidated (in the following we will refer to it as endotoxin tolerance).

Endotoxin tolerance is a transient state of low responsiveness to LPS which disappears within several days and is independent of antibodies to the applied endotoxin [56]. When endotoxin tolerance is induced in experimental animals or humans the first treatment with endotoxin provokes synthesis of cytokines. This reaction is practically absent upon subsequent treatment with endotoxin [58–60], in particular for TNF and IL-1. TNF and IL-1 were shown to induce tolerance to endotoxin and vice versa [61, 62]. Therefore, major characteristics of endotoxin tolerance seem to be the absence of cytokine synthesis (TNF, IL-1) upon LPS challenge and a markedly diminished reactivity towards TNF and IL-1 [62, 63].

The major cellular component for development of endotoxin tolerance is represented by macrophages which by an unknown mechanism become desensitized and fail to produce cytokines upon LPS challenge [49, 64, 65].

Based on several recent findings, it should be considered that low responsiveness to endotoxin reflects only part of endotoxin tolerance and that other mechanisms are in operation during its development. We have recently found that mice made tolerant to LPS with a single treatment contained a circulating activity in plasma, after challenge with LPS, which inhibited TNF-synthesis in the blood of normal mice [66]. This inhibitory activity was not present in the plasma of normal, LPS-challenged mice and was not identical with TGFβ or IL-10. Macrophages isolated from tolerant mice and transferred to normal mice substantially protected the recipients against an LD_{80} and, when stimulated with LPS *in vitro*, synthesized a protein which inhibited the synthesis of TNF by normal murine macrophages [67]. These findings suggest that macrophages from tolerant hosts do not become unresponsive to LPS, but rather alter their spectrum of products and synthesize factors inhibiting the synthesis and possibly the action of proinflammatory mediators such as TNF or IL-1. Such factors may represent future tools for interfering with endotoxin-induced reactions leading to the sepsis syndrome.

Acknowledgment

Part of the work described here, carried out in our laboratory, was supported by the Deutsche Forschungsgemeinschaft (Schm 74/13-1, 13-2, Schu 828/1–5), Fond der Chemischen Industrie (FUS) (BMBFKI9475/0; 01KV9507/5).

References

1   Rietschel ETh, Brade H, Holst O, Brade L, Müller-Loennis S, Mamat U, Zähringer U, Beckmann F, Seydel U, Brandenburg K et al (1996) Bacterial endotoxin: chemical constitution, biological recognition, host response, and immunological detoxification. In: ETh Rietschel, H Wagner (eds): *Pathology of septic shock, Curr Top Microbiol Immunol*, Vol 216. Springer-Verlag, Berlin, 40–81
2   Martich GD, Boujoukos AJ, Suffredini AF (1993) Response of man to endotoxin. *Immunobiology* 187: 403–416
3   Nauts HC (1989) Bacteria and cancer – antagonisms and benefits. *Cancer Surveys* 8: 713–723
4   Suffredini AF, Fromm RE, Parker MM, Brenner M, Kovacs JA, Wesley RA, Parrillo JE (1989) The cardiovascular response of normal humans to the administration of endotoxin. *The New Engl J Medicine* 321: 280–287

5   van Deventer SJH, Büller HR, ten Cate JW, Aarden LA, Hack CE, Sturk A (1990) Experimental endotoxemia in humans: analysis of cytokine release and coagulation, fibrinolytic, and complement pathways. *Blood* 76: 2520–2526

6   Suffredini AF, Shelhamer JH, Neumann RD, Brenner M, Baltaro RJ, Parrillo JE (1992) Pulmonary and oxygen transport effects of intravenously administered endotoxin in normal humans. *Am Rev Respir Dis* 145: 1398–1403

7   Suffredini AF, Harpel PC, Parrillo JE (1989) Promotion and subsequent inhibition of plasminogen activation after administration of intravenous endotoxin to normal subjects. *N Engl J Med* 320: 1165–1172

8   De La Cadena RA, Suffredini AF, Page JD, Pixley RA, Kaufman N, Parrillo JE, Colman RW (1993) Activation of the kallikrein-kinin system after endotoxin administration to normal human volunteers. *Blood* 81: 3313–3317

9   Moore FD, Moss NA, Revhaug A, Wilmore D, Mannick JA, Rodrick ML (1987) A single dose of endotoxin activates neutrophils without activating complement. *Surgery* 102: 200–205

10   Martich GD, Van Dervort AL, Danner RL, Suffredini AF (1992) Intravenous endotoxin administration to normal humans primes neutrophils for an enhanced respiratory burst. *Crit Care Med* 20: 100

11   Smith PD, Suffredini AF, Lamerson CL, Allen JB, McCartney-Frances N, Parvillo JE, Wahl SM (1988) Endotoxin administration to normal humans causes increased alveolar permeability and priming of alveolar macrophages to produce enhanced superoxide and IL-1 production. *Clin Res* 36: 374A

12   Foreman NK, Wang WC, Cullen EJ, Stidham GL, Pearson TA, Shenep JL (1991) Endotoxin shock after transfusion of contaminated red blood cells in a child with sickle cell disease. *Pediatr Inf Dis J* 10: 624–626

13   Da Silva AMT, Kaulbach HC, Chuidian FS, Lambert DR, Suffredini AF, Danner RL (1993) Brief report: shock and multiple-organ dysfunction after selfadministration of salmonella endotoxin. *N Engl J Med* 328: 1457–1460

14   Levin J, Poore TE, Neil BA, Zauber NP, Oser RS (1970) Detection of endotoxin in the blood of patients with sepsis due to gram-negative bacteria. *N Engl J Med* 283: 1313–1316

15   van Deventer SJH, Buller HR, ten Cate JW, Sturk A, Pauw W (1988) Endotoxaemia: an early predictor of septicaemia in febrile patients. *Lancet* 605–608

16   McCartney AC, Banks JG, Clements GB, Sleigh JD, Tehrani M, Ledingham JM (1983) Endotoxemia in septic shock: clinical and post mortem correlations. *Intens Care Med* 9: 117–122

17   Brandtzaeg P, Kierulf P, Gaustad P, Skulberg A, Bruun JN, Halvorsen S, Sorensen E (1989) Plasma endotoxin as a predictor of multiple organ failure and death in systemic meningococcal disease. *J Infect Dis* 159: 195–204

18   Danner RL, Elin RJ, Hosseini JM, Wesley RA, Reilly JM, Parillo JE (1991) Endotoxemia in human septic shock. *Chest* 99: 169–175

19   Ketchum PA, Parsonnet J, Stotts LS, Novitsky TJ, Schlain B, Bates DW (1997) Utiliza-

tion of a chromogenic Limulus amebocyte lysate blood assay in a multi-center study of sepsis. *J Endotox Res* 4: 9–16

20 Ulevitch RJ, Johnston AR, Weinstein DB (1979) New function for high density lipoproteins: their participation in intravascular reactions of bacterial lipopolysaccharides (LPS). *J Clin Invest* 64: 1516–1524

21 Levine DM, Parker TS, Donnelly TM, Walsh A, Rubin AL (1993) *In vivo* protection against endotoxin by plasma high density lipoprotein. *Proc Natl Acad Sci USA* 90: 12040–12044

22 Pajkrt D, Doran JE, Koster F, Lerch PG, Arnet B, Van der Poll T, ten Cate JW, van Deventer SJH (1996) Antiinflammatory effects of reconstituted high-density lipoprotein during human endotoxemia. *J Exp Med* 185: 1601–1608

23 Flegel WA, Wolpl A, Mannel DN, Northoff H (1989) Inhibition of endotoxin-induced activation of human monocytes by human lipoproteins. *Infect Immun* 57: 2237–2245

24 Navab M, Hough GP, Van Lenten BJ, Berliner JA, Fogelman AM (1988) Low density lipoproteins transfer bacterial lipopolysaccharides across endothelial monolayers in a biologically active form. *J Clin Invest* 81: 601–605

25 Netea MG, Demacker PN, Kullberg BJ, Boerman OC, Verschueren I, Stalenhoef AF, Van der Meer JW (1997) Low-density lipoprotein receptor-deficient mice are protected against lethal endotoxemia and severe gram-negative infections. *J Clin Invest* 97: 1366–1372

26 Morrison DC (1990) Diversity of mammalian macromolecules which bind to bacterial lipopolysaccharide. *Excerpta Med Int Cong Ser* 923: 183–189

27 Wright SD, Ramos RA, Tobias PS, Ulevitch RJ, Mathison JC (1990) CD14, a receptor for complexes of lipopolysaccharide (LPS) and LPS binding protein. *Science* 249: 1431–1433

28 Grunwald U, Kruger C, Schutt C (1993) Endotoxin-neutralizing capacity of soluble CD14 is a highly conserved specific function. *Circ Shock* 39: 220–225

29 Hailman E, Lichtenstein HS, Wurfel MM, Miller DS, Johnson DA, Kelley M, Busse LA, Zukowski MM, Wright SD (1994) Lipopolysaccharide (LPS)-binding protein accelerates the binding of LPS to CD14. *J Exp Med* 179: 269–277

30 Goyert SM, Ferrero E, Rettig WJ, Yenamandra AK, Obata F, LeBeau MM (1988) The CD14 monocyte differentiation antigen maps to a region encoding growth factors and receptors. *Science* 239: 497–500

31 Durieux JJ, Vita N, Popescu O, Guette F, Calzadawack J, Munker R, Schmidt RE, Lupker J, Ferrara P, Ziegler-Heitbrock HWL, et al (1994) The two soluble forms of the lipopolysaccharide receptor, CD14: characterization and release by normal human monocytes. *Eur J Immunol* 24: 2006–2012

32 Frey EA, Miller DS, Jahr TG, Sundan A, Bazil V, Espevik T, Finlay BB, Wright SD (1992) Soluble CD14 participates in the response of cells to lipopolysaccharide. *J Exp Med* 176: 1665–1671

33 Pugin J, Schürer-Maly CC, Leturcq D, Moriarty A, Ulevitch RJ, Tobias PS (1993) Lipopolysaccharide activation of human endothelial and epithelial cells is mediated by

lipopolysaccharide-binding protein and soluble CD14. *Proc Natl Acad Sci USA* 90: 2744–2748

34   Leturcq DJ, Moriarty AM, Talbott G, Winn RK, Martin TR, Ulevitch RJ (1996) Antibodies against CD14 protect primates from endotoxin-induced shock. *J Clin Invest* 98: 1533–1538

35   Ferrero E, Jiao D, Tsuberi BZ, Tesio L, Rong GW, Haziot A, Goyert SM (1993) Transgenic mice expressing human CD14 are hypersensitive to lipopolysaccharide. *Proc Natl Acad Sci USA* 90: 2380–2384

36   Haziot A, Ferrero E, Kontgen F, Hijiya N, Yamamoto S, Silver J, Stewart CL, Goyert SM (1996) Resistance to endotoxin shock and reduced dissemination of gram negative bacteria in CD14 deficient mice. *Immunity* 4: 407–414

37   Haziot A, Rong GW, Lin XY, Silver J, Goyert SM (1995) Recombinant soluble CD14 prevents mortality in mice treated with endotoxin (lipopolysaccharide). *J Immunol* 154: 6529–6532

38   Tobias PS, Soldau K, Ulevitch RJ (1989) Identification of a lipid A binding site in the acute phase reactant lipopolysaccharide binding protein. *J Biol Chem* 264: 10867–10871

39   Schumann RR, Kirschning C, Unbehaun A, Aberle H, Knopf HP, Ulevitch RJ, Herrmann F (1996) Lipopolysaccharide binding protein (LBP) is a secretory class 1 acute phase protein requiring binding of the transcription factor STAT-3, C/EBPb, and AP-1. *Mol Cell Biol* 16: 3490–3503

40   Kirschning C, Unbehaun A, Lamping N, Pfeil D, Herrmann F, Schumann RR (1997) Control of transcriptional activation of the lipopolysaccharide binding protein (LBP) gene by pro-inflammatory cytokines. *Cyt Mol Therapy* 3: 59–62

41   Kirschning CJ, Hallatschek W, Lamping N, Reuter D, Pfeil D, Schumann RR (1997) Transcriptional activation of the acute phase protein lipopolysaccharide binding protein (LBP) involves transcription factors (STAT-3, C/EBP, and AP-1). In: E Faist (ed): *The immune consequences of trauma, shock and sepsis. Mechanisms and therapeutic approaches.* Monduzzi Editore, Bologna, 807–810

42   Lamping N, Hoess A, Yu B, Park TC, Kirschning CJ, Pfeil D, Reuter D, Wright SD, Herrmann F, Schumann RR (1996) Effects of site directed mutagenesis of basic residues (Arg 94, Lys 95, Lys 99) of lipopolysaccharide (LPS) binding protein on binding and transfer of LPS and subsequent immune cell activation. *J Immunol* 157: 4648–4656

43   Hailman E, Albers JJ, Wolfbauer G, Tu AY, Wright SD (1996) Neutralization and transfer of lipopolysaccharide by phospholipid transfer protein. *J Biol Chem* 271: 12172–12178

44   Park CT, Wright SD (1996) Plasma lipopolysaccharide-binding protein is found associated with a particle containing apolipoprotein A-I, phospholipid, and factor H-related proteins. *J Biol Chem* 271: 18054–18060

45   Agellon LB, Quinet EM, Gillette TG, Drayna DT, Brown ML, Tall AR (1990) Organization of the human cholesteryl ester transfer protein gene. *Biochemistry* 29: 1372–1376

46   Day JR, Albers JJ, Lofton-Day CE, Gilbert TL, Ching AFT, Grand FJ, O'Hara PJ, Mar-

covina SM, Adolphson JL (1994) Complete cDNA encoding human phospholipid trans-fer protein from human endothelial cells. *J Biol Chem* 269: 9388–9391

47   Hubaceck JA, Buchler C, Aslandinis C, Schmitz G (1997) The genomic organization of the genes for human lipopolysaccharide binding protein (LBP) and bactericidal perme-ability increasing protein (BPI) is highly conserved. *Biochem Biophys Res Commun* 236: 427–430

48   Kirschning CJ, Au-Young J, Lamping N, Reuter D, Pfeil D, Seilhamer J, Schumann RR (1997) Similar organization of the lipopolysaccharide binding protein and phospholipid transfer protein (PLTP). Genes suggest a common gene family of lipid binding proteins. *Genomics* 46: 416–425

49   Mathison JC, Tobias PS, Wolfson E, Ulevitch RJ (1992) Plasma lipopolysaccharide (LPS) binding protein. A key component in macrophage recognition of gram negative LPS. *J Immunol* 149: 200–206

50   Schumann RR, Leong SR, Flaggs GW, Gray PW, Wright SD, Mathison JC, Tobias PS, Ulevitch RJ (1990) Structure and function of lipopolysaccharide binding protein. *Sci-ence* 249: 1429–1431

51   Grunwald U, Fan XL, Jack RS, Workalemahu G, Kallies A, Stelter F, Schütt C (1996) Monocytes can phagocytose gram negative bacteria by a CD14 dependent mechanism. *J Immunol* 157: 4119–4125

52   Gallay P, Heumann D, Le RD, Barras C, Glauser MP (1994) Mode of action of anti-lipopolysaccharide binding protein antibodies for prevention of endotoxemic shock in mice. *Proc Natl Acad Sci USA* 91: 7922–7926

53   Lamping N, Dettmer R, Schröder NWJ, Pfeil D, Hallatschek W, Burger R, Schumann RR (1998) LPS-binding protein protects mice from septic shock caused by LPS or gram-negative bacteria. *J Clin Invest* 101: 2065–2071

54   Jack RS, Fan X, Bernheiden M, Rune G, Ehlers M, Weber A, Kirsch G, Mentel R, Fürll B, Freudenberg M et al (1997) Lipopolysaccharide-binding protein is reguired to com-bat a murine gram-negative bacterial infection. *Nature* 389: 742–745

55   Wurfel MM, Monks BG, Ingalls R, Dedrick R, Delude R, Zhou D, Lamping N, Schu-mann RR, Thieringer R, Fenton MJ, et al (1997) Targeted deletion of the LBP gene leads to profound suppression of LPS responses *ex vivo* while *in vivo* responses remain intact. *J Exp Med* 186: 2051–2056

56   Johnston CA, Greisman SE (1985) Mechanism of endotoxin tolerance. In: LB Hinshaw (ed): *Handbook of endotoxin, Vol 2: Pathophysiology of endotoxin*. Elsevier, Amster-dam, New York, Oxford, 359–391

57   Schade FU, Flach R, Flohé S, Majetschak M, Kreuzfelder E, Domínguez-Fernández E, Börgermann J, Reuter M, Obertacke U (1998) *Endotoxin tolerance*. Marcel Dekker Inc; *in press*

58   Flohé S, Heinrich PC, Schneider J, Wendel A, Flohe L (1991) Time course of IL-6 and TNF alpha release during endotoxin-induced endotoxin tolerance in rats. *Biochem Pharmacol* 41: 1607–1614

59   Mathison JC, Wolfson E, Ulevitch RJ (1988) Participation of tumor necrosis factor in

the mediation of gram negative bacterial lipopolysaccharide-induced injury in rabbits. *J Clin Invest* 81: 1925–1937

60   Mackensen A, Galanos C, Wehr U, Engelhardt R (1992) Endotoxin tolerance: regulation of cytokine production and cellular changes in response to endotoxin application in cancer patients. *Eur Cytokine Netw* 3: 571–579

61   Henricson BE, Neta R, Vogel SN (1991) An interleukin-1 receptor antagonist blocks lipopolysaccharide-induced colony-stimulating factor production and early endotoxin tolerance. *Infect Immun* 59: 1188–1191

62   Fraker DL, Stovroff MC, Merino MJ, Norton JA (1988) Tolerance to tumor necrosis factor in rats and the relationship to endotoxin tolerance and toxicity. *J Exp Med* 168: 95–105

63   Galanos C, Freudenberg M, Katschinski T, Salomoa R, Mossmann H Kumazawa Y (1992) Tumor necrosis factor and host response to endotoxin. In: JL Ryan, DC Morrison (eds): *Bacterial endotoxic lipopolysaccharides*. CRC Press, Boca Raton, 75–104

64   Mathison JC, Virca GD, Wolfson E, Tobias PS, Glaser K, Ulevitch RJ (1990) Adaptation to bacterial lipopolysaccharide controls lipopolysaccharide-induced tumor necrosis factor production in rabbit macrophages. *J Clin Invest* 85: 1108–1118

65   Freudenberg MA, Galanos C (1988) Induction of tolerance to lipopolysaccharide (LPS)-D-galactosamine lethality by pretreatment with LPS is mediated by macrophages. *Infect Immun* 56: 1352–1357

66   Schade FU, Schlegel J, Hofmann K, Brade H, Flach R (1996) Endotoxin-tolerant mice produce an inhibitor of tumor necrosis factor-synthesis. *J Endotox Res* 3: 455–462

67   Flach R, Schade FU (1997) Peritoneal macrophages from endotoxin-tolerant mice produce an inhibitor of tumor necrosis factor α synthesis and protect against endotoxin shock. *J Endotox Res* 4: 241–250

68   Zanetti G, Glauser MP, Baumgartner JD (1993) Anti-endotoxin antibodies and other inhibitors of endotoxin. *New Horizons* 1:110–119

Acute lung inflammation in septic shock of the cytokine release induced by bacterial superantigens

Brigitte Neumann and Bernhard Holzmann

Department of Surgery, Klinikum rechts der Isar, Technical University of Munich, Ismaninger Str. 22, D-81675 Munich, Germany

Superantigens – mechanisms of action

A group of bacterial and viral proteins termed superantigens share the ability to associate with T cell receptor (TCR) and major histocompatibility complex (MHC) class II molecules, generating unique multimeric protein complexes that trigger polyclonal T cell activation [1–4]. Members of the superantigen family include bacterial exotoxins like staphylococcal enterotoxins and toxic shock syndrome toxin-1 (TSST-1), proteins encoded by viral genomes, and retroviral products from mouse mammary tumor viruses [1, 5, 6]. The mechanisms by which superantigens stimulate T cells differ from those of conventional antigens, which require endocytosis and proteolytic processing for presentation of MHC-bound antigenic peptides to T lymphocytes. In contrast, superantigens interact with MHC class II molecules as intact proteins at a site distinct from the peptide binding groove without conformational changes of MHC proteins or superantigens occurring upon complex formation (Fig. 1) [7–13]. The superantigen binding region of MHC class II proteins seems to be conserved among different mammalian haplotypes since superantigens bind to murine, rat, and human class II molecules [3, 14].

Individual superantigens may differ in their relative affinity to class II molecules as was shown for staphylococcal enterotoxin A (SEA) and TSST-1 which bind class II proteins with higher affinity than does staphylococcal enterotoxin B (SEB) [2, 14, 15]. The mechanisms of superantigen binding to MHC class II molecules may also vary. Thus, SEA contains two distinct MHC class II binding domains with both the N-terminal and C-terminal site of the superantigens mediating MHC class II association [16–18]. On SEA, the N-terminal domain is homologous to the single binding site of SEB mediating low affinity interactions with the class II α-chain, while the C-terminal site of SEA contacts the class II β-chain with high affinity [16, 17]. Furthermore, alternative superantigen-binding proteins have been described for staphylococcal enterotoxin C (SEC), which in addition binds to vascular cell adhesion molecule-1 (VCAM-1) [19, 20]. The function of superantigen presentation to T cells by non-MHC class II proteins, however, is currently unknown.

Cytokines in Severe Sepsis and Septic Shock, edited by H. Redl and G. Schlag[†]

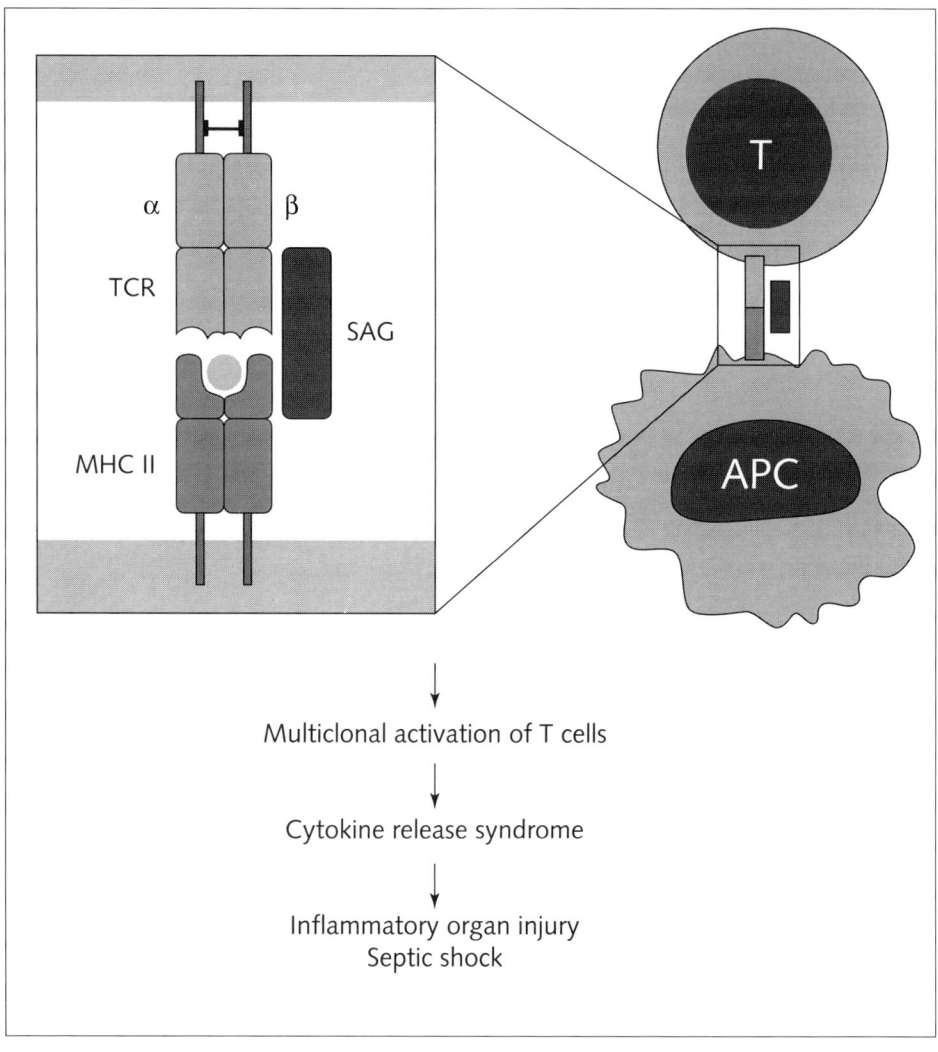

Figure 1
Model for the induction of acute hyperinflammation by bacterial superantigens (SAG).
TCR, T cell receptor; APC, antigen-presenting cell

On T lymphocytes superantigens bind to conserved regions of the TCR β subunit, which are encoded by specific Vβ gene segments, thereby rendering T cell recognition of superantigens independent of the clonal specificity of the TCR [2, 21–23]. Interestingly, superantigens may also form complexes with TCR Vβ segments in the absence of MHC class II proteins [23]. Depending on the Vβ-specificity of a given superantigen and the number of individual Vβ segments per genome, superantigens may therefore interact with as many as 2 to 5% of peripheral T cells, which contrasts with a frequency of 1×10^{-4} to 1×10^{-5} for recognition of foreign MHC or peptide antigens, respectively. Thus, the immune reaction to superantigens is characterized as a multiclonal, yet TCR Vβ-selective, T cell response.

Acute response to superantigen challenge *in vivo*

Challenge of the immune system with bacterial superantigens such as SEB results in a complex pattern of concomitant and sequential responses of T lymphocytes. Acute hyperactivation of CD4+ and CD8+ T cells is followed by early cellular depletion, Vβ-selective clonal expansion, late cellular deletion, and distinct levels of long-lasting and ligand-specific anergy [4]. Functional alterations of superantigen-responsive T cells have been summarized in a recent review [4]. In addition, a transient dysfunction of antigen-presenting cells (APC) that is mediated by T cell-derived cyclosporin A (CsA)-sensitive cytokines has been described 24–48 h after administration of SEB to mice [4].

The immediate response of peripheral T cells to *in vivo* administration of superantigens, however, is characterized by cellular hyperactivation (Fig. 1). Upon SEB exposure, a selective loss of cell surface L-selectin on TCR Vβ8-expressing T cells within 10 to 15 min after injection is followed by initiation of T helper 1 (Th1)- and Th2-type cytokine gene transcription in CD4+ and CD8+ T cells [24, 25]. Systemic release of cytokines including TNFα, IL-1, IL-2, IL-4, IL-6, and IFN-γ is observed in sera of SEB-challenged mice within 1 to 4 h [25–27]. Administration of superantigens to mice induces rapid weight loss and death at high doses probably due to systemic action of TNF and lymphotoxin [5, 28]. The LD_{50} of superantigens is reduced about 100-fold in mice due to sensitization by D-galactosamine, blockage of glucocorticoid receptors, inhibition of the inducible nitric oxide synthetase, or coinjection of endotoxin [26, 29–32].

Lethal shock in sensitized mice challenged with superantigens like SEB is clearly dependent on the presence of T cells, because CsA-treated mice and severe combined immunodeficiency disease (SCID) mice, but not T cell repopulated SCID mice, are protected from toxic effects of SEB [26]. Furthermore, MHC class II-deficient mice were shown to be resistant to septic shock induced by SEA or SEB [31]. Additional studies have demonstrated that lethal SEB shock is dependent on the presence of T cell-derived TNFα, the 55 kDa receptor for TNF, and ICAM-1 [26, 33–35]. It is interesting to note that although primarily activating mononuclear phagocytes, administration of endotoxin to mice provokes a similar, but not identical, cascade of cytokines with TNFα and the 55 kDa receptor for TNF acting as principal mediators of systemic inflammation, multiorgan failure, and lethal septic shock in sensitized animals [33, 34, 36–38].

Induction of acute lung inflammation by superantigens

Analysis of putative pathogenic mechanisms of T cell-dependent septic shock revealed that administration of SEB results in acute inflammatory lung injury that is characterized by marked leukocyte infiltration, endothelial cell injury, and increased vascular permeability [39]. Thus, pathological alterations of lungs following superantigen exposure are similar to those observed after administration of endotoxin [40]. Independent of the superantigen applied (SEA or SEB), lung infiltrating leukocytes consist of granulocytes, mononuclear phagocytes, and NK cells, with granulocytes representing the major fraction (Fig. 2) [39]. In contrast to superantigen treatment, endotoxin does not induce infiltration of natural killer (NK) cells [39]. Superantigen stimulation does not induce recruitment of T cells that are also recognized by the NK1.1 Ab as was shown by double-marker flow cytometry and analysis of NK1.1 T cell-deficient β2 microglobulin knockout mice ([39] and our unpublished observations). NK1.1 T cells produce large amounts of cytokines and express a restricted repertoire of TCRs with more than 50% of them using the SEB-binding Vβ8 segment [39]. In addition, following superantigen challenge the number of leukocytes increases in bronchioalveolar lavage fluid (Tab. 1) as well as in liver and kidney (our unpublished observations). Independent studies have also shown recruitment of neutrophils and mononuclear phagocytes into the peritoneal cavity of SEB-treated mice [41, 42]. Concomitant with organ infiltration, leukocytes are depleted in large numbers from the blood circulation (Tab. 1).

Leukocyte lung infiltration induced by superantigens was shown to depend on the presence and activation of T cells. Thus, in nude mice challenged with SEA, leukocyte recruitment was not detectable (Tab. 2) and pretreament of mice with CsA completely blocked SEB-triggered lung leukocyte accumulation (our unpublished observations). Previously, it was shown that CsA markedly enhances the elimination of peripheral SEB-reactive T cells such that up to 90% of the targeted Vβ subpopulations are deleted [43]. In addition to T lymphocytes, neutrophils also respond to CsA exposure. It has been reported that in neutrophils inhibition of calcineurin by CsA leads to increased cell adhesion mediated by integrins [44]. These findings may explain the elevated numbers of neutrophils in lungs following CsA-treatment of mice (our unpublished observations).

Neutrophils have been implicated as cellular mediators of acute lung injury characteristic of adult respiratory distress syndrome (ARDS). Clinical observations as well as animal models of ARDS have demonstrated that sequestration of large numbers of neutrophils in the lung microvasculature is linked to the development of lung capillary leak syndrome [45–51]. Moreover, animal models have shown that depletion of neutrophils attenuates lung damage induced by microembolization, complement activation, endotoxin, or TNF [47–50]. It therefore appears likely that neutrophils also contribute to lung injury following administration of bacterial superantigens.

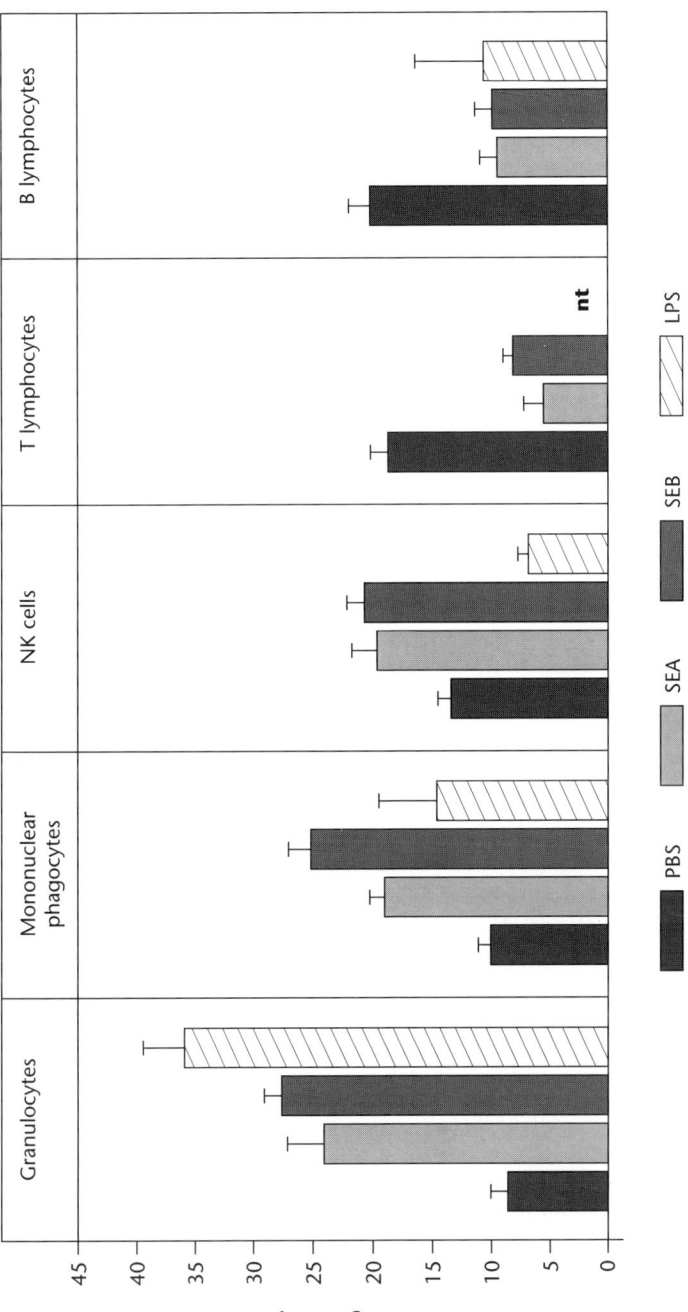

Figure 2

SEA, SEB, and endotoxin induce infiltration of different leukocyte subpopulations into lungs.
C57BL/6 mice were injected with 50 μg superantigen (SEA or SEB) or 10 μg endotoxin (LPS) i. p. and lungs were removed 6 h later after extensive perfusion with phosphate buffered saline (PBS). Single-cell suspensions were prepared by collagenase digestion of lung tissue and infiltrating leukocytes were examined by two-color flow cytometry analysis. Leukocytes were defined by expression of the leukocyte common antigen CD45. Results are presented as percentage of all CD45+ cells (mean ± s.e.m.) and are derived from 5 to 15 independent animals in each group.

Table 1 - Leukocyte numbers in peripheral blood and bronchioalveolar lavage fluid

	Control	6 h SEB
Peripheral blood	$6.1 \pm 0.4 \times 10^6$	$2.6 \pm 0.3 \times 10^6$
Bronchioalveolar lavage	$45.3 \pm 13.1 \times 10^3$	$97.8 \pm 11.2 \times 10^3$

C57BL/6 mice were injected with 50 µg SEB i.p. and blood or bronchioalveolar lavage was collected 6 h later. Results are presented as mean ± SD of total cell numbers (n = 11 for peripheral blood samples and n = 4 for bronchioalveolar lavage).

Although neutrophils are clearly capable of mediating acute lung injury, clinical observations showing that patients who are severely neutropenic can still develop ARDS provide evidence for neutrophil-independent mechanisms of lung injury [52, 53]. Animal models have supported this hypothesis and have implicated macrophages as alternative effector cells, which release toxic oxygen and L-arginine-derived products [54, 55]. Based on these reports it is conceivable that mononuclear phagocytes may act in concert with neutrophils to damage tissue and to induce vascular permeability changes. Thus, superantigen-dependent recruitment of mononuclear phagocytes to the lung may be of pathogenic significance.

TNF has been identified as a principal mediator of septic shock. Thus, death of mice treated with endotoxin and D-galactosamine or injected with lethal doses of Gram-negative bacteria is prevented by antibodies against TNF [37, 56] or genetic ablation of the 55 kDa TNF-receptor [33, 34]. When injected as a recombinant cytokine, TNF is sufficient to induce acute lung inflammation that is dependent on the presence of the 55 kDa TNF-receptor [57]. The role of TNF in septic lung injury is further emphasized by reports showing that antibodies against TNF partially block endotoxin-triggered neutrophil infiltration of lungs [58]. However, following administration of the bacterial superantigen SEB the lung capillary leak syndrome is not inhibited by neutralizing TNF antibodies (Fig. 3). These results may be explained by the release of multiple mediators in response to SEB that exhibit redundant functions in the development of inflammatory organ injury. In superantigen-dependent septic shock the lack of TNF activity may therefore be compensated by alternative inflammatory cytokines such as IL-1 and IFN-γ suggesting that septic lung injury may result from the activity of a complex pattern of mediators rather than a single inflammatory cytokine.

Table 2 - Subpopulations of lung-infiltrating leukocytes in SEA-challenged mice

Leukocyte subsets	Marker	C57BL/6		Balb/c nu/nu		
		Control	SEA	Control	SEA	LPS
Granulocytes	Gr-1+	8.4 ± 1.5	24.0 ± 3.1	10.9 ± 0.6	11.2 ± 1.8	52.6 ± 3.0
Mononuclear phagocytes	Mac-3+	9.9 ± 1.0	19.0 ± 1.2	13.1 ± 3.8	13.9 ± 6.3	51.2 ± 0.7
NK cells, T cell subset	NK1.1+	13.1 ± 1.2	19.5 ± 2.1	n.a.	n.a.	n.a.
T lymphocytes	Thy1.2+ or CD3+	18.5 ± 1.4	5.2 ± 1.7	0	0	0
B lymphocytes	B220+	19.9 ± 1.8	9.2 ± 1.5	23.4 ± 2.5	23.0 ± 2.3	0.5 ± 0.5

C57BL/6 or Balb/c nu/nu mice were injected with 50 µg SEA or 10 µg LPS i.p. and lungs were removed 6 h later after extensive perfusion with PBS. Single-cell suspensions were prepared by collagenase digestion of lung tissue and infiltrating leukocyte subsets were identified by two-color flow cytometry analysis. Leukocytes were defined by expression of the leukocyte common antigen CD45. Results are presented as percentage of CD45+ cells (mean ± s.e.m.) and are derived from 3 to 15 independent animals in each group. n.a., not applicable.

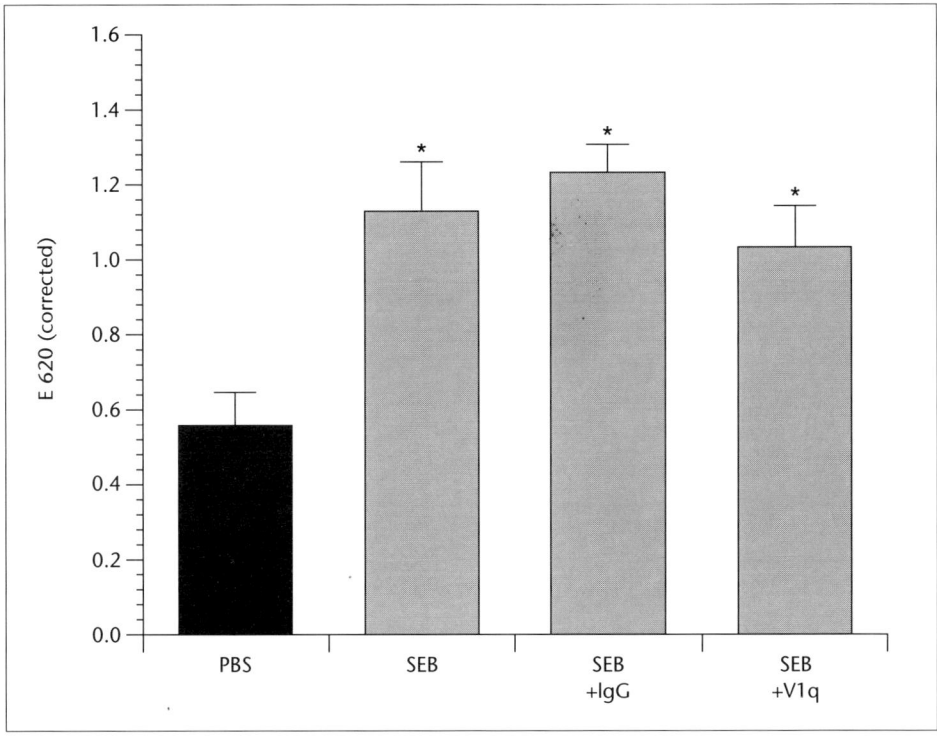

Figure 3
Increased lung vascular permeability induced by SEB is independent of TNF.
C57BL/6 mice were injected with 270 μg neutralizing anti-TNF Ab (V1q) [26, 107] or rat IgG
and 2 h later challenged with 50 μg SEB i.p. (grey bars) or PBS (black bar). Lungs were
removed 6 h later after extensive perfusion with PBS. Mice were injected i.v. with Evans blue
30 min before termination of the experiment. Evans blue binds to serum albumin and its dis-
tribution was used as a marker for the transcapillary flux of macromolecules. Evans blue in
lung homogenates was quantified by a dual wavelength spectrophotometric method [39].
Increased absorbance (E_{620}) indicates increased vascular permeability.
*p < 0.005

In vivo activation of granulocytes following superantigen administration

Neutrophil activation results in endothelial cell injury *in vitro* and injection of pre-activated neutrophils into the lung vasculature directly induces lung capillary leak *in vivo* by elastase-dependent mechanisms [59, 60]. The pathogenic role of elastase in acute lung injury was also demonstrated in endotoxin-treated mice [61]. More-

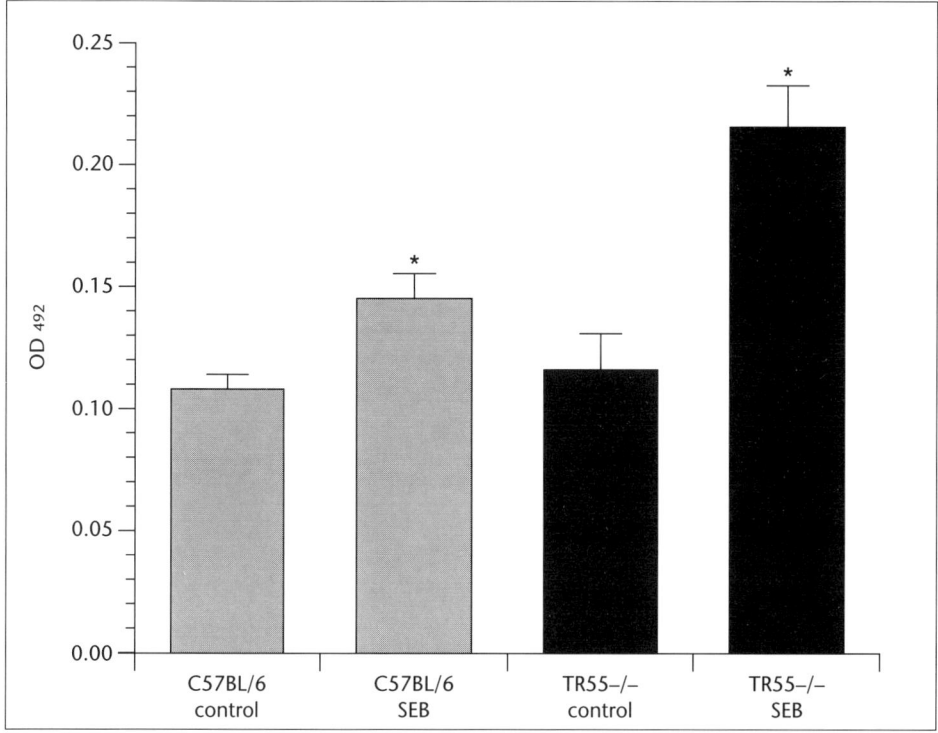

Figure 4
Increased serine protease activity in C57BL/6 and 55 kDa TNF receptor-deficient mice is induced by SEB.
Cellular serine protease activity was analysed in peripheral blood leukocytes of C57BL/6 (grey bars) and 55 kDa TNF receptor deficient mice (TR55–/–) (black bars) 6 h after SEB challenge. Leukocytes were lysed by sonication and cellular content of serine proteases was measured photometrically after incubation of cell lysates with FTC-casein overnight at 37°C. Increased OD_{492} indicates increased protease activity.
$*p < 0.01$

over, clinical observations as well as animal models of ARDS have documented accumulation of neutrophil proteases in bronchioalveolar lavage fluid and serum [45, 46, 62–67]. The tissue-destroying capacity of neutrophil proteases such as elastase may be further enhanced by reactive oxygen metabolites that were shown to inactivate tissue proteinase inhibitors by oxidation of critical methionine residues [68–70]. Consistently, previous findings have demonstrated an important role of reactive oxygen metabolites in lung damage induced by immune complexes [55, 71].

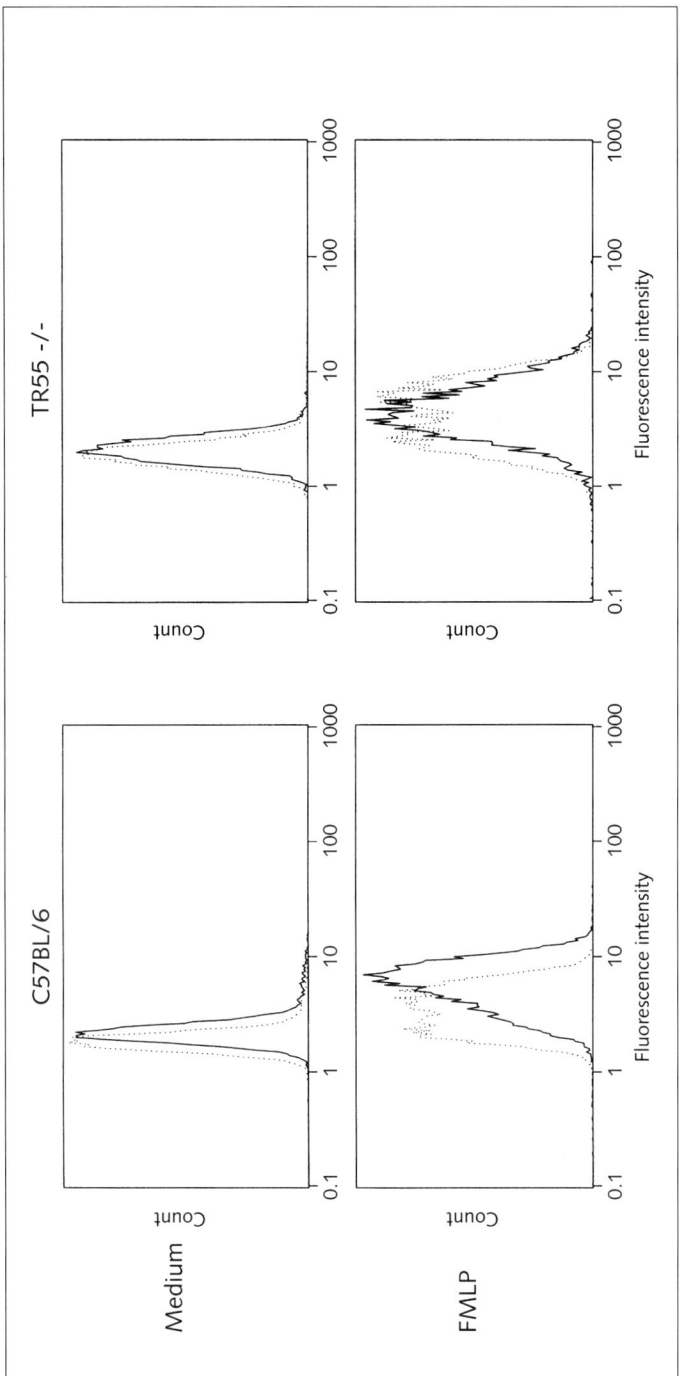

Figure 5

SEB challenge of C57BL/6, but not 55 kDa TNF receptor-deficient mice is associated with priming of granulocytes for increased oxidant production.

Peripheral blood cells were collected 6 h after injection of SEB (solid lines) or PBS (dotted lines) and leukocytes were stimulated for 20 min at 37°C with the indicated reagents. Generation of reactive oxygen metabolites was examined by flow cytometry using the fluorescence dye dihydrorhodamine 123. Histograms are derived from granulocytes of a single mouse and are representative of six experiments yielding similar results.

Following superantigen exposure, increased serine protease activity was demonstrated in circulating leukocytes (Fig. 4). Elevated elastase mRNA levels and increased cellular protease activity were also reported for endotoxin-treated neutrophils [72]. In addition, we have demonstrated that SEB challenge of mice augments production of reactive oxygen metabolites by circulating granulocytes stimulated with formyl-methionine-leucine-phenylalanine (FMLP) (Fig. 5) [39]. Interestingly, TNFα enhanced oxidant production of granulocytes from SEB-treated, but not from control mice suggesting that the systemic response to SEB increases granulocyte sensitivity to TNF-mediated signals [39]. This conculsion was supported by our finding that granulocytes of SEB-treated TNF receptor p55 knockout mice failed to respond with an increased production of reactive oxygen metabolites upon secondary *in vitro* stimulation (Fig. 5). However, induction of cellular protease activity by administration of SEB was not affected by TNF receptor p55 deficiency (Fig. 4). Consistent with these results, previous studies have indicated that TNF may increase the oxidative burst reaction of neutrophils primed by various stimuli [73–76]. Together, these findings indicate a distinct function for the 55 kDa TNF receptor in enhancing granulocyte production of reactive oxygen metabolites, but not of serine proteases.

Additional evidence for *in vivo* activation of granulocytes after SEB challenge was provided by elevated expression of Mac-1 on circulating cells, whereas cell surface levels of L-selectin were downregulated [39]. Interestingly, in trauma patients developing ARDS, neutrophils circulating in the pulmonary artery also showed increased oxygen radical production and elevated Mac-1 expression [77]. Putative *in vivo* mediators for the inverse regulation of Mac-1 and L-selectin on granulocytes include inflammatory cytokines like TNF or IL-1 [78–80]. However, induction of Mac-1 and downregulation of L-selectin in TNF receptor p55-deficient mice was not altered as compared to wildtype mice suggesting the existence of additional mediators that may regulate distinct aspects of neutrophil activation in septic shock (our unpublished observations). Together, the systemic response of granulocytes to hyperinflammation induced by bacterial superantigens is consistent with the model that the recruitment of pre-activated / primed neutrophils to the lung and possibly other tissues may be critical for the development of organ injury in septic shock.

Mechanisms of leukocyte recruitment in septic organ injury

In different experimental models development of inflammatory organ injury requires cellular interactions mediated by leukocyte and endothelial adhesion molecules. Central to the processes of inflammation is a dramatic increase in endothelial cell surface expression of adhesion molecules such as P- and E-selectin, VCAM-1, and ICAM-1 [81]. Blockage of E-selectin, P-selectin, or L-selectin as well as inhibition of the integrins VLA-4 and LFA-1, and the adhesion molecule ICAM-1 were shown to protect against lung injury induced by deposition of immune complexes or complement activation [82–87]. In SEB-treated mice, the immunglobulin-related adhesion molecules VCAM-1 and ICAM-1 were shown to be upregulated both at the protein and mRNA level ([39] and our unpublished observations). Administration of SEB also resulted in a strong induction of P-selectin mRNA in the majority of lung vessels, whereas elevated expression of E-selectin transcripts was only detectable in a few scattered endothelial cells [39].

Chemokines are involved in a variety of immune and inflammatory responses acting primarily as chemoattractants and activators of specific leukocyte subsets. In patients, development of ARDS and ARDS-related mortality correlate with high pulmonary levels of the C-X-C chemokine IL-8 [88–90]. Neutralization of IL-8 prevents neutrophil recruitment to the lung in rabbit endotoxin models [91, 92]. In the mouse, macrophage inflammatory protein-2 (MIP-2) and cytokine-induced neutrophil chemoattractant (KC) potently activate neutrophils via the murine IL-8 receptor homologue [93, 94]. KC increases Mac-1 expression and respiratory burst activity on neutrophils and stimulates neutrophil influx into lungs when administered intratracheally [93, 95]. Neutralizing antibodies against KC or MIP-2 markedly inhibit neutrophil accumulation in lungs and reduce vascular leakage following intratracheal instillation of endotoxin [95–97]. Upon challenge of mice with SEB, mRNA levels of KC and MIP-2 are upregulated (Fig. 6) suggesting a role of these C-X-C chemokines in superantigen-induced lung inflammation and vascular injury.

Studies in animal models have also indicated a potential role of C-C chemokines in lung pathology and sepsis. Following administration of SEB, mRNA levels of macrophage chemotactic protein-1 (MCP-1) were induced about 80-fold, while MIP-1α was only weakly upregulated (Fig. 6). In contrast, the C-C chemokine regulated upon activation, normally T cell expressed and secreted (RANTES) that is chemotactic for monocytes, CD4+ T lymphocytes, eosinophils, and basophils [98], was not induced after SEB challenge (Fig. 6). Administration of superantigens and endotoxin therefore appears to result in distinct patterns of chemokine induction since RANTES expression was elevated in endotoxic shock and antibody neutralization of RANTES reduced the infiltration of mononuclear phagocytes after endotoxin injection [99]. In murine endotoxemia, MIP-1α also appears to be involved in acute lung injury [100]. Pretreatment with neutralizing MIP-1α antibodies prevents capillary leakage as well as neutrophil and macrophage influx in lungs after endotoxin challenge [100]. Clinical observations revealed that Gram-negative and Gram-positive infections resulting in sepsis are associated with elevated serum levels of MCP-1 [101]. During lethal or sublethal bacteremia in baboons, MCP-1 was released and the increase of plasma levels correlated with those of IL-8 [102]. In mice, neutralization of MCP-1 significantly increased endotoxin-induced mortality as well as serum TNF and IL-12 levels, while administration of recombinant MCP-1 protein resulted in elevated IL-10 serum levels and protected mice from lethal

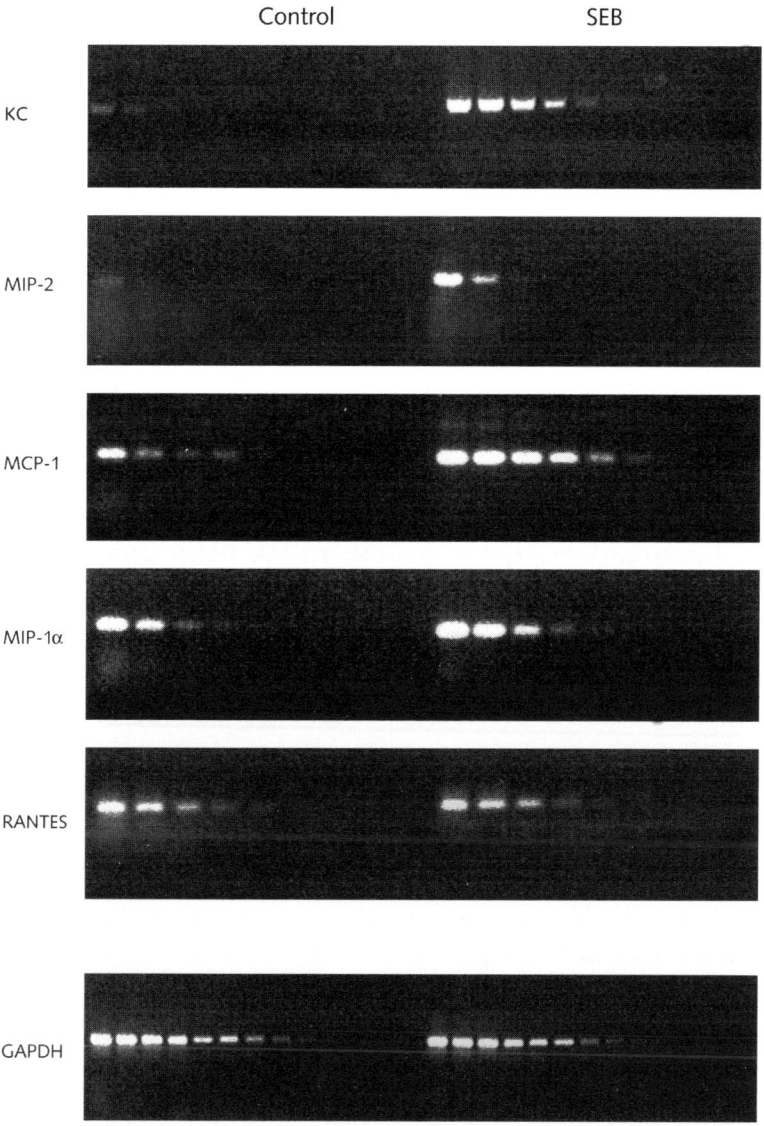

Figure 6
Rapid induction of lung chemokine expression following SEB administration.
Total RNA was isolated from lungs of C57BL/6 control mice or 6 h after SEB challenge and reverse transcribed. Serial cDNA dilutions (1:3) were used as template for PCR amplifications detecting expression of the chemokines KC, MIP-2, MCP-1, MIP-1α, and RANTES. PCR reactions for glyceraldehyde 3-phosphate dehydrogenase (GAPDH) were included in each case as an internal standard and to control for contamination with genomic DNA.

endotoxemia [103]. In a rat IgA immune complex model of alveolitis, which is characterized by mononuclear phagocyte-dependent lung injury, however, infusion of neutralizing MCP-1 antibodies reduced both accumulation of mononuclear phagocytes and vascular damage in lung [104]. Consistent with a role of MCP-1 in the pathogenesis of monocyte-dependent inflammatory lung injury, MCP-1 was shown to function as a chemoattractant for monocytes, but not neutrophils, and to induce a respiratory burst reaction in monocytes [105, 106]. In summary, these results provide evidence for an *in vivo* crosstalk between cytokines and chemokines such as MCP-1 which, dependent on the inflammatory stimulus, may either promote or attenuate organ injury.

Summary

Superantigens stimulate T lymphocytes at high frequency by interacting with specific TCR Vβ segments. Challenge of mice with bacterial superantigens such as staphylococcal enterotoxin B (SEB) induces the systemic release of cytokines resulting in septic shock and death of sensitized animals. Analysis of the putative pathogenic mechanisms of T cell-dependent septic shock revealed that administration of SEB results in acute inflammatory lung injury characterized by a marked increase in vascular permeability. SEB-induced lung capillary leakage was independent of TNF. Injury was associated with the recruitment of leukocytes, induction of cell adhesion molecules including VCAM-1, ICAM-1, and P-selectin, and increased production of C-X-C and C-C chemokines such as KC and MCP-1 in the lung. Infiltrating leukocytes consisted of granulocytes, mononuclear phagocytes and NK cells with granulocytes representing the major fraction. Consistent with a role of neutrophils as cellular mediators of inflammatory organ injury, activation of circulating granulocytes in SEB-treated mice was demonstrated by elevated levels of cell surface Mac-1, downregulation of L-selectin, and increased production of toxic oxygen metabolites and serine proteases. Interestingly, *in vivo* granulocyte priming for enhanced production of oxidants upon secondary *in vitro* stimulation was dependent on the 55 kDa TNF receptor. Together, these results suggest that acute inflammatory lung injury may contribute to the pathogenesis of T cell-dependent lethal shock in mice challenged with bacterial superantigens and indicate both common and distinct pathogenic mechanisms of lung injury induced by a large number of distinct inflammatory stimuli.

Acknowledgments
This work was supported by a grant from the Deutsche Forschungsgemeinschaft to the Clinical Research group "Immunsuppression und postoperative sepsis".

References

1 Acha-Orbea H, Held W, Waanders GA, Shakhov AN, Scarpellino L, Lees RK, Mac-Donald HR (1993) Exogenous and endogenous mouse mammary tumor virus super-antigens. *Immunol Rev* 131: 5–25

2 Herman A, Kappler JM, Marrack P, Pullen AM (1991) Superantigens: mechanisms of T-cell stimulation and role in immune responses. *Annu Rev Immunol* 9: 745–772

3 Herrmann T, MacDonald HR (1991) T cell recognition of superantigens. *Curr Top Microbiol Immunol* 174: 21–38

4 Heeg K, Miethke T, Wagner H (1996) Superantigen-mediated lethal shock: the functional state of ligand-reactive T cells. *Curr Top Microbiol Immunol* 216: 83–100

5 Marrack P, Kappler J (1990) The staphylococcal enterotoxins and their relatives. *Science* 248: 705–711

6 Marrack P, Winslow GM, Choi Y, Scherer M, Pullen A, White J, Kappler JW (1993) The bacterial and mouse mammary tumor virus superantigens; two different families of proteins with the same functions *Immunol Rev* 131: 79–92

7 Carlsson R, Fischer H, Sjögren HO (1988) Binding of staphylococcal enterotoxin A to accessory cells is a requirement for its ability to acivate human T cells. *J Immunol* 140: 2484–2488

8 Mollick JA, Cook RG, Rich RR (1989) Class II MHC molecules are specific receptors for staphylococcus enterotoxin A. *Science* 244: 817–820

9 Torres BA, Griggs ND, Johnson HM (1993) Bacterial and retroviral superantigens share a common binding region on class II MHC antigens. *Nature* 364: 152–154

10 Thibodeau J, Labrecque N, Denis F, Huber BT, Sekaly RP (1994) Binding sites for bacterial and endogenous retroviral superantigens can be dissociated on major histocompatibility complex class II molecules. *J Exp Med* 179: 1029–1034

11 Mottershead DG, Hsu PN, Urban RG, Strominger JL, Huber BT (1995) Direct binding of the Mtv7 superantigen (Mls-1) to soluble MHC class II molecules. *Immunity* 2: 149– 154

12 Jardetzky TS, Brown JH, Gorga JC, Stern LJ, Urban RG, Chi Y, Stauffacher C, Strominger JL, Wiley DC (1994) Three-dimensional structure of a human class II histocompatibility molecule comlexed with superantigen. *Nature* 368: 711–718

13 Dellabona P, Peccoud J, Kappler JW, Marrack P, Benoist C, Mathis D (1990) Superantigens interact with MHC class II molecules outside of the antigen groove. *Cell* 62: 1115–1121

14 Fraser JD (1989) High-affinity binding of staphylococcal enterotoxins A and B to HLA-DR. *Nature* 339: 221–223

15 Scholl PR, Diez A, Geha RS (1989) Staphylococcal enterotoxin B and toxic shock syndrome toxin-1 bind to distinct sites on HLA-DR and HLA-DQ molecules. *J Immunol* 143: 2583–2588

16 Abrahamsen L, Dohlsten M, Segren S, Björk P, Jonsson E, Kalland T (1995) Characterization of two distinct MHC class II binding sites in the superantigen staphylococcal enterotoxin A. *EMBO J* 14: 2978–2986

17 Hudson KR, Tiedemann RE, Urban RG, Lowe SC, Strominger JL, Fraser JD (1995) Staphylococcal enterotoxin A has two cooperative binding sites on major histocompatibility complex class II. *J Exp Med* 182: 711–720

18 Kozono H, Parker D, White J, Marrack P, Kappler J (1995) Multiple binding sites for bacterial superantigens on soluble class II MHC molecules. *Immunity* 3: 187–196

19 Cantor H, Crump AL, Raman VK, Liu H, Markowitz JS, Grusby MJ, Glimcher LH (1993) Immunoregulatory effects of superantigens: interactions of staphylococcal enterotoxins with host MHC and non-MHC products. *Immunol Rev* 131: 27–42

20 Avery AC, Markowitz JS, Grusby MJ, Glimcher LH, Cantor H (1994) Activation of T cells by superantigen in class II-negative mice. *J Immunol* 153: 4853–4861

21 Fleischer B, Schrezenmeier H (1988) T cell stimulation by staphylococcal enterotoxins. Clonally variable response and requirement for major histocompatibility complex class II molecules on accessory or target cells. *J Exp Med* 167: 1697–1707

22 Irwin MJ, Hudson KR, Ames KT, Fraser JD, Gascoigne NRJ (1993) T-cell receptor β-chain binding to enterotoxin superantigens. *Immunol Rev* 131: 61–78

23 Seth A, Stern LJ, Ottenhoff THM, Engel I, Owen MJ, Lamb JR, Klausner RD, Wiley D (1994) Binary and ternary complexes between T cell receptor, class II MHC and superantigen *in vitro. Nature* 369: 324–327

24 Miethke T, Wahl C, Holzmann B, Heeg K, Wagner H (1993) Bacterial superantigens induce rapid and TCR Vβ-selective downregulation of L-selectin (gp90^{Mel14}) *in vivo. J Immunol* 151: 6777–6782

25 Gaus H, Miethke T, Wagner H, Heeg K (1994) Superantigen-induced anergy of Vβ8+ CD4+ T cells induces functional but nonproliferative T cells *in vivo. Immunology* 83: 333–340

26 Miethke T, Wahl C, Heeg K, Echtenacher B, Krammer PH, Wagner H (1992) T-cell mediated lethal shock triggered in mice by the superantigen staphylococcal enterotoxin B: critical role of tumor necrosis factor. *J Exp Med* 175: 91–98

27 Miethke T, Wahl C, Regele D, Gaus H, Heeg K, Wagner H (1993) Superantigen mediated shock: a cytokine release syndrome. *Immunobiology* 189: 270–284

28 Aroeira LS, Williams O, Lozano EG, Martinez-A C (1994) Age-dependent changes in the response to staphylococcal enterotoxin B. *Int Immunol* 6: 1555–1560

29 Florquin S, Amraoui Z, Dubois C, Decuyper J, Goldman M (1994) The protective role of endogenously synthesized nitric oxide in staphylococcal enterotoxin B-induced shock in mice. *J Exp Med* 180: 1153–1158

30 Gonzalo JA, Gonzalez-Garcia A, Martinez C, Kroemer G (1993) Glucocorticoid-mediated control of the activation and clonal deletion of peripheral T cells *in vivo. J Exp Med* 177: 1239–1246

31 Stiles BG, Bavari S, Krakauer T, Ulrich RG (1993) Toxicity of staphylococcal enterotoxins potentiated by lipopolysaccharide: Major histocompatibility complex class II molecule dependency and cytokine release. *Infect Immun* 61: 5333–5338

32 Blank C, Luz A, Bendigs S, Erdmann A, Wagner H, Heeg K (1997) Superantigen and endotoxin synergize in the induction of lethal shock. *Eur J Immunol* 27: 825–833

33   Pfeffer K, Matsuyama T, Kündig TM, Wakeham A, Kishihara K, Shahinian A, Wiegmann K, Ohashi PS, Krönke M, Mak TW (1993) Mice deficient for the 55-kd tumor necrosis factor receptor are resistant to endotoxic shock, yet succumb to L monocytogenes infection. *Cell* 73: 457–467

34   Rothe J, Lesslauer W, Lötscher H, Lang Y, Koebel P, Köntgen F, Althage A, Zinkernagel R, Steinmetz M, Bluethmann H (1993) Mice lacking the tumour necrosis factor receptor 1 are resistant to TNF-mediated toxicity but highly susceptible to infection by Listeria monocytogenens. *Nature* 364: 798–802

35   Xu H, Gonzalo JA, Pierre YS, Williams IR, Kupper TS, Cotran RS, Springer TA, Gutierrez Ramos JC (1994) Leukocytosis and resistance to septic shock in intercellular adhesion molecule 1-deficient mice. *J Exp Med* 180: 95–109

36   Freudenberg MA, Keppler D, Galanos C (1986) Requirement for lipopolysaccharide-responsive macrophages in galactosamine-induced sensitization to endotoxin. *Infect Immun* 51: 891–895

37   Beutler B, Milsark IW, Cerami A (1985) Passive immunization against cachectin/tumor necrosis factor protects mice from lethal effect of endotoxin. *Science* 229: 869–871

38   Tracey KJ, Beutler B, Lowry SF, Merryweather J, Wolpe S, Milsark IW, Hariri RJ, Fahey III TJ, Zentella A, Albert JD et al (1986) Shock and tissue injury induced by recombinant human cachectin. *Science* 234: 470–474

39   Neumann B, Engelhardt B, Wagner H, Holzmann B (1997) Induction of acute inflammatory lung injury by staphylococcal enterotoxin B. *J Immunol* 158: 1862–1871

40   Brigham KL, Meyrick B (1986) Endotoxin and lung injury. *Am Rev Respir Dis* 133: 913–927

41   DeGrendele HC, Estess P, Siegelman MH (1997) Requirement for CD44 in activated T cell extravasation into an inflammatory site. *Science* 278: 672–675

42   Mohamadzadeh M, DeGrendele H, Arizpe H, Estess P, Siegelman M (1998) Proinflammatory stimuli regulate endothelial hyaluronan expression and CD44/HA-dependent primary adhesion. *J Clin Invest* 101: 97–108

43   Vanier LE, Prud'homme GJ (1992) Cyclosporin A markedly enhances superantigen-induced peripheral T cell deletion and inhibits anergy induction. *J Exp Med* 176: 37–46

44   Lawson MA, Maxfield FR (1995) Ca^{2+}- and calcineurin-dependent recycling of an integrin to the front of migrating neutrophils. *Nature* 377: 75–79

45   Windsor ACJ, Mullen PG, Fowler AA, Sugerman HJ (1993) Role of the neutrophil in adult respiratory distress syndrome. *Br J Surg* 80: 10–17

46   Weiland JE, Davis WB, Holter JF, Mohammed JR, Dorinsky PM, Gadek JE (1986) Lung neutrophils in the adult respiratory distress syndrome: clinical and pathophysiologic significance. *Am Rev Respir Dis* 133: 218–225

47   Heflin AC, Brigham KL (1981) Prevention by granulocyte depletion of increased vascular permeability of sheep lung following endotoxemia. *J Clin Invest* 68: 1253–1260

48   Johnson A, Malik AB (1980) Effect of granulocytopenia on extravascular lung water content after microembolization. *Am Rev Respir Dis* 122: 561–566

49   Stephens KE, Ishizaka A, Wu ZH, Larrick JW, Raffin TA (1988) Granulocyte depletion

prevents tumor necrosis factor-mediated acute lung injury in guinea pigs. *Am Rev Respir Dis* 138: 1300–1307

50 Till GO, Johnson KJ, Kunkel R, Ward PA (1982) Intravascular activation of complement and acute lung injury: dependency on neutrophils and toxic oxygen metabolites. *J Clin Invest* 69: 1126–1135

51 Welsh CH, Lien DC, Worthen GS, Henson PM, Weil JV (1989) Endotoxin-pretreated neutrophils increase pulmonary vascular permeability in dogs. *J Appl Physiol* 66: 112–119

52 Maunder RJ, Hackman RC, Riff E, Albert RK, Springmeyer SC (1986) Occurrence of the adult respiratory distress syndrome in neutropenic patients. *Am Rev Respir Dis* 133: 313–316

53 Ognibene FP, Martin SE, Parker MM, Schlesinger T, Roach P, Burch C, Shelhamer JH, Parrillo JE (1986) Adult respiratory distress syndrome in patients with severe neutropenia. *New Engl J Med* 315: 547–551

54 Mulligan MS, Warren JS, Smith CW, Anderson DC, Yeh CG, Rudolph AR, Ward PA (1992) Lung injury after deposition of IgA immune complexes, Requirements for CD18 and L-arginine. *J Immunol* 148: 3086–3092

55 Johnson KJ, Ward PA, Kunkel RG, Wilson BS (1986) Mediation of IgA induced lung injury in the rat. Role of macrophages and reactive oxygen products. *Lab Invest* 54: 499–506

56 Tracey KJ, Fong Y, Hesse DG, Manogue KR, Lee AT, Kuo GC, Lowry SF, Cerami A (1987) Anti-cachectin/TNF monoclonal antibodies prevent septic shock during lethal bacteraemia. *Nature* 330: 662–664

57 Neumann B, Machleidt T, Lifka A, Pfeffer K, Vestweber D, Mak TW, Holzmann B, Krönke M (1996) Crucial role of 55-kilodalton TNF receptor in TNF-induced adhesion molecule expression and leukocyte organ infiltration. *J Immunol* 156: 1587–1593

58 Remick DG, Strieter RM, Eskandari MK, Nguyen DT, Genord MA, Raiford CL, Kunkel SL (1990) Role of tumor necrosis factor-α in lipopolysaccharide-induced pathologic alterations. *Am J Pathol* 136: 49–60

59 Anderson BO, Brown JM, Bensard DD, Grosso MA, Banerjee A, Patt A, Whitman GJR, Harken AH (1990) Reversible lung neutrophil accumulation can cause lung injury by elastase-mediated mechanisms. *Surgery* 108: 262–268

60 Smedly LA, Tonnesen MG, Sandhaus RA, Haslett C, Guthrie LA, Johnston RB, Henson PM, Worthen GS (1986) Neutrophil-mediated injury to endothelial cells. Enhancement by endotoxin and essential role of neutrophil elastase. *J Clin Invest* 77: 1233–1243

61 Sakamaki F, Ishizaka A, Urano T, Sayama K, Nakamura H, Terashima T, Waki Y, Tasaka S, Hasegawa N, Sato K et al (1996) Effect of a specific neutrophil elastase inhibitor, ONO-5046, on endotoxin-induced acute lung injury. *Am J Respir Crit Care Med* 153: 391–397

62 Ricou B, Nicod L, Lacraz S, Welgus HG, Suter PM, Dayer JM (1996) Matrix metalloproteinases and TIMP in acute respiratory distress syndrome. *Am J Respir Crit Care Med* 154: 346–352

63   Torii K, Iida KI, Miyazaki Y, Saga S, Kondoh Y, Taniguchi H, Taki F, Takagi K, Matsuyama M, Suzuki R (1997) Higher concentrations of matrix metalloproteinases in bronchoalveolar lavage fluid of patients with adult respiratory distress syndrome. *Am J Respir Crit Care Med* 155: 43–46

64   Delclaux C, d'Ortho MP, Delacourt C, Lebargy F, Brun-Buisson C, Brochard L, Lemaire F, Lafuma C, Harf A (1997) Gelatinases in epithelial lining fluid of patients with adult respiratory distress syndrome. *Am J Physiol* 272: L442–L451

65   Redl H, Schlag G, Bahrami S, Schade U, Ceska M, Stütz P (1991) Plasma neutrophil-activating peptide-1/interleukin-8 and neutrophil elastase in a primate bacteremia model. *J Infect Dis* 164: 383–388

66   Gando S, Nakanishi Y, Kameue T, Nanzaki S (1995) Soluble thrombomodulin increases in patients with disseminated intravascular coagulation and in those with multiple organ dysfunction syndrome after trauma: Role of neutrophil elastase. *J Trauma* 39: 660–664

67   Duswald KH, Jochum M, Schramm W, Fritz H (1985) Released granulocytic elastase: An indicator of pathobiochemical alterations in septicemia after abdominal surgery. *Surgery* 98: 892–899

68   Reddy VY, Desrochers PE, Pizzo SV, Gonias SL, Sahakian JA, Levine RL, Weiss SJ (1994) Oxidative dissociation of human α2-macroglobulin tetramers into dysfunctional dimers. *J Biol Chem* 269: 4683–4691

69   Weiss SJ, Regiani S (1984) Neutrophils degrade subendothelial matrices in the presence of α1-proteinase inhibitor: cooperative use of lysosomal proteinases and oxygen metabolites. *J Clin Invest* 73: 1297–1303

70   Ossanna PJ, Test ST, Matheson NR, Regiani S, Weiss SJ (1986) Oxidative regulation of neutrophil elastase-alpha-1-proteinase inhibitor interactions. *J Clin Invest* 77: 1939–1951

71   Johnson KJ, Ward PA (1981) Role of oxygen metabolites in immune complex injury of lung. *J Immunol* 126: 2365–2369

72   Hart DHL (1984) Polymorphonuclear leukocyte elastase activity is increased by ba-cterial lipopolysaccharide: a response inhibited by glucocorticoids. *Blood* 63: 421–426

73   Ottonello L, Morone MP, Dapino P, Dallegri F (1995) Tumour necrosis factor alpha-induced oxidative burst in neutrophils adherent to fibronectin: effects of cyclic AMP-elevating agents. *Br J Haematol* 91: 566–570

74   Dusi S, Bianca VD, Donini M, Nadalini KA, Rossi F (1996) Mechanisms of stimulation of the respiratory burst by TNF in nonadherent neutrophils Its independence of lipidic transmembrane signaling and dependence on protein tyrosine phosphorylation and cytoskeleton. *J Immunol* 157: 4615–4623

75   Klebanoff SJ, Vadas MA, Harlan JM, Sparks LH, Gamble JR, Agosti JM, Waltersdorph AM (1986) Stimulation of neutrophils by tumor necrosis factor. *J Immunol* 136: 4220–4225

76   Berkow RL, Wang D, Larrick JW, Dodson RW, Howard TH (1987) Enhancement of

neutrophil superoxide production by preincubation with recombinant human tumor necrosis factor. *J Immunol* 139: 3783–3791

77 Simms HH, D'Amico R (1991) Increased PMN CD11b/CD18 expression following post-traumatic ARDS. *J Surg Res* 50: 362–367

78 Kishimoto TK, Jutila MA, Berg EL, Butcher EC (1989) Neutrophil Mac-1 and MEL-14 adhesion proteins inversely regulated by chemotactic factors. *Science* 245: 1238–1241

79 Bainton DF, Miller LJ, Kishimoto TK, Springer TA (1987) Leukocyte adhesion receptors are stored in peroxidase-negative granules of human neutrophils. *J Exp Med* 166: 1641–1653

80 Miller LJ, Bainton DF, Borregaard N, Springer TA (1987) Stimulated mobilization of monocyte Mac-1 and p150,95 adhesion proteins from an intracellular vesicular compartment to the cell surface. *J Clin Invest* 80: 535–544

81 Bevilacqua MP (1993) Endothelial-leukocyte adhesion molecules. *Annu Rev Immunol* 11: 767–804

82 Mulligan MS, Varani J, Dame MK, Lane CL, Smith CW, Anderson DC, Ward PA (1991) Role of endothelial-leukocyte adhesion molecule 1 (ELAM-1) in neutrophil-mediated lung injury in rats. *J Clin Invest* 88: 1396–1406

83 Mulligan MS, Watson SR, Fennie C, Ward PA (1993) Protective effects of selectin chimeras in neutrophil-mediated lung injury. *J Immunol* 151: 6410–6417

84 Mulligan MS, Smith CW, Anderson DC, Todd RF, Miyasaka M, Tamatani T, Issekutz TB, Ward PA (1993) Role of leukocyte adhesion molecules in complement-induced lung injury. *J Immunol* 150: 2401–2406

85 Mulligan MS, Polley MJ, Bayer RJ, Nunn MF, Paulson JC, Ward PA (1992) Neutrophil-dependent acute lung injury: requirement for P-selectin (GMP-140). *J Clin Invest* 90: 1600–1607

86 Mulligan MS, Wilson GP, Todd RF, Smith CW, Anderson DC, Varani J, Issekutz TB, Miyasaka M, Tamatani T, Myasaka M (1993) Role of β_1, β_2 integrins and ICAM-1 in lung injury after deposition of IgG and IgA immune complexes. *J Immunol* 150: 2407–2417

87 Mulligan MS, Miyasaka M, Tamatani T, Jones ML, Ward PA (1994) Requirement for L-selectin in neutrophil-mediated lung injury in rats. *J Immunol* 152: 832–840

88 Miller EJ, Cohen AB, Nagao S, Griffith D, Maunder RJ, Martin TR, Weiner-Kronish JP, Sticherling M, Chrisophers E, Matthay MA (1992) Elevated levels of NAP-1/interleukin-8 are present in the airspaces of patients with the adult respiratory distress syndrome and are associated with increased mortality. *Am Rev Respir Dis* 146: 427–432

89 Miller EJ, Cohen AB, Matthay MA (1996) Increased interleukin-8 concentrations in the pulmonary edema fluid of patients with acute respiratory distress syndrome from sepsis. *Crit Care Med* 24: 1448–1454

90 Donnelly SC, Strieter RM, Kunkel SL, Walz A, Robertson CR, Carter DC, Grant IS, Pollok AJ, Haslett C (1993) Interleukin-8 and development of adult respiratory distress syndrome in at-risk patient groups. *Lancet* 341: 643–647

91 Courtney Broaddus V, Boylan AM, Hoeffel JM, Kim KJ, Sadick M, Chuntharapai A,

Hebert CA (1994) Neutralization of IL-8 inhibits neutrophil influx in a rabbit model of endotoxin-induced pleurisy. *J Immunol* 152: 2960–2967

92 Yokoi K, Mukaida N, Harada A, Watanabe Y, Matsushima K (1997) Prevention of endotoxemia-induced acute respiratory distress syndrome-like lung injury in rabbits by a monoclonal antibody to IL-8. *Lab Invest* 76: 375–384

93 Bozic CR, Kolakowski LF, Gerard NP, Garcia-Rodriguez C, von Uexkull-Guldenband C, Conklyn MJ, Breslow R, Showell HJ, Gerard C (1995) Expression and biologic characterization of the murine chemokine KC. *J Immunol* 154: 6048–6057

94 Lee J, Cacalano G, Camerato T, Toy K, Moore MW, Wood WI (1995) Chemokine binding and activities mediated by the mouse IL-8 receptor. *J Immunol* 155: 2158–2164

95 Frevert CW, Huang S, Danaee H, Paulauskis JD, Kobzik L (1995) Functional characterization of the rat chemokine KC and its importance in neutrophil recruitment in a rat model of pulmonary inflammation. *J Immunol* 154: 335–344

96 Schmal H, Shanley TP, Jones ML, Friedl HP, Ward PA (1996) Role for macrophage inflammatory protein-2 in lipopolysaccharide-induced lung injury in rats. *J Immunol* 156: 1963–1972

97 Ulich TR, Howard SC, Remick DG, Wittwer A, Yi ES, Yin S, Guo K, Welply JK, Williams JH (1995) Intratracheal administration of endotoxin and cytokines VI Antiserum to CINC inhibits acute inflammation. *Am J Physiol* 268: L245–L250

98 Baggiolini M, Dewald B, Moser B (1994) Interleukin-8 and related chemotactic cytokines – CXC and CC chemokines. *Adv Immunol* 55: 97–179

99 VanOtteren GM, Strieter RM, Kunkel SL, Paine R, Greenberger MJ, Danforth JM, Burdick MD, Standiford TJ (1995) Compartmentalized expression of RANTES in a murine model of endotoxemia. *J Immunol* 154: 1900–1908

100 Standiford TJ, Kunkel SL, Lukacs NW, Greenberger MJ, Danforth JM, Kunkel RG, Strieter RM (1995) Macrophage inflammatory protein-1α mediates lung leukocyte recruitment, lung capillary leak, and early mortality in murine endotoxemia. *J Immunol* 155: 1515–1524

101 Bossink AW, Paemen L, Jansen PM, Hack CE, Thijs LG, van Damme J (1995) Plasma levels of the chemokines monocyte chemotactic proteins-1 and -2 are elevated in human sepsis. *Blood* 86: 3841–3847

102 Jansen PM, van Damme J, Put W, de Jong IW, Taylor FB, Hack CE (1995) Monocyte chemotactic protein 1 is released during lethal and sublethal bacteremia in baboons. *J Infect Dis* 171: 1640–1642

103 Zisman DA, Kunkel SL, Strieter RM, Tsai WC, Bucknell K, Wilkowski J, Standiford TJ (1997) MCP-1 protects mice in lethal endotoxemia. *J Clin Invest* 99: 2832–2836

104 Jones ML, Mulligan MS, Flory CM, Ward PA, Warren JS (1992) Potential role of monocyte chemoattractant protein 1/JE in monocyte/macrophage-dependent IgA immune complex alveolitis in the rat. *J Immunol* 149: 2147–2154

105 Jiang Y, Beller DI, Frendl G, Graves DT (1992) Monocyte chemoattractant protein-1 regulates adhesion molecule expression and cytokine production in human monocytes. *J Immunol* 148: 2423–2428

106 Rollins BJ, Walz A, Baggiolini M (1991) Recombinant human MCP-1/JE induces chemotaxis, calcium flux, and the respiratory burst in human monocytes. *Blood* 78: 1112–1116

107 Echtenacher B, Falk W, Männel DN, Krammer PH (1990) Requirement of endogenous tumor necrosis factor/cachectin for recovery from experimental peritonitis. *J Immunol* 145: 3762–3766

Lipopolysaccharide signaling pathways and their role in the development of the systemic inflammatory response syndrome

David J. Hackam[1,2], Sergio Grinstein[2] and Ori D. Rotstein[1]

[1]Department of Surgery, The Toronto Hospital, 200 Elizabeth Street, Toronto, Ontario, M5G 2C4, Canada
[2]Division of Cell Biology, The Hospital for Sick Children, 555 University Avenue, Toronto, Ontario M5G 1X8, Canada

Introduction

The development of the "systemic inflammatory response syndrome" (SIRS) is associated with significant morbidity and causes over 175,000 deaths annually in the United States [1, 2]. Up to 50% of these cases are due to a generalized activation of the immune syndrome related to Gram-negative bacterial infection. The glycolipid surface component of Gram-negative bacteria called lipopolysaccharide (LPS) is central to the development of SIRS and MODS (multiple organ dysfunction syndrome) [3]. While not intrinsically toxic to tissue, LPS acts by inducing myeloid and/or non-myeloid cells to express a variety of pro-inflammatory genes whose products result in the initiation and propagation of SIRS [4]. The elucidation of the signaling mechanisms underlying the activation of cells by LPS has not only improved our understanding of the pathogenesis of SIRS and MODS, but has also provided insight into the development of novel therapeutic modalities.

This chapter will focus on the biology of endotoxin signaling, with a view to understanding the cellular basis for the inflammatory response and the extension of these findings to clinical practice.

Cellular mechanisms of lipopolysaccharide signaling

Structure of lipopolysaccharide

LPS is a complex glycolipid expressed in the outer membrane of all Gram-negative bacteria [4]. It is composed of two chemically distinct regions. The first consists of a hydrophilic segment of repeating polysaccharides and O-antigen structures, while the second consists of a hydrophobic domain known as lipid-A. Structural diversity among the various lipopolysaccharide molecules of different Gram-negative bacteria is due to variations in the O-antigen polysaccharides. The hydrophobic core is considerably more conserved. For example, a single core structure exists for the *Sal-*

Cytokines in Severe Sepsis and Septic Shock, edited by H. Redl and G. Schlag[†]

monella serotypes and only six core structures have been identified for over one hundred different serotypes of *Escherichia coli* [5]. It has been well documented that the biological activity of lipopolysaccharide is dependent upon the lipid core [6]. Takada and colleagues, for instance, showed that synthetic lipid A had full endo-toxic activity [7]. Hence, recognition of the lipid A component by cells most likely represents the initial step in LPS-induced cellular responses. The receptors mediating this recognition, and the ensuing signaling events, are central in the pathogenesis of the septic response.

LPS binding protein

The recognition of LPS binding protein (LBP) as the protein cofactor contributing to LPS signaling represented a significant development in determining how LPS stimulates cells. LBP was identified by showing that the binding of LPS to high-density lipoproteins was markedly reduced in acute phase compared to normal serum, due to the formation of a stable complex between LPS and acute phase proteins [8]. Fractionation of serum revealed the presence of a 60kDa glycoprotein that was responsible for complexing the LPS; this molecule was subsequently named LBP. The complete primary structure of human LBP was subsequently deduced by Ule-vitch and others from cDNA cloning [9].

LBP is synthesized predominantly in hepatocytes as a single polypeptide, and released into the blood as a 60 kDa glycoprotein [10]. Its synthesis is under the control of cytokines and steroid hormones [10], and it behaves as an acute phase protein. *In vitro* studies have shown that LBP binds to LPS via the lipid A portion of the molecule [11] and is unaffected by the O-antigen polysaccharide segments of the protein. Similar studies have also indicated that the Kd for LPS-LBP binding is in the nanomolar range and that the stoichiometry is 1:1 [11].

The functional properties of LBP on lipopolysaccharide-induced cell activation were convincingly demonstrated by Mathison and colleagues [12]. Measurements of LPS-induced tumor necrosis factor (TNF) production showed that the presence of LBP markedly lowered the threshold stimulatory concentration of LPS, and significantly enhanced the rate of TNF production over a range of LPS concentrations [12]. Other investigators have shown that LBP enhances the effects of LPS on the induction of other cytokines [13], as well as on nitric oxide production [14]. LBP also enhances LPS-induced upregulation of integrin function and arachidonic acid metabolism in neutrophils [15]. Convincing evidence for the role of LBP in mediating the effects of endotoxin was provided by Schumann and colleagues [9]. This group demonstrated that immunodepletion of LBP from plasma significantly reduced LPS-induced cell activation [9].

LBP shares amino acid sequence homology with another LPS/lipid A binding protein, namely bactericidal/permeability increasing protein BPI [16]. BPI is a

50 kDa protein localized in neutrophil granules which binds to LPS via lipid A [17]. Despite similarities in primary structure and ability to bind LPS, the biological activities of LBP and BPI differ markedly [16]. For instance, rather than being stimulatory, BPI neutralizes the ability of isolated LPS to activate cells. In addition, BPI is directly bactericidal when it binds LPS on bacteria whereas LBP functions as an opsonin.

Receptors for lipopolysaccharide

A variety of cell surface molecules have been demonstrated to bind LPS and therefore have been implicated in the signaling cascade. These molecules include membrane-bound CD14, a 70–80 kDa membrane protein, integrins (CD11a/CD18, CDllb/CD18, CD11c/CD18) and the scavenger receptor. Current studies have demonstrated that membrane-bound CD14 is the most physiologically significant receptor regarding LPS signaling.

CD14

CD14 is a 55 kDa glycoprotein which is present in two forms: In cells of myeloid lineage, it is expressed as a glycosylphosphatidyl inositol (GPI) linked protein anchored to the plasma membrane. In serum, CD14 is present as a soluble glycoprotein lacking the GPI anchor [18]. The human CD14 gene is located on chromosome five in a region containing genes for several growth factors or growth factor receptors. While this suggested that CD14 might also function as a receptor, definitive evidence was provided by the studies of Wright and colleagues [19]. This group showed that the binding of LPS-LBP- coated erythrocytes to the surface of human monocytes was markedly reduced in the presence of anti-CD14 monoclonal antibodies but not with antibodies to other surface proteins [19]. Moreover, addition of anti-CD14 antibodies to whole blood completely prevented LPS-induced cytokine release under physiologically relevant LPS concentrations [19].

Although CD14 mediates attachment of LPS-bearing opsonized with LBP to the cell surface it does not appear to result in phagocytosis of the particle [20]. However, Gallay et al. [21] demonstrated that CD14 mediates uptake of isolated LPS into human monocytes. Kitchens et al. [22] showed that CD14-dependent uptake of LPS by THP-1 cells occurred independently of the ability of CD14 to signal cell activation. This functional independence of LPS uptake and LPS-mediated activation suggested the concept that CD14 might function with additional proteins to form a functional LPS receptor.

It appears that the major function of CD14 as a LPS/LBP receptor is to facilitate macrophage activation at very low levels of LPS [23]. For example, macrophages from patients with paroxysmal nocturnal hemoglinuria, which lack CD14, require as much as 10,000-fold greater LPS concentrations for activation than do CD14-positive cells [24]. The level of CD14 on the plasmalemma is regulated. It increases during monocyte differentiation and is responsive to cytokines such as interferon gamma [25]. In addition, circulating LPS can alter the expression of CD14 on monocytes: freshly isolated cells undergo upregulation of surface CD14 in response to LPS [26] while tissue macrophages display a loss of CD14 [27]. Part of the regulation of surface CD14 may be mediated by shedding of the receptor from the cell surface. Monocytes spontaneously shed a soluble form of CD14 into culture supernatants. This molecule is approximately 48 kDa and lacks the GPI anchor, suggesting that it was proteolytically cleaved from the membrane.

How can CD14, which does not directly communicate with the cytoplasm, stimulate cells in response to LPS/LBP binding? Studies by Lee, Ulevitch and co-workers examined 70Z/3 cells, a murine pre-B cell line that is LPS responsive but does not express CD14 [28, 29]. They determined that after transfecting 70Z/3 cells with GPI-linked human CD14, the amount of LPS required to stimulate these cells was 1000-fold less than that for the parental lines [28], and that the maximum increase in sensitivity to LPS required LBP. Further, transfection of 70Z/3 cells with a hybrid receptor consisting of CD14 with the transmembrane domain and intracellular tail of tissue factor resulted in similar levels of LPS-induced activation compared with the GPI-linked form [29]. Taken together, these findings indicate that CD14, while not directly responsible for the initiation of signaling, might be part of a membrane-associated receptor complex. Extracellular interactions between the LPS-CD14 complex and other transmembrnae proteins might then initiate transmembrane signaling.

The 70–80 kDa LPS receptor

The identification of additional LPS binding receptors has been facilitated by the use of radioiodinated derivatives of LPS which cross-link with other proteins upon UV irradiation [30]. Lee, Morrison, and colleagues identified a membrane protein of 70–80 kDa which interacted with the lipid A moiety of LPS [31, 32]. This protein is expressed on the surface of lymphoid cells, and contributes to cell activation upon binding to LPS (see [33] for a recent review). Interestingly, this protein was also shown to bind other molecules, including surface peptidoglycan of Gram-positive bacteria, bacterial lipoteichoic acid, and heparin, indicating that it possesses functions in addition to LPS binding. Recently, Dziarski demonstrated that this protein is cell-bound albumin, although the molecular mechanisms by which albumin interacts with the cell surface remain to be elucidated.

The integrins

Integrins are adhesion molecules which play important roles in phagocyte adherence and migration. They are heterodimeric proteins consisting of non-covalently associated α and β subunits generally of 150 and 100 kDa respectively. Both α and β subunits are transmembrane glycoproteins. Interaction of integrins with ligand depends on the divalent cations Ca^{2+} or Mg^{2+} [34], which bind to the extracellular domains of the α subunits. Interestingly, studies by Wright and Jong showed that antibodies to the alpha or beta subunits of the CD11/CD18 integrin inhibited binding of LPS-coated erythrocytes to monocytes [35]. This indicated a role for integrins in binding endotoxin. Recent studies have suggested that these receptors may participate in LPS-mediated cell activation. Chateau et al. demonstrated that antibodies against CD11b inhibited the oxidative response developed by differentiated U937 cells in response to the O-antigen component of endotoxin [36]. Studies by Ingalls et al. have provided insight into the molecular basis of LPS signaling through the CD11/CD18 receptor [37]. They determined that CHO cells, which were transfected with a mutation of the integrin lacking the cytoplasmic tail, exhibited normal LPS-induced signaling, yet were unable to mediate integrin dependent phagocytosis [37]. This suggested that while full length CD11/CD18 is required for phagocytosis, LPS activation does not require the cytoplasmic domains, suggesting that it may activate cells by presenting endotoxin to other downstream signaling molecules. Activation of surface integrins in myeloid cells by LPS may have significant proinflammatory effects, including induction of inducible nitric oxide synthase (iNOS) protein and nitric oxide production [38]. A potential basis for integrin-mediated LPS signaling may be through direct interaction of the integrin with CD14, as was recently demonstrated using resonance energy transfer techniques [39]. A definitive role for CD11/CD18 in LPS signaling remains controversial, as macrophages from CD11/CD18-deficient patients demonstrated normal amounts of IL-1 and TNF in response to LPS when compared to control patients [27]. It is notworthy that other adhesion molecules may conribute to the activation response. Malhotra et al. recently showed that interaction of LPS with cell surface L-selectin results in activation of human neutrophils as demonstrated by superoxide production [40].

The scavenger receptor

The scavenger receptor (ScR) is a surface molecule capable of binding to acetyl-low density lipoproteins. It is expressed on the surface of a variety of cells including hepatocytes and macrophages, where it participates in clearance and detoxification of circulating lipids [35]. Cross linking studies demonstrated that the ScR could bind to the lipid A core of endotoxin, suggesting that it may participate in LPS signaling. This hypothesis was initially refuted by evidence from Hampton et al. [41], who showed that blockade of these receptors with lipoproteins had no effect on TNF release by RAW macrophages after exposure to LPS [41]. More recent studies however have indicated that ScR's may participate in endotoxin signaling. Shynra et al. [42] showed that endotoxin binds specifically to the ScR of Kupffer cells, and that this binding was independent of cations, susceptible to proteases, and was competitive with acetylated low density lipoprotein [42]. Levels of ScR are under the influence of the inflammatory microenvironment. Roselaar et al. [43] showed that LPS-induced TNF production produced a significant, reversible, reduction in ScR mRNA in Swiss Webster mice [43]. What role might ScR have in the cellular response to endotoxin? To address this, Haworth et al. [44] recently studied LPS signaling in macrophages obtained from ScR knockout mice. They showed that mice lacking the receptor where more susceptible to endotoxic shock and produced more TNF and IL-6 in response to LPS compared to wild-type controls. The authors therefore hypothesized that ScR plays a protective role in host defense by scavenging LPS and reducing the release of proinflammatory cytokines [44].

Transmembrane signaling induced by lipopolysaccharide

After interacting with surface receptor, lipopolysaccharide induces a profound cellular activation characterized by the induction of proinflammatory genes and the release of cytokines. The precise mechanisms by which LPS-induced cell activation occurs remain incompletely understood, although significant progress has been achieved in this area over the past several years. Specifically, the interaction of molecular constituents of signaling cascades known to be present in myeloid cells have been shown to mediate the signaling response. These will be reviewed below.

Protein tyrosine kinases
Biochemical and functional considerations

Weinstein and colleagues first showed that LPS treatment of macrophages increased protein tyrosine phosphorylation (PTK), and identified mitogen-activated protein kinase (MAPK) isoforms as targets (see below) [45, 46]. This effect was rapid and could be inhibited by various protein tyrosine kinase inhibitors, including herbimycin A [46] and tyrphostin-25 [47]. Cellular activation is likely dependent upon the induction of tyrosine phosphorylation by MAPK. For instance, Beaty et al. showed that LPS treatment of monocytes resulted in a concentration dependent increase in tyrosine phosphorylation which preceded a rise in TNF and IL-6 mRNA and protein synthesis. Further, tyrosine phosphorylation may directly regulate cytokine production, since inhibitors of PTKs inhibited expression of TNF, IL-1 and IL-6 [48–50]. There is compelling evidence that these studies may have *in vivo* significance. Since TNF is known to be a central mediator of endotoxemia, Novogrodsky et al. investigated the effect of inhibitors of the tyrphostin AG126 on outcome in mice injected with LPS [48]. Pre-treatment with tyrphostin significantly reduced the 5-day mortality in LPS-treated mice compared with control mice exposed to LPS alone. This beneficial effect correlated with reduced TNF production by macrophages derived from treated mice.

A role for Src family kinases?

How might CD14 activation initiate tyrosine kinase activity? One possible mechanism involves the Src family of non-receptor tyrosine kinases. These proteins interact with a variety of cell surface receptors, and play a central role in propagating signals from binding by immunoglobulin receptors and integrins. Five out of nine members of the Src gene family kinases have been identified in phagocytic cells: Src, Fyn, Fgr, Hck, and Lyn [51]. Importantly, immunoprecipitation of the CD14 receptor from CD14-stimulated cells coprecipitated several Src family members, including *lyn*, *hck* and *fgr* [52]. Subsequent investigation revealed that only *lyn* was directly coupled to CD14, while all three tyrosine kinases were activated following exposure of cells to LPS. Convincing evidence that Src family members participate in the signaling cascade is found in studies in which inhibition of *hck* expression by the use of anti-sense oligonucleotides [53] resulted in decreased TNF and IL-1 production [53, 54]. The exact mechanism whereby CD14, which lacks a cytoplasmic tail, associates with these molecules remains unclear. It is likely that the LPS-CD14 complex must interact with another membrane component which might serve to transduce the signal across the plasma membrane. In support of this concept, Vasselon et al. recently showed that responsiveness of human monocytes to LPS was abolished by trypsin, which was shown to digest a cell surface protein distinct from CD14 [55]. Recent studies have examined the role of Src family members, which could interact with such surface proteins, in more detail. To directly determine whether *hck*, *fgr*, and *lyn* are required, Meng and colleagues generated null mutations of all three kinases in a single mouse strain [56]. They found that macrophages cultured from these mice express normal levels of CD14 and no other Src-family kinases were detected. Interestingly, although the total protein phosphorylation level was greatly reduced in macrophages derived from the mutant mice, functional analysis indicated that both peritoneal and bone marrow macrophages had no defects in LPS-induced cytokine production. Moreover, the activation of MAP kinases was also normal. This evidence strongly argues against a direct role for Src family kinases in LPS initiated signal transduction [56]. It is likely, therefore, that a variety of parallel pathways participate in the signaling response and the requirement for Src kinases may not be complete for all of them.

A role for MAPK family members

The underlying processes by which tyrosine phosphorylation might signal cellular activation has been extensively examined in a variety of systems over the past several years. The mitogen-activated protein kinase family are ser/thr kinases which play key roles in the regulation of pathways governing many cellular processes, cell proliferation, and cell differentiation. Most protein kinases are in an inactive state until phosphorylation induces kinase activity. MAPKs require dual and mixed phosphorylation for their activation, i.e. threonine and tyrosine residues must be phosphorylated to achieve enzymatic activity. These phosphorylations are catalyzed by dual specificity protein kinases called MAP kinase kinases (MAPKK or MEK) [57]. The primary amino acid sequences around the threonine/tyrosine phosphorylation sites of MAPKs are highly conserved [58].

A specific role of LPS on activation of these signaling intermediates has recently been established. Using stably-transfected 70Z/3 cells expressing human CD14, Han et al. showed that LPS-CD14 binding resulted in activation of the MAPK isoform p38 [59]. p38 is distinct from the 44 or 40 kDa isoforms of MAPK, and is closely related to the product of the HOG1 gene in yeast [60]. p38 may also be relevant in non-transfected cells, as several authors have shown that LPS-stimulation of neutrophils results in a marked activation of the kinase [61, 62] in a concentration dependent manner. The functional importance of p38 in LPS-induced signaling has been elucidated using the specific inhibitor SB 203580 [4-4(fluorophenyl)-2-(4-methylsulfinylphenyl)-5-(4-pyridyl)imidazole]. This compound was demonstrated to be a potent inhibitor of LPS-induced cytokine production *in vivo* in a variety of studies [63,64], confirming the functional relevance of p38 activation to endotoxin signaling. Various authors have also shown that LPS stimulation increases tyrosine phosphorylation and augments the activity of other MAP kinase isoforms, including p42/p44 (ERK 1/2) in murine monocyte cell lines, murine peritoneal macrophages, and human peripheral monocytes [45, 60, 65–67]. Worth noting is that activation of these proteins may not be an absolute requirement for cytokine production. In support of this, Swantek et al. recently showed that although LPS induces the activation of MEKs 1-4 and their downstream targets ERK1/2, MEK activation was not required for LPS-induced cytokine release [68].

Other kinases

In addition to the molecules described above, additional signaling molecules have been shown to mediate LPS-induced cell activation. Emerging evidence points to a role for the lipid molecule phosphatidylinositol (PtdIns) and its phosphorylated derivatives, collectively referred to as phosphoinositides (PIs), in the signaling events which occur downstream of CD14. The inositol ring which forms the head group of the PtdIns is a highly versatile structure that can be modified at several sites. Phosphorylation at one or a combination of positions (3′, 4′ or 5′) generates a set of five unique stereoisomers that appear to function as intracellular signaling molecules. An important mediator of these reactions is PI 3-kinase, which has been implicated in LPS mediated signaling. In human peripheral blood monocytes exposed to LPS, PI 3-kinase activity underwent an immediate elevation which correlated with increased levels of the enzymatic product PtdIns 3,4,5-triphosphate [69]. Activation of PI 3-kinase involved signaling through CD14 as antibodies to CD14 abrogated the increase in PtdIns production [69]. The degree to which the signaling process depends on these molecules remains to be established.

Recently, homologues of the p42 and p44 isoforms of the MAP kinases have been described, namely the stress activated protein kinases (SAPKs) or alternatively the c-jun N-terminal kinases (JNKs). These molecules are essential components of signaling cascades in response to a number of cellular stresses including inflammatory cytokines, heat and chemical shock, ultraviolet irradiation, osmotic stress and ischemia [70]. Emerging evidence has indicated that these molecules also become activated upon endotoxin stimulation [68, 71]. A major thrust of current research is the identification and function of the major intermediates of the SAPK cascades and their physiological function.

Tyrosine phosphorylation and cytokine expression

How does activation of this signaling cascade by LPS result in production of inflammatory cytokines? The transcription factor NF-κB is known to be translocated to the nucleus in LPS-stimulated macrophages, where it plays an important role in the generation of proinflammatory mediators. A specific link between the LPS-induced *raf*/MEK/MAPK cascade and NF-κB activity was demonstrated by Li et al. This group showed that raf activation resulted in phosphorylation of the inhibitory chaperone IκB, leading to release and nuclear translocation of NF-κB [72]. It is noteworthy that other transcription factors become activated and translocate to the nucleus upon LPS stimulation. Han et al. recently showed that LPS-induced p38 activation resulted in transactivation of the myocyte-enhancer factor 2 (MEF2) group of transcription factors [73], which regulate the transcription of a variety of proinflammatory genes.

The phospholipase C/Calcium/Protein kinase C (PKC) axis

The role of phospholipase C

One of the most important signal transduction cascades in many cell types involves activation of phospholipase C (PLC) and the hydrolysis of its substrate phosphatidylinositol tris-phosphate. Not surprisingly, the role of this cascade in LPS-mediated signal transduction has generated significant interest, often with conflicting results. Two main types of PLC have been detected in leukocytes: PLCβ and PLCγ. These isoforms have similar catalytic activity, but differ in their mode of action. Both types of PLC cleave phosphatidylinositol tris-phosphate, releasing diacylglycerol (DAG) and inositol 1,4,5-trisphosphate (IP$_3$). In the case of PLCβ, the quiescent enzyme is activated by guanine nucleotide binding proteins (G-proteins). By contrast, PLCγ activation occurs independent of G proteins and is activated by receptors that are themselves tyrosine kinases or are associated with such kinases. Phosphorylation of PLCγ on tyrosine residues results in its activation, a process that is terminated by phosphotyrosine phosphatases. In LPS-stimulated cells, there is evidence that one or both of these types of PLC might contribute to cellular activation. For instance, studies reporting an inhibitory effect of pertussis toxin have implicated a role for G proteins in mediating LPS-stimulated cell activation [74, 75], while the accumulation of tyrosine phosphorylated proteins is known to occur following LPS stimulation (see above).

Recent studies have provided evidence suggesting that PLC lies downstream of the CD14 receptor. For instance, NF-κB activation in CD14 transfected CHO cells occurred during incubation with DAG analogues or phospholipase C, even without LPS stimulation [76]. Moreover, pharmacological inhibition of phospholipase C markedly reduced the LPS-dependent production of DAG as well as LPS-induced NF-κB activation [76]. These results indicated that the production of DAG by PLC was upstream of NF-κB activation in response to a CD14-mediated LPS stimulus. It is noteworthy that other authors have failed to detect PLC activation following LPS stimulation [77].

The role of PKC

Independent of the type of specific PLC activated, stimulation results in a similar cascade of events. The most relevent consequence of the release of diacylglycerol is the activation of PKC, a family of calcium and phospholipid-dependent serine/threonine kinases. Multiple isoforms of PKC have been described, which differ in the extent of their dependence on calcium and lipid, as well as their tissue and subcellular distribution. PKC exerts pleiotropic effects on many aspects of cell activation, implying that it could participate in LPS-mediated signaling. Several substrates of PKC have been shown to undergo increased protein phosphorylation and plasma membrane translocation in response to LPS: 68 kDa [78], 66 kDa [79] and 140 kDa [80] proteins in murine peritoneal macrophages and a 79 kDa protein in human peripheral monocytes [81]. Recent reports have demonstrated that LPS stimulation increases the activity of many PKC isoforms, with particular isoforms having specific functional significance. For instance, PKC-ε was recently shown to be the predominant isoform activated upon LPS stimulation, and inhibition of PKC-ε was sufficient to reduce the entire PKC response [82]. PKC-ζ was shown to become specifically activated upon LPS stimulation of a variety of myeloid cells, including human peripheral blood monocytes and the cell lines U937 and THP-1 [83]. Interestingly, preincubation of monocytes with the inhibitor wortmannin, or transfection with dominant negative PI 3-kinase, abrogated LPS-induced activation of PKC-ζ, implying that the activity of this isoform lies downstream of PI 3-kinase [83]. Adding to this controversy are recent reports showing that pharmacological inhibition of PKC markedly attenuates LPS-induced cytokine release [84].

The role of IP$_3$

The other product of phosphoinositide hydrolysis, IP$_3$, acts primarily as a messenger in the pathway leading to an increased cytosolic calcium concentration ($[Ca^{2+}]_i$).

IP$_3$ enters the endoplasmic reticulum or a specialized subcompartment thereof, called the calciosome. Binding of IP$_3$ promotes the release of calcium from within these endomembrane stores, which signals the opening of plasmalemmal calcium channels which leads to a sustained rise in [Ca^{2+}]$_i$. A number of reports describe increases in [Ca^{2+}]$_i$ in response to LPS [85, 86], while others find minimal or no changes [87].

Other signaling cascades

Phospholipase A$_2$

Following exposure to LPS, activation of phospholipase A$_2$ (PLA$_2$) has been shown to occur both *in vitro* and *in vivo*. PLA$_2$ is a family of enzymes that catalyze the hydrolysis of phosphatidylcholine and/or phosphatidlyethanolamine. Typically, they cleave position *sn*-2 of the phospholipid, where arachidonate is most frequently located. The free arachidonate generated can then be used by the lipooxygenase and cyclooxygenase pathways to generate other second messengers. Three general types of PLA$_2$ have been described which can be separated into calcium-dependent and calcium-independent. The calcium-dependent molecules can be subdivided into two groups: cytosolic (cPLA$_2$) and secretory (sPLA$_2$, present in secretory granules). There is convincing evidence that LPS activates cPLA$_2$ and also induces the secretion of sPLA$_2$ in leukocytes. In human neutrophils, PLA$_2$ is activated many-fold within minutes of addition of LPS (C4-57) and cPLA$_2$ becomes phosphorylated in the process [88]. Recent evidence has suggested that PLA$_2$ participates in endotoxin-mediated signaling. For instance, experiments performed in mice deficient in the PLA$_2$ receptor showed a decreased LPS-induced TNF and IL-1 production after LPS injection [89]. Importantly, this was associated with longer survival after endotoxin challenge in mutant mice compared to wild-type controls [89].

Phospholipase D

In addition to PLA$_2$ and PLC, stimulation of leukocytes is also associated with activation of phospholipase D (PLD). PLD catalyses the hydrolysis of phosphatidylcholine to choline and phosphatidic acid (PA), the latter of which functions as a second messenger in a variety of cellular processes. Since PA is a major source of diacylglycerol, PLD can indirectly support continued stimulation of PKC. PA can also exert direct effects. These include activation of the NADPH oxidase responsible for the respiratory burst [90], and modulation of GTPase activity [91]. PLD may contribute to the transduction of signals generated by LPS, as inhibition of PA was shown to be protective against endotoxic shock *in vivo* [92]. These observations suggest that PLD can be stimulated by LPS and may participate in the biological effects of endotoxin.

Therapeutic modulation of LPS signaling

The signaling pathways described above provide insight into potential sites whereby the host immune response may be manipulated by therapeutic agents in an attempt to treat SIRS. In general terms, such sites may be viewed as those which alter the interaction of macrophages with LPS/LBP, those which impair normal intracellular signaling, and those that alter the activity of the liberated cytokines. Progress in each of these areas will be described below.

Strategies which attempted to prevent the interaction of LPS with macrophages have involved neutralizing or binding LPS with specific antibodies. Clinical trials using anti-LPS antibodies directed against the conserved lipid A portion of LPS have yielded disappointing results. This is in part related to the fact that only approximately 40% of patients with clinical SIRS actually have Gram-negative infection as an underlying cause [93]. However, of the patients with documented Gram-negative bacteremia who were followed to hospital discharge or death, there was a statistically significant improved likelihood of being discharged alive in antibody treated patients compared to placebo treated controls [93]. As an alternative strategy, CD14 has been shown to inhibit TNF production in monocytes/macrophages by binding LPS [94]. However, the utility of this approach in preventing the septic response is unclear, as soluble CD14 facilitates the response to LPS in cells which lack a CD14 receptor, such as endothelial cells [95].

Other strategies have attempted to protect the patient form endotoxemia by disrupting the intracellular signaling cascade. As described above, agents which impair tyrosine kinases or preclude normal PLA_2 activity have been shown to improve outcome in experimental models of sepsis [96], suggesting the potential for clinical efficacy. Recently, Bernard and colleagues reported the use of the cyclooxygenase inhibitor ibuprofen in the treatment of sepsis [97]. They determined that ibuprofen-treated patients had significant reductions in circulating levels of prostacyclin and thromboxane as well as decreased fever, tachycardia, oxygen consumption and lactic acidosis. However, there was no improvement in the development of shock or the acute respiratory distress syndrome, nor in survival.

The third approach attempts to prevent the activity of the cytokines, either by neutralizing them or interfering with their receptors. Significant effort was exerted to neutralize the effects of TNF, initially by using anti-TNF antibodies [98]. While initial results were somewhat encouraging, longterm antibody usage has inherent risks of antigenicity. For this reason, chimeric TNF inhibitor proteins, consisting of the extracellular domain of a TNF receptor spliced to a portion of an IgG heavy chain have been developed for TNF neutralization [99]. When expressed at high levels *in vivo*, experimental animals become blind to TNF, and are thus LPS resistant. However, clinical use of this reagent in patients with septic shock was extremely disappointing, as treatment with the chimeric protein did not reduce mortality [100]. Moreover, higher doses appeared to be associated with increased mortality.

Summary

This discussion has attempted to overview the cellular processes whereby LPS interacts with cells, induces their activation, and generates molecules which participate in the inflammatory response. While understanding these pathways has led to the development of innovative strategies, the complexity of the patient population studied and the redundancy of much of the signaling pathways during inflammation has precluded successful intervention to this point. Clearly, however, careful consideration of the strategies as part of multi-modal therapy may someday prove fruitful.

References

1   Parillo JE (1993) Pathogenetic mechanisms of septic shock. *N Engl J Med* 328: 1471–1477

2   Stone R (1994) Search for sepsis drugs goes on despite past failures. *Science* 64: 365–367

3   Glauser MP, Zanetti G, Baumgartner JD, Cohen J (1991) Septic shock: pathogenesis. *Lancet* 338: 732–736

4   Ulevitch RJ, Tobias PS (1995) Receptor dependent mechanisms of cell stimulation by bacterial endotoxin. *Annu Rev Immunol* 13: 437–457

5   Jansson P, Lindberg AA, Lindberg B, Wollin R (1981) Structural studies on the hexose region of the core in lipopolysaccharide from Enterobactereaceae. *Eur J Biochem* 115: 571–577

6   Rietschel ET, Kirikae T, Schade FU, Mamat U, Schmidt G, Loppnow H, Ulmer AJ, Zahringer U, Seydel U, di Padova F et al (1994) Bacterial endotoxin: molecular relationships of structure to activity and function. *FASEB J* 8: 217–225

7   Takada H, Kotani S (1989) Structural requirements of lipid A for endotoxicity and other biological activities. *CRC Crit Rev Microbiol* 16: 477–525

8   Tobias PS, Soldau K, Ulevitch RJ (1986) Isolation of a lipopolysaccharide-binding acute phase reactant from rabbit serum. *J Exp Med* 164: 777–793

9   Schumann RR, Leong SR, Flaggs GW, Gray PW, Wright SD, Mathison JC, Tobias PS, Ulevitch RJ (1990) Structure and function of lipopolysaccharide binding protein. *Science* 249: 1429–1433

10 Grube BJ, Cochrane CG, Ye RD, Ulevitch RJ, Tobias PS (1994) Cytokine and dexamethasone regulation of lipopolysaccharide binding protein (LBP) expression in human hepatoma (HepG2) cells. *J Biol Chem* 269: 8477–8482

11 Tobias PS, Soldau K, Ulevitch RJ (1989) Identification of a lipid A binding site in the acute phase reactant lipopolysaccharide binding protein. *J Biol Chem* 264: 10867–10871

12 Mathison JC, Tobias PS, Wolfson E, Ulevitch RJ (1992) Plasma lipopolysaccharide bind-

ing protein: a key component in macrophage recognition of Gram-negative lipopolysaccharide (LPS). *J Immunol* 149: 200–206

13　Martin TR, Mathison JC, Tobias PS, Maunder RJ, Ulevitch RJ (1992) Lipopolysaccharide binding protein enhances the responsiveness of alveolar macrophages to bacterial lipopolysaccharide: implications for cytokine production in normal and injured lungs. *J Clin Invest* 90: 2209–2219

14　Corradin SB, Mauel J, Ulevitch RJ, Tobias PS (1992) Enhancement of murine macrophage binding of and response to bacterial lipopolysaccharide (LPS) by LPS-binding protein. *J Leukocyte Biol* 52: 363–368

15　Surette ME, Palmantier R, Gosselin J, Borgeat P (1993) Lipopolysaccharides prime whole human blood and isolated nautrophils for the increased synthesis of 5-lipoxygenase products by enhancing arachidonic acid availability: involvement of the CD14 antigen. *J Exp Med* 178: 1347–1355

16　Elsbach P, Weiss J (1993) Bactericidal/permeability increasing protein and host defense against Gram-negative bacteria and endotoxin. *Curr Opin Immunol* 5: 103–107

17　Dziarski R (1991) Demonstration of peptidoglycan-binding sites on lymphocytes and macrophages by photoaffinity cross-linking. *J Biol Chem* 266: 4713–4718

18　Bazil V, Horejsi V, Baudys M, Kristopova H, Strominger J, Kostka W, Hilgert I (1986) Biochemical characterization of a soluble form of the 53-kDa monocyte surface antigen. *Eur J Immunol* 16: 1583–1589

19　Wright SD, Ramos RA, Tobias PS, Ulevitch RJ, Mathison JC (1990) CD14, a receptor for complexes of lipopolysaccharide (LPS) and LPS binding protein. *Science* 249: 1431–1433

20　Wright SD, Tobias PS, Ulevitch RJ, Ramos RA (1989) Lipopolysaccharide (LPS) binding protein opsonizes LPS-bearing particles for recognition by a novel receptor on macrophages. *J Exp Med* 170: 1231–1241

21　Gallay P, Jongeneel CV, Barras C, Burnier M, Baumgartner JD, Glauser MP, Heumann D (1993) Short time exposure to lipopolysaccharide is sufficient to activate human monocytes. *J Immunol* 150: 5086–5093

22　Kitchens RL, Ulevitch RJ, Munford RS (1992) Lipopolysaccharide (LPS) partial structure inhibit responses to LPS in a human macrophage cell line without inhibiting LPS uptake by a CD14-mediated pathway. *J Exp Med* 176: 485–494

23　Lee J, Kato K, Tobias PS, Kirkland TN, Ulevitch RJ (1992) Transfection of CD14 into 70Z/3 cells dramatically enhances the sensitivity to complexes of lipopolysaccharide (LPS) and LPS binding protein. *J Exp Med* 175: 1697–1705

24　Duchow J, Marchant A, Crusiaux A, Husson C, Alonso-Vega C, DeGroote D, Neve P, Goldman M (1993) Impaired phagocyte responses to lipopolysaccharide in paroxysomal nocturnal hemoglobinuria. *Infect Immun* 61: 4280–4285

25　Landmann R, Wesp M, Ludwig C, Obrist R, Knusli C, Obrecht JP (1990) Recombinant interferon gamma upregulates *in vivo* and downregulates *in vitro* monocyte CD14 expression in cancer patients. *Cancer Immunol Immunother* 31: 292–296

26   Birkenmaier C, Hong YS, Horn JK (1992) Modulation of endotoxin receptor (CD14) in septic patients. *J Trauma* 32: 473–479

27   Wright SD, Detmers PA, Aida Y, Adamoski R, Anderson DC, Chad Z, Kabbash LG, Pabst MJ (1990) CD18-deficient cells respond to lipopolysaccharide *in vitro*. *J Immunol* 144: 2566–2571

28   Lee JD, Kato K, Tobias PS, Kirkland TN, Ulevitch RJ (1992) Transfection of CD14 into 70Z/3 cells dramatically enchances the sensitivity to complexes of lipopolysaccharide (LPS) binding protein. *J Exp Med* 175: 485–494

29   Lee JD, Kravchenko VV, Kirkland TN, Han J, Mackman N, Moriarty A, Leturcq D, Tobias PS, Ulevitch RJ (1993) GPI anchored or integral membrane forms of CD14 mediate identical cellular responses to endotoxin. *Proc Natl Acad Sci USA* 90: 9930–9934

30   Tobias PS, Soldau K, Kline L, Lee J, Kato K, Martin TR, Ulevitch RJ (1993) Crosslinking of lipopolysaccharide to CD14 on THP-1 cells mediated by lipopolysaccharide binding protein. *J Immunol* 150: 3011–3021

31   Lee M, Morrison DC (1988) Specific endotoxic lipopolysaccharide binding proteins on murine splenocytes. I. Detection of lipopolysaccharide binding sites on splenocytes and splenocyte subpopulations. *J Immunol* 141: 996–1005

32   Lee M, Morrison DC (1988) Endotoxic lipopolysaccharide binding proteins on murine splenocytes. II. Membrane localization and binding characteristics. *J Immunol* 141: 1006–1011

33   Ulevitch RJ (1993) Recognition of bacterial endotoxins by receptor dependent mechanisms. *Adv Immunol* 53: 267–289

34   Imhof BA, Dunon D (1995) Leukocyte migration and adhesion. *Adv Immunol* 58: 345–416

35   Wright SD, Jong MTC (1986) Adhesion promoting receptors on human macrophages recognize E. coli by binding to lipopolysaccharide. *J Exp Med* 164: 1876–1888

36   Chateau MT, Caravano R (1997) The oxidative burst triggered by Salmonella typhimurium in differentiated U937 cells requires complement and a complete bacterial lipopolysaccharide. *FEMS Immunol Med Microbiol* 17: 57–66

37   Ingalls RR, Arnaout MA, Golenbock DT (1997) Outside-in signaling by lipopolysaccharide through a tailless integrin. *J Immunol* 159: 433–438

38   Matsuno R, Aramaki Y, Arima H, Adachi Y, Ohno N, Yadomae T, Tsuchiya S (1998) Contribution of CR3 to nitric oxide production from macrophages stimulated with high-dose of LPS. *Biochem Biophys Res Comm* 244: 115–119

39   Zarewych DM, Kindzelskii AL, Todd RF, 3rd, Petty HR (1996) LPS induces CD14 association with complement receptor type 3, which is reversed by neutrophil adhesion. *J Immunol* 156: 430–433

40   Malhotra R, Priest R, Bird MI (1996) Role for L-selectin in lipopolysaccharide induced activation of neutrophils. *Biochem J* 320: 589–593

41   Hampton RY, Raetz CRH (1991) Macrophage catabolism of lipid A is regulated by endotoxin stimulation. *J Biol Chem* 266: 19499–19503

42 Shnyra A, Lindberg AA (1995) Scavenger receptor pathway for lipopolysaccharide binding to Kupffer and endothelial liver cells *in vitro*. *Infect Immun* 63: 865–873

43 Roselaar SE, Daugherty A (1997) Lipopolysaccharide decreases scavenger receptor mRNA *in vivo*. *J Interferon Cytok Res* 17: 573–579

44 Haworth R, Platt N, Keshav S, Hughes D, Darley E, Suzuki H, Kurihara Y, Kodama T, Gordon S (1997) The macrophage scavenger receptor type A is expressed by activated macrophages and protects the host against lethal endotoxic shock. *J Exp Med* 186: 1431–1439

45 Weinstein SL, Sanghera JS, Lemke K, DeFranco AL, Pelech SL (1992) Bacterial lipopolysaccharide induces tyrosine phosphorylation and activation of mitogen activated protein kinase in macrophages. *J Biol Chem* 267: 14955–14962

46 Weinstein SL, Gold MR, DeFranco AL (1991) Bacterial lipopolysaccharide stimulates protein tyrosine phosphorylation in macrophages. *Proc Natl Acad Sci USA* 88: 4148–4152

47 Glaser KB, Sung A, Bauer J, Weichman BM (1993) Regulation of protein tyrosine phosphorylation and modulation by selective protein tyrosine kinase inhibitors. *Biochem Pharmacol* 45: 711–721

48 Novogrodsky A, Vanichkin A, Patya M, Gazit A, Osherov N, Levitzki A (1994) Prevention of lipopolysaccharide induced lethal toxicity by tyrosine kinase inhibitors. *Science* 264: 1319–1322

49 Shapira L, Takashiba S, Champagne C, Amar S, Van Dyke TE (1994) Involvement of protein kinase C and protein tyrosine kinase in lipopolysaccharide induced TNF and IL-1 production by human monocytes. *J Immunol* 153: 1818–1824

50 Geng Y, Zhang B, Lotz M (1993) Protein tyrosine kinase activation is required for lipopolysaccharide induction of cytokines in human blood monocytes. *J Immunol* 151: 6692–6700

51 Huang M, Indik ZK, Brass LF, Hoxie JA, Schreiber AD, Brugge JS (1992) Activation of Fc gamma RII induces tyrosine phosphorylation of multiple proteins including Fc gamma RII. *J Biol Chem* 267: 5467–5473

52 Stefanova I, Corcoran ML, Horak EM, Wahl LM, Bolen JB, Horak ID (1993) lipopolysaccharide induces activation of CD14 associated protein tyrosine kinase p53/56 lyn. *J Biol Chem* 268: 20725–20728

53 English BK, Ihle JN, Myracle A, Yi T (1993) Hck tyrosine kinase activity modulates tumour necrosis factor production by murine macrophages. *J Exp Med* 178: 1017–1022

54 English BK, Orlicek SL, Mei Z, Meals EA (1997) Bacterial LPS and IFN-gamma trigger the tyrosine phosphorylation of vav in macrophages: evidence for involvement of the hck tyrosine kinase. *J Leukocyte Biol* 62: 859–864

55 Vasselon T, Pironkova R, Detmers PA (1997) Sensitive responses of leukocytes to lipopolysaccharide require a protein distinct from CD14 at the cell surface. *J Immunol* 159: 4498–4505

56 Meng F, Lowell CA (1997) Lipopolysaccharide (LPS)-induced macrophage activation

and signal transduction in the absence of Src-family kinases *Hck, Fgr,* and *Lyn. J Exp Med* 185: 1661–1670

57 Davis RJ (1993) The mitogen activated protein kinase signal transduction pathway. *J Biol Chem* 268: 14553–14556

58 Nishida E, Gotoh Y (1993) The MAP kinase cascade is essential for diverse signal transduction pathways. *Trends Biochem Sci* 18: 128–131

59 Han J, Lee JD, Tobias PS, Ulevitch RJ (1993) Endotoxin induces rapid protein tyrosine phosphorylation in 70Z/3 cells expressing CD14. *J Biol Chem* 268: 25009–25014

60 Han J, Lee JD, Bibbs L, Ulevitch RJ (1994) A MAP kinase targeted by endotoxin and hyperosmolarity in mammalian cells. *Science* 265: 808–811

61 Nahas N, Molski TF, Fernandez GA, Sha'afi RI (1996) Tyrosine phosphorylation and activation of a new mitogen-activated protein (MAP)-kinase cascade in human neutrophils stimulated with various agonists. *Biochem J* 318: 247–253

62 Nick JA, Avdi NJ, Gerwins P, Johnson GL, Worthen GS (1996) Activation of a p38 mitogen-activated protein kinase in human neutrophils by lipopolysaccharide. *J Immunol* 156: 4867–4875

63 Badger AM, Bradbeer JN, Votta B, Lee JC, Adams JL, Griswold DE (1996) Pharmacological profile of SB 203580, a selective inhibitor of cytokine suppressive binding protein/p38 kinase, in animal models of arthritis, bone resorption, endotoxin shock and immune function. *J Pharm Exp Ther* 279: 1453–1461

64 Lee JC, Young PR (1996) Role of CSB/p38/RK stress response kinase in LPS and cytokine signaling mechanisms. *J Leukocyte Biol* 59: 152–157

65 Liu MK, Herrera-Velit P, Brownsey RW et al (1994) CD14 dependent activation of protein kinase C and mitogen activated protein kinases (p42 and p44) in human monocytes treated with bacterial lipopolysaccharide. *J Immunol* 153: 2642–2652

66 Dong Z, Qi X, Fidler IJ (1993) Tyrosine phosphorylation of mitogen activated protein kinases is necessary for activation of murine macrophages by natural and synthetic bacterial products. *J Exp Med* 177: 1071–1077

67 Schumann RR, Pfeil D, Lamping N, Kirschning C, Scherzinger G, Schlag P, Karawajew L, Herrmann F (1996) Lipopolysaccharide induces the rapid tyrosine phosphorylation of the mitogen-activated protein kinases erk-1 and p38 in cultured human vascular endothelial cells requiring the presence of soluble CD14. *Blood* 87: 2805–2814

68 Swantek JL, Cobb MH, Geppert TD (1997) Jun N-terminal kinase/stress-activated protein kinase (JNK/SAPK) is required for lipopolysaccharide stimulation of tumor necrosis factor alpha (TNF-alpha) translation: glucocorticoids inhibit TNF-alpha translation by blocking JNK/SAPK. *Mol Cell Biol* 17: 6274–6282

69 Herrera-Velit P, Reiner NE (1996) Bacterial lipopolysaccharide induces the association and coordinate activation of p53/56lyn and phosphatidylinositol 3-kinase in human monocytes. *J Immunol* 156: 1157–1165

70 Paul A, Wilson S, Belham CM, Robinson CJ, Scott PH, Gould GW, Plevin R (1997) Stress activated protein kinases: activation, regulation and function. *Cell Signaling* 9: 403–410

71   Sanghera JS, Weinstein SL, Aluwalia M, Girn J, Pelech SL (1996) Activation of multiple proline-directed kinases by bacterial lipopolysaccharide in murine macrophages. *J Immunol* 156: 4457–4465

72   Li S, Sedivy JM (1993) Raf-1 protein kinase activates the NF-kappaB transcription factor by dissociating the cytoplasmic NF-kappaB-IkappaB complex. *Proc Natl Acad Sci USA* 90: 9247–9251

73   Han J, Jiang Y, Li Z, Kravchenko VV, Ulevitch RJ (1997) Activation of the transcription factor MEF2C by the MAP kinase p38 in inflammation. *Nature* 386: 296–299

74   Jakway JP, DeFranco AL (1986) Pertussis toxin inhibition of B cell and macrophage responses to bacterial lipopolysaccharide. *Science* 234: 743–746

75   Zhang X, Morrison DC (1993) Pertussis toxin sensitive factor differentially regulates lipopolysaccharide induced tumor necrosis factor alpha and nitric oxide production in mouse peritoneal macrophages. *J Immunol* 150: 1011–1018

76   Yamamoto H, Hanada K, Nishijima M (1997) Involvement of diacylglycerol production in activation of nuclear factor kappaB by a CD14-mediated lipopolysaccharide stimulus. *Biochem J* 325: 223–228

77   Dieter P, Fitzke E (1995) Differential regulation of phospholipase D and phospholipase C by protein kinase C-beta and -delta in liver macrophages. *Cell Signaling* 7: 687–694

78   Rosen A, Nairn AC, Greengard P (1988) Bacterial lipopolysaccharide regulates the phosphorylation of the 68kDa protein kinase C substrate in macrophages. *J Biol Chem* 264: 9118–9121

79   Nakano M, Saito S, Nakano Y, Yamasu H, Matsuura M, Shinomiya H (1993) Intracellular protein tyrosine phosphorylation in murine peritoneal macrophages in response to bacterial lipopolysaccharide (LPS): effects of kinase inhibitors and LPS induced tolerance. *Immunobiol* 187: 272–282

80   Shinji H, Akagawa KS, Tsuji M, Maeda M, Yamada R, Matsuura K, Yamamoto S, Yoshida T (1997) Lipopolysaccharide-induced biphasic inositol 1,4,5-trisphosphate response and tyrosine phosphorylation of 140-kilodalton protein in mouse peritoneal macrophages. *J Immunol* 158: 1370–1376

81   Bakouche O, Moreau JL, Lachman LB (1992) Secretion of IL-1: Role of protein kinase C. *J Immunol* 148: 84–91

82   Shapira L, Sylvia VL, Halabi A, Soskolne WA, Van Dyke TE, Dean DD, Boyan BD, Schwartz Z (1997) Bacterial lipopolysaccharide induces early and late activation of protein kinase C in inflammatory macrophages by selective activation of PKC-epsilon. *Biochem Biophys Res Com* 240: 629–634

83   Herrera-Velit P, Knutson KL, Reiner NE (1997) Phosphatidylinositol 3-kinase-dependent activation of protein kinase C-zeta in bacterial lipopolysaccharide-treated human monocytes. *J Biol Chem* 272: 16445–16452

84   Paul A, Pendreigh RH, Plevin R (1995) Protein kinase C and tyrosine kinase pathways regulate lipopolysaccharide-induced nitric oxide synthase activity in RAW 264.7 murine macrophages. *Br J Pharm* 114: 482–488

85   Letari O, Nicosia S, Chiavaroli C, Vacher P, Schlegel W (1991) Activation by bacterial

LPS causes changes in the cytosolic free calcium concentration in single peritoneal macrophages. *J Immunol* 147: 980–983

86 Waga I, Nakamura M, Honda Z, Ishiguro S, Shimizu T (1993) Two distinct signal transduction pathways for the activation of macrophages and neutrophils by endotoxin. *Biochem Biophys Res Comm* 197: 465–472

87 Martin TR, Mathison JC, Tobias PS, Moriarty A, Ulevitch RJ (1992) LPS-binding protein enhances the responsiveness of alveoalr macrophages to bacterial LPS. *J Clin Invest* 90: 2209–2215

88 Doerfler ME, Weiss J, Cjark JD, Elsbach P (1994) Bacterial LPS primes human neutrophils for enhanced release of arachidonic acid and causes phosphorylation of cPLA$_2$. *J Clin Invest* 93: 1583–1591

89 Hanasaki K, Yokota Y, Ishizaki J, Itoh T, Arita H (1997) Resistance to endotoxic shock in phospholipase A2 receptor-deficient mice. *J Biol Chem* 272: 32792–32797

90 Bauldry SA, Bass DA, Cousart SL, MacCall CE (1991) TNF priming of phospholipase D in human neutrophils: correlation between phosphatidic acid production and the respiratory burst. *J Biol Chem* 266: 4173–4179

91 Billah MM (1993) Phospholipase D and cell signaling. Curr Opin Immunol 5: 114–123

92 Rice GC, Brown PA, Nelson RJ, Bianco JA, Singer JW, Bursten S (1994) Protection from endotoxic shock in mice by inhibition of phosphatidic acid. *Proc Natl Acad Sci USA* 91: 3857–3861

93 Ziegler EJ, Fisher CJ, Jr., Sprung CL, Straube RC, Sadoff JC, Foulke GE, Wortel CH, Fink MP, Dellinger RP, Teng NN et al (1991) Treatment of Gram-negative bacteremia and septic shock with HA-1A human monoclonal antibody against endotoxin. A randomized, double-blind, placebo-controlled trial. The HA-1A Sepsis Study Group. *N Eng J Med* 324: 429–436

94 Haziot A, Rong G, Bazil V, Silver J, Goyert SM (1994) Recombinant soluble CD14 inhibits LPS-induced tumor necrosis factor alpha production by cells in whole blood. *J Immunol* 152: 5868–5876

95 Frey EA, Miller DS, Jahr TG, Sundan A, Bazil V, Espevik T, Finlay BB, Wright SD (1992) Soluble CD14 participates in the response of cells to lipopolysaccharide. *J Exp Med* 176: 1665–1671

96 Ziegler EJ, Fisher CJ, Sprung CL, Straube RC, Sadoff JC, Foulke GE, Wortel DH, Fink MP, Dellinger RP, Teng MM et al (1991) Treatment of Gram-negative bacteremia and septic shock with HA-1A monoclonal antibodies against endotoxin. *N Eng J Med* 324: 429–436

97 Bernard GR, Wheeler AP, Russell JA, Schein R, Summer WR, Steinberg KP, Fulkerson WJ, Wright PE, Christman BW, Dupont WD et al (1997) The effects of ibuprofen on the physiology and survival of patients with sepsis. The Ibuprofen in Sepsis Study Group. *N Eng J Med* 336: 912–918

98 Exley AR, Cohen J, Buurman W, Owen R, Hanson G, Lumley J, Aulakh JM, Bodmer M, Riddell A, Stephens S et al (1990) Monoclonal antibody to TNF in severe septic shock. *Lancet* 335: 1275–1277

99   Peppel K, Crawford D, Beutler B (1991) A tumor necrosis factor (TNF) receptor-IgG
     heavy chain chimeric protein as a bivalent antagonist of TNF activity. *J Exp Med* 174:
     1483–1489
100 Fisher CJ, Jr., Agosti JM, Opal SM, Lowry SF, Balk RA, Sadoff JC, Abraham E, Schein
     RM, Benjamin E (1996) Treatment of septic shock with the tumor necrosis factor recep-
     tor:Fc fusion protein. The Soluble TNF Receptor Sepsis Study Group. *N Engl J Med*
     334: 1697–1702

Predisposing factors: effect of sex, nutritional factors and age on immunity following shock and sepsis

René Zellweger[1,2], Alfred Ayala[1,2] and Irshad H. Chaudry[1,2,3]*

[1]Center for Surgical Research and [2]Departments of Surgery, [3]Molecular Pharmacology, Physiology and Biotechnology, Brown University School of Medicine and Rhode Island Hospital, Providence, RI 02903, USA; *Present address: Department of Trauma Surgery, University of Zurich, 8091 Zurich, Switzerland

General introduction

Research from numerous laboratories throughout the world now indicates that many, if not all, of the physiological, metabolic, and immunological responses to trauma, sepsis and cancer are not mediated directly by bacteria or their toxins, or by tumor cells, but rather by groups of host-derived polypeptide molecules which are produced in response to these stimuli and have collectively been called cytokines [1–4]. These molecules work together with classic stress hormones and with other humoral mediators to orchestrate and coordinate the cellular response to critical illnesses. The central role occupied by these polypeptide signals has challenged past teachings and prompted a rethinking of traditional approaches for treating the host with severe infections. New knowledge delineating how these key polypeptide molecules control the catabolic response to stress states has been generated at a staggering pace. From an evolutionary standpoint, these biological responses are the result of a process that favors survival of the fittest in the struggle to survive and preserve the species. Ironically, these polypeptide mediators, which clearly orchestrate many of the appropriate and beneficial responses to these catabolic diseases (i.e. fever, tachycardia, and acute-phase protein synthesis), can also initiate detrimental physiological responses, such as hypotension, organ failure, cachexia, and death [5–7].

In the case of tumor necrosis factor (TNF), it has been suggested that excessive production of this particular cytokine during severe sepsis may serve as an endogenous "self-destruct mechanism" with the purpose of eliminating wounded members of the herd or the host with lethal sepsis or advanced incurable cancer to ensure survival of the fittest. In selected patients with infections, the TNF concentration in the bloodstream is a predictor of survival [8–11].

One school of thought is that cytokines are produced locally within tissues and are designed to control cellular metabolism in a paracrine or autocrine fashion [4, 12]. Only when excess production occurs, leading to spillover into the systemic circulation, are their effects harmful [13]. It remains unclear why, under certain cir-

Cytokines in Severe Sepsis and Septic Shock, edited by H. Redl and G. Schlag[†]

cumstances, tighter control of cytokine signals does not exist and why under those conditions they may be responsible for the death of the host after overwhelming microbial invasion.

Cytokines bind to specific membrane receptors that are expressed on the surface of virtually all cells. Binding to the receptor affects a variety of intracellular responses that result from complex signal transduction pathways activated by specific cytokine receptors [3, 14]. Different portions of the signal transduction pathways appear to be represented in different cells. Accordingly, different tissues respond to cytokines in different ways. Therefore a particular interleukin may stimulate amino acid transport *in vitro* in one cell type but not in another [14–16]. Further understanding of these intracellular signaling pathways may lead to the development of therapies designed to block specific cytokine effects.

A growing interest in cytokine biology has led to productive collaborations between clinicians, basic scientists, and industry. Clinical trials designed to determine whether a role exists for cytokine blockade with monoclonal antibodies or receptor antagonists in critically ill patients are in progress, the overall benefits of which should be measured in terms of a reduction in major complications and improved survival. However, as the clinical and scientific collaborations have evolved, by bringing forth new therapies for patients with severe trauma, shock or sepsis, it has become apparent, due to the failure of a number of the early clinical trials [17–28], that much more needs to be understood about the pathobiology of these states. In this regard, the predisposition of the animal or patient population with respect to gender, nutritional status or age, has, until recently, not been a common component actively addressed either in experimental animal studies examining the immune response following shock or sepsis, nor in clinical trials. To a degree, our lack of understanding of how these variables affect the immune response following trauma, shock and sepsis may explain, at least in part, why some of these initial exciting new therapeutic approaches were not efficacious clinically. This chapter is, therefore, aimed at briefly reviewing the current information on these predisposing states and what the findings have been as to their contributions to the altered immune status encountered following shock, traumatic injury or the onset of sepsis. We do not, however, intend this as a review of immune process or their mediators (i.e. cytokine, prostanoids, NO, O_2, etc.), as these are covered extensively in other parts of this book.

Influence of sex on the immune system

Sex differences in the susceptibility to and morbidity from sepsis have been observed in several clinical and epidemiological studies [29–31]. The alterations in endocrine and immune functions have been investigated primarily using male laboratory animals. Immune function in normal males and females has been reported to be influenced by sex-steroids [32–33]. In this regard, it appears that better maintained immune functions in females are not only due to physiologic levels of female sex-steroids, but also at least in part due to the lower levels of immunosuppressive androgenic hormones [34–35]. A number of clinical and experimental studies have shown the suppressive effects of androgens on immunity [34–38]. Recent immuno-logical studies suggest beneficial effects of prior testosterone depletion by castration on splenocyte immune function after soft-tissue trauma and hemorrhagic shock [39–40]. The suppressive effects of androgens on immunity have been observed on normal immune functions as well as in autoimmune diseases [35–37, 41]. Studies also indicate a predominance of diverse autoimmune diseases such as systemic lupus erythematosus, Hashimoto's thyroiditis, rheumatoid arthritis and primary biliary cirrhosis in females [42–43]. Cell-mediated immune responses also appear to exhib-it sexual dimorphism [44]. Thymocytes and lymphocytes from normal female mice respond more vigorously to exogenous and allogeneic antigens than do cells from male mice [45].

Since 1898, when Calzolari [46] demonstrated that castration of adult male rab-bits resulted in an increase in thymic mass, it has been known that sexual hormones can affect the immune system. In recent years, it has become apparent from a large number of experimental studies that sex-linked hormonal factors may influence immune response and modify the expression of autoimmunity in animals as well as in humans [47]. Studies have shown that both the humoral and cell-mediated immune responses are more prominent in females than in males [44, 48, 49]. In both human and animal models [50–51], circulating concentrations of the major immunoglobulin classes (IgG, IgM, IgA) in females far exceeded those concentra-tions found in males of the same species, age, and physiological conditions when challenged with antigens such as polio, bovine serum albumin or hemagglutinin. This difference was reflected not only as higher titers of antibody, but also as a more sustained primary and secondary response in females than in males [52]. Increased plasma concentrations of prolactin in females are associated with increased T helper and T cytotoxic lymphocyte activity [53]. The increased T helper and T cytotoxic lymphocyte activity results in an increased cell-mediated immune response, accom-panied by an increase in humoral immunity (i.e. T helper cell-mediated B cell pro-duction of immunoglobulin). Prolactin has been demonstrated to have stimulatory effects on the immune system, and may be a key hormone contributing to the dichotomy seen in the immune response between females and males [54–56]. Recent work suggests a significant depression of cytokine release from macrophages of male mice harvested from either the peritoneal cavity or the spleen of septic mice at 24 h after the onset of sepsis [57–58]. Development of such an immune depres-sion during late sepsis may translate into decreased ability to ward off microbial pathogens which, in turn, contributes to increased morbidity and mortality under these conditions. Treatment of septic animals with either prolactin or metoclo-pramide (which is known to elevate prolactin levels [59]) immediately after the onset of sepsis resulted in significantly increased innate and inducible IL-1β, IL-6 and TNFα gene expression in both splenic and peritoneal macrophage populations [60]. Moreover, prolactin administration following hemorrhagic shock improved macrophage cytokine release capacity and decreased mortality from subsequent sepsis [61]. The physiological release of prolactin from the pituitary fluctuates in a pulsatide circadian fashion, as do glucocorticoids, and is further modulated by behavioral and environmental stimuli, the reproductive cycle, steroid hormones, neurotransmitters, immunoregulatory cytokines, and various drugs. Further studies [54, 55, 62–65] support the view that hormones of the endocrine system (i.e. pro-lactin, progesterone, the adrenal glucocorticoids, growth hormones, and endoge-nous opioids) are intimately involved in immunological sexual dimorphism [54, 55, 62–65].

Gram-negative bacterial sepsis and the ensuing multiple organ failure remain the leading cause of morbidity and mortality following trauma [66–68]. McGowan et al. [31] found in their pioneering study of bacteremia more males suffering from sepsis than females. Barrow and Herndon [69] compared the fre-quency of mortality in boys and girls between the ages of one and 15 years after severe thermal injury (≥ 30% body surface area) and noted a significantly higher mortality rate in males. Bone [29] analyzed four severe sepsis studies and found that 60% to 65% of the patients were males. Experimental studies have demon-strated that the link between cell and organ dysfunction associated with multiple organ failure lies in the initial presentation of sepsis [70–71]. The early (1–4 h) systemic inflammatory response results from the activation of macrophages to produce a number of pro-inflammatory cytokines, including IL-1β, IL-6 and TNFα [72–74]. These activated macrophages have been implicated as exocrine mediators involved in initiating and developing cell and organ dysfunction during sepsis [5, 75, 76]. The development of macrophage dysfunction or hyporespon-siveness in late sepsis, may profoundly reduce the animals ability to ward off the lethal effects of sepsis.

Nutritional status and immune functions

It is well known that the patient's nutritional status and nutrient intake can alter cytokine production. Cytokines initiate the acute-phase response, induce changes in substrate flow and use, and cause weight loss and fever. Cytokines control the altered substrate metabolism that develops in trauma, sepsis, and cancer. It is becoming increasingly clear that the derangements in nutrient metabolism that develop in each of these disease states are strikingly similar and are at least partly mediated by cytokines.

Nutrition is a critical determinant of immunocompetence and risk of illness. Young children with protein-energy malnutrition exhibit increased mortality and morbidity, due largely to infectious disease. Recent work has demonstrated that undernourished individuals have impaired immune responses. The most consistent abnormalities are seen in cell-mediated immunity, complement system, phagocytes, mucosal secretory antibody response, and antibody affinity. Malnutrition is associated with a number of acute and chronic sequelae. One of the most frequent complications is infection. Due to its widespread occurrence, nutritional deficiency is the commonest cause of immunodeficiency worldwide. Although much of the initial work on nutrition and immunity was done on young children in developing countries, the general principle that nutrition is a critical determinant of immunocompetence is applicable universally. For instance, in patients with a variety of diseases, such as cancer and Crohn's inflammatory bowel disease, nutritional deficiencies further complicate the picture and increase the risk of infectious complications.

Epidemiological studies have documented the adverse effect of protein-energy malnutrition (PEM) on morbidity and mortality [77–80]. Chandra et al. [77, 79, 81, 82] have performed several studies in undernourished children and found that pathological examination of tissues from children dying of PEM showed the frequent presence of several opportunistic microorganisms including *Pneumocystis carinii*. Lymphoid tissues show a significant atrophy; the size of the thymus is reduced. Histologically, there is a loss of thymic corticomedullary differentiation, there are fewer lymphoid cell, and the Hassal bodies are enlarged, degenerated, and occasionally, calcified. In the spleen, there is a loss of lymphoid cells around small blood vessels. In the lymph node, the thymus-dependent areas show depletion of lymphoid cells. Several aspects of cell-mediated immunity are significantly altered by PEM. Delayed cutaneous hypersensitivity responses both to recall and new antigens are markedly depressed. One plausible reason for reduced cell-mediated immunity in PEM is the reduction in the number of fully mature differentiated T-lymphocytes. The use of monoclonal antibodies and of flow cytometric methods showed that the number of CD4+ T-helper cells was decreased markedly, often to values less than 50% of controls. The change in the number of suppressor T cells (CD8+) is less marked. Thus, the helper/suppressor ratio is significantly decreased. Lymphocyte proliferation and synthesis of DNA are reduced. Antibody responses were among the first set of immune indices examined in PEM and showed that antibody affinity is decreased along with decreased secretory IgA antibody levels after immunization with viral antigens. This may have several clinical implications, including an increased frequency of septicemia in undernourished children. The process of phagocytosis is also affected in PEM. Although the ingestion of particles by phagocytes is intact, subsequent metabolic activation and destruction of bacteria is reduced. The levels of complement, an essential opsonin, and activity of most complement components are decreased by PEM. Moreover, recent work in man and animal has demonstrated that the production of interleukin-1 is decreased in PEM [81].

Micronutrients

Observations in laboratory animals deprived of various dietary elements and findings in patients with a given nutrient deficiency have confirmed the crucial role of several vitamins and trace elements in immunocompetence [83]. Deficiencies of pyridoxine, folic acid, vitamin A, vitamin C and vitamin E result in impaired cell-mediated immunity and reduced antibody responses. Vitamin B6 deficiency results in a decreased lymphocyte stimulation response to mitogens such as phytohemagglutinin. A moderate increase in vitamin A or beta-carotene intake enhances immune response and affords partial protection against the development of certain tumors in animals. Zinc deficiency, both acquired and inherited, is associated with lymphoid atrophy, decreased cutaneous delayed hypersensitivity responses and homograft rejection, and lower thymic hormone activity. Moreover, there are a reduced number of antibody-forming cells in the spleen and impaired T-killer cell activity. In addition, wound healing is impaired. Excess zinc also depresses neutrophil function and lymphocyte responses [84]. Deficiency of iron is the commonest nutritional problem worldwide, even in industrialized countries. Studies have shown that free iron is necessary for bacterial growth since removal of iron with the help of lactoferrin or other chelating agents reduced bacterial multiplication, particularly in the presence of specific antibody [81]. Iron is, however, needed by neutrophils and lymphocytes for optimal function. Response to tetanus toxoid and herpes simplex antigens was low in iron-deficiency subjects and iron therapy resulted in a significant improvement in their response [81]. There are many molecular explanations for impaired lymphocyte and neutrophil function in iron deficiency, including the deficiency of myeloperoxidase and ribonucleotidyl reductase. T-lymphocytes constitute approximately 80% of the circulating pool of lymphocytes. In PEM, there is a sharp reduction in the proportion and absolute number of these cells and there is a correlation with weight deficit [81].

In certain segments of the population, such as the elderly and smokers, activity of the immune indexes can be increased through dietary supplementation with micronutrients, and there may be a rationale to increase selected recommended dietary allowances for the general population.

Dietary fat

The activity of the immune system may also be enhanced with decreases in total fat intake or lessened with increases in total fat intake, particularly of the *n*-3 type. In the past decade, several studies have been conducted to examine the effects of amount and type of dietary fat on the human immune response. In two separate studies conducted in a metabolic suite, the proliferation of peripheral blood lymphocytes increased significantly in men and women in response to mitogens specific for T and B cells when the fat content of the diets was reduced from 30% or 40% of energy to 25% of energy [85, 86]. An increase in lymphocyte proliferation and the secretion of interleukin 1 (IL-1) was also observed in a group of elderly subjects when fat intake was reduced from 36% to 27% of energy [87]. The lowering of fat intake from 32% to 22% of energy increased natural killer cell activity in a group of healthy men [88]. This increase in natural killer activity was prevented by the daily additional intake of 15 g safflower oil but not coconut oil.

Whether *n*-6 polyunsaturated fatty acids (PUFA's) are more inhibitory than saturated fatty acids, as seen in animal studies, is not clear from the limited studies conducted in humans. The available data suggest that a moderate increase in the intake on *n*-6 PUFAs in a diet containing > 30% of energy from total fat and with adequate amounts of antioxidant nutrients should not have any adverse effects on immune response. However, such an increase may suppress immune response in individuals with low antioxidant-nutrient status who are consuming high-fat diets [89]. Because of the recommendations made by some groups that the intake of *n*-3 PUFAs should be increased to improve cardiovascular health, several studies have been conducted in the past few years to examine the effects of these fatty acids on immune response. Adding 18 g fish oil, equivalent to 5 g eicosapentaenoic acid plus docosahexaenoic acid, to the diets of nine healthy subjects for six weeks inhibited several indexes of immune response including neutrophil chemotaxis and secretion of IL-1, IL-2, and tumor necrosis factor [90, 91]. Further preliminary clinical studies showed that fish-oil (i.e. *n*-3 PUFA) supplementation had a restorative effect on the depressed cellular immunity of patients in intensive-care units [92] and of patients after major surgery [93, 94]. A recent prospective clinical study in burn patients has shown that the use of a diet containing fish oil significantly reduced wound infection, shortened hospital stay and lowered mortality rates compared with other standard enteral formulations [95]. Similar results have recently been reported by Daly et al. [96], who found that patients placed on enteral diets containing fish-oil after major elective surgery demonstrated not only improved *in vitro* lymphocyte mitogenic responses but also fewer infection/wound complications and decreased length of hospital stay. Barton et al. [97] reported that Kupffer cells taken from septic animals prefed for five days and then postfed for seven days with a Menhaden-oil (*n*-3 PUFA) diet produced lower levels of PGE_2, which correlated positively with increased survival after a septic challenge. These studies support the notion that the *n*-3 PUFA diet alters eicosanoid biosynthesis, and that this is one of the mechanisms responsible for the immunoprotective effects reported above.

Other studies indicate that many indexes of immune response are inhibited by supplementation with fish oils, and the time taken for the inhibition to occur as well as for it to be overcome after discontinuation of fish oil supplementation varies with the different indexes of immune response [90, 91]. Inhibition of lymphocyte proliferation caused by fish oil supplementation could be overcome with increased intake of vitamin E [98].

The net effect of dietary fat on immune response is an outcome of the interaction and balance between several factors including total fat, type of fat, the ratios between different fatty acids, chain length, degree of unsaturation, duration of feeding, and antioxidant-nutrient status. Because several other micronutrients can affect immune status, indexes of immune response cannot be used to detect essential fatty acid nutritional status except under rare deficiency conditions. However, the amount of total fat in the diet and the ratios between different fatty acid classes can be used to modulate human immune response. The existing immunological data support the current recommendations by the American Heart Association to decrease fat intake to 30% of energy with 10% of energy each from saturated, monounsaturated, and polyunsaturated fatty acids. On the lower end, $\geq 20\%$ of energy from fat is needed for health maintenance and work efficiency in healthy adult populations [99].

Vitamins

Recent, well-controlled human intervention studies found that clinically important immune responses were improved when amounts of vitamin C, vitamin E, or β-carotene higher than the recommended dietary allowance (RDA) were consumed in healthy populations [100]. For example, in a placebo-controlled, double-blind intervention study conducted in a metabolic ward, responses on delayed-type hypersensitivity (DTH) skin tests, an important index of overall immune function, were significantly reduced in a group of healthy men when their vitamin C intake was reduced from 250 to 5, 10 or 20 mg/day for 60 days. In another placebo-controlled, double-blind study, incidence of post-race infections in marathon runners was twice as high as in those not taking vitamin C supplements compared with runners who took ≈ 1 g vitamin C/day [101]. Data from a large national survey found that forced expiratory lung volume, a clinically important index of lung function, was significantly greater in individuals consuming ≈ 178 mg vitamin C/day compared with those consuming the RDA for vitamin C [102].

Diet and lifestyle

Lifestyle and environmental factors can adversely affect both the status of essential nutrients and immune responses. For example, tissue concentrations of vitamin C, vitamin E, β-carotene, vitamin B-6, and folate are lower in smokers than the corresponding values in nonsmokers. Smokers have elevated neutrophil-oxidation activity, which may reduce antioxidant-nutrient status. In one trial, the activity of neutrophils from smokers was restored to normal with β-carotene supplementation (40 mg/day) [103]. In another study, supplementation of β-carotene (30 mg/day) reduced the number of precancerous oral leukoplakia lesions, and at the same time, natural killer cell functions were significantly enhanced [104].

Diet and aging

The elderly are another group at risk for decreased immune responses. In fact, DHT responses at the time of hospitalization of elderly persons can be used to predict death. The incidence of death was 30 times higher in those with negative responses to all seven recall antigens compared with those who had at least one positive response [105]. DTH responses were significantly enhanced in a separate placebo-controlled study in which healthy elderly subjects took a multivitamin and mineral tablet for one year [106]. Chandra [107] showed a significant decrease in number of sick days and in use of antibiotics, as well as an increase in antibody response to the flu vaccine, in a group of healthy elderly subjects who supplemented their diets with a multivitamin that contained 100% of the RDA of most vitamins and moderately higher amounts of vitamin C (80 mg/day), vitamin E (44 mg/day), and β-carotene (16 mg/day). Thus, it appears that to maintain their immune responses at an optimum, healthy elderly persons may need higher amounts of certain essential micronutrients than their usual dietary intake and the current RDA recommendations. Furthermore, these amounts for the elderly are higher than the amounts needed by younger adults.

The many observations on the interactions between nutrition and immunity have led to several practical applications. For example, the outcome of surgical patients can be predicted on the basis of preoperative assessment of nutritional status and of immunocompetence. Practicing surgeons should become knowledgeable about the potential strategies involving the use of cytokine antagonists and specialized nutritional regimens as potential new treatment options because these therapies may become an integral part of the care of critically ill surgical patients in the next decade.

Research to date suggests that several dietary components, both essential and non-essential, can affect human immune response. The intake of these nutrients can be modulated to regulate the activity of the immune system. Scrimshaw et al [108] in 1959 reviewed the literature linking malnutrition and immune response and reported, "Many of the important infections of human populations are rendered more serious in their consequences by the presence of malnutrition." Beisel [109] coined the acronym NAIDS to depict *nutritionally acquired immune deficiency syndrome* and reported that a combination of infection and malnutrition in children with NAIDS accounted for > 40 000 deaths/day in underdeveloped countries, plus countless other deaths of adults with NAIDS in modern hospitals. Several other chronic diseases including cardiovascular disease, cancer, and arthritis also have their roots in disorders of the immune system. Nonetheless, several nutrients, including vitamins, minerals, and amino acids, influence the activity of immune cells to infections.

The immune system during aging (endocrine effects)

Changes in body composition are known to occur with aging. Specifically a decrease in lean body mass and an increase in fat mass are both characteristic of the aging process. Alterations in hormonal status and immune modulators of metabolism (i.e. cytokines), and thus in body composition, may occur among the elderly and contribute to the loss of lean body mass. In males, peak lean body mass (LBM) occurs during the mid-thirties, after which there is a continued, gradual decline [110]. Women maintain their peak LBM until the early fifties, after which they also begin to lose LBM, but at a slower rate than men [111]. Loss of LBM is reflected by a proportional loss of diaphragm muscle mass and muscle strength. The clinical implication of decreased LBM is increased susceptibility to respiratory complications among the elderly, as expiratory muscle weakness renders coughing ineffective [112].

Host derived mediators which may contribute to various states of predisposition to immune suppression

Thus far we have attempted to provide a general overview of three of the most common categories of predisposition encountered in the traumatized, shock and/or septic patient/animal population. However, while a number of mediators have been mentioned, as stated in the introduction, one of the main hypotheses as to why the shock, injured and/or septic patient/animal develops multiple organ failure is considered to be due to the altered host-mediated response to the initial traumatic and/or infectious insult and not due to a direct action of the microbes or their toxins. In view of this, it is worthwhile to briefly discuss some of the mediators which may be contributing in these different states of predisposition in somewhat more detail.

Several major components of the immune system (immunoglobulins, cytokines), as well as other factors that may influence immune function (i.e. many hormones), are all proteins. Normal functioning of the immune system requires rapid division and proliferation of the immune cells. Therefore, a decreased efficiency of protein metabolism, such as that which occurs during aging, could decrease the production of substances essential for normal functioning of the immune system. Conversely, activation of the immune system by illness may increase protein turnover in the elderly and place a higher demand on an already reduced LBM. Some of the primary hormones implicated in these changes associated with aging include growth hormone, prolactin, the androgens, insulin, cortisol, and the thyroid hormones. In this respect, some of the above mentioned hormones have an anabolic role while others are catabolic, which may account for some of the impact on the immune response of the aged, as well as normal, animal or patient.

Growth hormone (GH) is a potent anabolic agent that stimulates protein synthesis and cell growth and improves nitrogen balance while reducing stored and circulating lipids [113]. Interestingly, increasing evidence suggests that lymphocytes also synthesize de novo and secrete an immunoreactive GH that is similar, if not identical, in terms of bioactivity, antigenicity, and molecular weight, to that produced by cells of the anterior pituitary [114]. The production of GH can be altered under various physiological conditions. Exercise, for example, acts as a powerful stimulus to increase serum GH concentrations. There is also abundant evidence that GH secretion declines with advancing age after reaching maximal secretion at puberty [115–119]. After age 40, GH secretion by the anterior pituitary gland tends to decline [115, 117, 119]. It has been estimated that as many as 50% of individuals over 65 are partially or totally deficient in GH [115].

Prolactin, which is secreted by the anterior pituitary gland, can be classified as one of the GH-related hormones, since its major effects are promotion of growth and differentiation of target tissues (primarily breast and ovary). Studies in rats have indicated that plasma levels of prolactin seem to increase during aging; this finding is also consistent with the observed increase in body fat, perhaps related to increased prolactin levels among the elderly [120].

Testosterone is quantitatively the primary androgen. The difference in plasma testosterone levels between males and females (0.6 vs. 0.03 mg/dl, respectively) seems to account for the fact that the female begins her adult life with a LBM only two-thirds that of a male [121]. Male testosterone secretion peaks at approximately age 22 and declines steadily thereafter, consistent with the decrease in muscle mass that occurs with advancing age [110].

Insulin. The net effect of insulin is to increase both muscle mass and fat mass during times of fuel excess. It has recently been reported that the well-recognized insulin resistance observed in the elderly is due to a small decrease in pancreatic insulin output as well as to a small decline in peripheral tissue response to insulin [122]. Given the known physiological effects that insulin produces, a decrease in insulin effect during aging would be consistent with the decrease in LBM and muscle activity observed in the elderly.

Glucocorticoids (cortisone and cortisol) inhibit protein synthesis and stimulate protein degradation in skeletal muscle, resulting in net protein catabolism and decreased muscle mass. Circulating plasma glucocorticoid levels have been reported either to increase (in rats) [123] or remain unchanged (in humans) [124] during aging.

Thyroid hormones. The thyroid hormones themselves act to increase both protein synthesis and degradation, however, T_3 is also required for GH synthesis by the pituitary. Serum T_4 levels probably do not change with age, and it is unknown whether there is an age-related change in reverse T_3.

Cytokines. In addition to the influence of the classic neuroendocrine hormones on body composition, there is also considerable evidence supporting the notion that endogenous products of the immune system, the cytokines, also mediate LBM changes resulting from injury, inflammation and perhaps aging. In recent years, increased attention has been paid to the effects of aging on the production of cytokines. It has been suggested that dysregulation of cytokines may be partly responsible for the increased morbidity and mortality rates and the subtle presentation of infection in the elderly. Peterson et al. [125], however, found no differences in TNFα, IL-6, IL-10 and TGFβ serum levels from elderly (mean age of 80 years) as compared to the levels of these cytokines in younger controls (mean age of 30 years). Levels of IL-10 in serum were found to be higher in young females than in young males or elderly females [98]. Mooradian et al. [126] found that levels of IL-1 and TNFα were elevated in the serum of elderly patients with underlying medical conditions but not in the serum of healthy elderly controls. Gon et al. [127] demonstrated lower concentrations of G-CSF, GM-CSF, TNFα, IL-8 and MIP-1α in sera from elderly patients with bacterial pneumonia in the acute phase of disease, and an impaired ability of monocytes from normal healthy elderly subjects to produce the above mediators. These results may suggest, at least in part, the characteristic features of host defense mechanisms of the elderly with bacterial infections. The difference in cytokine levels in healthy elderly patients in the studies carried out by Peterson et al. [125] and Gon et al. [126] are unclear, however, they could partly be explained due to different methodologies used for the measurement of cytokines . For instance, Peterson et al. [125] determined cytokine levels by bioassay whereas Gon et al. [126] used quantitative enzyme immunoassays. The hypothesis that "successful aging" is associated with normal production of TNFα, IL-6, IL-10, and TGFβ is not entirely proven and needs further investigation. Studies are currently underway to explore the relationships between hormonal and cytokine changes during exercise and their potential benefit in terms of body composition among the elderly. Given that the elderly comprise an increasingly larger segment of the world population, it would be highly desirable to demonstrate, through a physiological intervention such as exercise, that body composition, and ultimately functional capacity, can be improved and maintained as people age.

Summary and conclusions

Numerous predisposing factors such as the sex, age, preexisting diseases, and nutritional status, as well as the socioeconomic background of the host, can influence the susceptibility to sepsis following trauma and shock. Sex differences in the susceptibility to and morbidity from sepsis have been observed in several clinical and epidemiological studies as well as in experimental studies. It appears that estrogen and/or low testosterone is responsible for better immunity in young females following trauma and sepsis whereas testosterone and/or low estradiol appear to be responsible for the immunosuppression which is observed in males of similar age under those conditions. Evidence is also available which indicates that if the host is protein-energy malnourished, he/she is more susceptible to sepsis and the ensuing septic complications. Moreover, micronutrient deficiency and the type of fat in the diet can also adversely affect the immune responses. Vitamin supplementation particularly during aging appear to be helpful for decreasing the morbidity following trauma and sepsis. The changes in growth hormone, prolactin, testosterone, glucocorticoids, insulin and sex hormones with aging can all influence cytokine production and consequently immune responses. In view of this, experimental studies dealing with the effects of shock or sepsis should consider not only the age of the animal but also the sex (particularly the different state of the estrous cycle in females) on immunity. Thus, there are several predisposing factors which can influence the host response to trauma and sepsis. Appropriate recognition and identification of those factors should be helpful for the care and better management of the traumatized host.

Acknowledgments

This work was supported by MSPHS grant RO1 GM 37127 and R29 GM 46354.

References

1   Chaudry IH, Ayala A (1992) *Immunological aspects of hemorrhage.* Medical Intelligence Unit, R.G. Landes Company, Austin, TX, 1–132
2   Schlag G, Redl H (1996) Mediators of injury and inflammation. *World J Surg* 20: 406–410
3   Redl H, Schlag G, Paul G, Bahrami S, Buurman WA, Strieter RM, Kunkel SL, Davies J, Foulkes R (1996) Endogenous modulators of TNF and IL-1 response are under partial control of TNF in baboon bacteremia. *Am J Physiol* 271: R1193–R1198
4   Molly RG, Mannick JA, Rodrick ML (1993) Cytokines, sepsis and immunomodulation. *Br J Surg* 80: 289–297
5   Tracey KJ, Beutler B, Lowry SF, Merryweather J, Wolpe S, Milsark IW, Haririr J, Fahey TJ, III, Zentella A, Albert JD, Shires GT, Cerami A (1986) Shock and tissue injury induced by recombinant human cachectin. *Science* 234: 470–474
6   Tracey Kj, Lowry SF, Cerami A. (1988) Cachectin/TNF-apha in septic shock and septic adult respiratory distress syndrome. *Am Rev Respir Dis* 138: 1377–1379
7   Baue AE (1994) Multiple organ failure, multiple organ dysfunction syndrome, and the systemic inflammatory response syndrome – Where do we stand? *Shock* 2: 385–397

8   Marano MA, Fong Y, Moldawer LL, Wei H, Calvano SE, Tracey KJ, Barie PS, Manogue K, Cerami A, Shires GT, Lowry SF (1990) Serum cachectin/TNF in critically ill patients with burns correlates with infection and mortality. *Surg Gynecol Obstet* 170: 32–38

9   Calandra T, Baumgartner JD, Grau GE, Wu MM, Lambert PH, Schellekens J, Verhoef J, Glauser MP (1990) Prognostic values of tumor necrosis factor/cachectin, interlukin-1, interferon-alpha, and interferon-gamma in the serum of patients with septic shock. *J Infect Dis* 161: 982–987

10 Offner F, Philippe J, Vogelaers D, Colardyn F, Baele G, Baudrihaye M, Vermeulen A (1990) Serum tumor necrosis factor levels in patients with infectious disease and septic shock. *J Lab Clin Med* 116: 100–105

11 Waage A, Halstensen A, Espevik T (1987) Association between tumor necrosis factor in serum and fatal outcome in patients with meningococcal disease. *Lancet* I: 355–357

12 Leist TP, Frei K, Kam-Hansen S, Zinkernagel RM, Fontano A (1993) Tumor necrosis factor alpha in cerebrospinal fluid during bacterial, but not, viral meningitis. *J Exp Med* 167: 1743–1748

13 Cerami A (1992) Inflammatory cytokines. *Clin Immunol Immunopathol* 62: S3–S10

14 Goldsmith MF (1991) Excitement over immunomodulation inundates clinical research meetings. *JAMA* 21: 2768–2769, 2773

15 Wang R (1997) R: CD28 Ligation prevents bacterial toxin-induced septic shock in mice by inducing IL-10 expression. *J Immunol* 158: 2856–2861

16 Redl H, Schlag G (1996) Animal models as the basis of pharmacologic intervention in trauma and sepsis patients. *World J Surg* 20: 487–492

17 Bone RC, Fisher CJ, Clemmer TP, Slotman GJ, Metz CA, Balk RA (1987) A controlled trial of high-dose methylprednisolone in the treatment of severe sepsis and septic shock. *N Engl J Med* 317: 653–658

18 Veterans Administration Systemic Sepsis Cooperative Group (1987) Effect of high-dose glucocorticoid therapy on mortality in patients with clinical signs of systemic sepsis. *N Engl J Med* 317: 659–665

19 Ziegler EJ, Fisher CJ, Sprung CL, Fisher CJ Jr., Sprung CL, Straube RC, Sadoff JC, Foulke GE, Wortel CH, Fink MP, Dellinger RP, Teng NN et al (1991) Treatment of gram-negative bacteremia and septic shock with HA-1A human monoclonal antibody against endotoxin: A randomized, double-blind, placebo-controlled trial. *N Engl J Med* 324: 429–436

20 Greenman, RL, Schein RMH, Martin MA, Wenzel RP, Macintyre NR, Emmanuel G, Chmel H, Kohler RB, McCarthy M, Plouffe J, et al (1991) A controlled clinical trial of E5 murine monoclonal IgM antibody to endotoxin in the treatment of gram-negative sepsis. *JAMA* 266: 1097–1102

21 Dhainaut JFA, Tenaillon A, LeTulzo Y, Schlemmer B, Solet JP, Wolff M, Holzapfel L, Zeni F, Dreyfuss D, Mira JP, et al (1994) Platelet-activating factor antagonist BN 52021 in the treatment of severe sepsis: A randomized, double-blind, placebo-controlled, multicenter clinical trial. *Crit Care Med* 22: 1720–1728

22 Fisher CJ, Dhainaut JFA, Opal SM, Prible JP, Balk RA, Slotman GJ, Iberti TJ, Rackow

EC, Shapiro MJ (1994) Recombinant human interleukin 1 receptor antagonist in the treatment of patients with sepsis syndrome. *JAMA* 271: 1836–1843

23 Bone RC, Balk RA, Fein AM, Perl TM, Wenzel RP, Reines HD, Quenzer RW, Iberti TJ, Macintyre N, Schein RM (1995) A second large controlled clinical study of E5 a monoclonal antibody to endotoxin: Results of a prospective, multicenter, randomized, controlled trial. *Crit Care Med* 23: 994–1006

24 Arbraham E, Wunderink R, Silverman H, Perl TM, Nasraway S, Levy H, Bone R, Wenzel RP, Balk P, Allred R et al (1995) Efficacy and safety of monoclonal antibody to human tumor necrosis factor α in patients with sepsis syndrome: A randomized, controlled, double-blind, multicenter clinical trial. *J Am Med Assoc* 273: 934–941

25 Cohen J, Carlet J (1996) INTERSEPT: An international, multicenter, placebo-controlled trial of monoclonal antibody to human tumor necrosis factor-α in patients with sepsis. *Crit Care Med* 24: 1431–1440

26 Fisher CJ, Agost JM, Opal SM, Lowry SF, Balk RA, Sadoff JC, Arbraham E, Schein RM, Benjamin E (1996) Treatment of septic shock with the tumor necrosis factor receptor: Fc fusion protein. *N Engl J Med* 334: 1697–1702

27 Abraham E, Glauser MP, Butler T, Garbino J, Gelmont D, Laterre PF, Kudsk K, Bruining HA, Otto C, Tobin E, Zwingelstein C, Lesslauer W, Leighton A (1997) P55 tumor necrosis factor receptor fusion protein in the treatment of patients with severe sepsis and septic shock: A randomized controlled multicenter trial. *JAMA* 277: 1531–1538

28 Bernard GR, Wheeler AP, Arons MM, Morris PE, Paz HL, Russell JA, Wright PE (1997) The effects of ibuprofen on the physiology and survival of patients with sepsis. *N Engl J Med* 336: 912–918

29 Bone RC (1992) Toward an epidemiology and natural history of SIRS (systemic inflammatory response syndrome). *JAMA* 268: 3452–3455.

30 Center for Disease Control: Mortality Patterns – United States, 1989. *Morbidity Mortality Wkly* Rpt 41 (1992): 121–125

31 McGowan JE, Barnes MW, Findland N (1975) Bacteremia at Boston City Hospital: occurrence and mortality during 12 selected years (1935–1972) with special reference to hospital-acquired cases. *J Infect Dis* 132: 316–335

32 Homo-Delarche F, Fitzpatrick R, Christeff N, Nunez EA, Bach JF, Dardenne M(1991) Sex steroids, glucocorticoids, stress and autoimmunity. *J Steroid Biochem Molec Biol* 40: 619–637

33 Zellweger R, Ayala A, Stein S, DeMaso CM, Chaudry IH (1995) Females in proestrus state tolerate sepsis better than males. *Surg Forum* 46: 65–67.

34 Wichmann MW, Ayala A, Chaudry IH (1997) Male sex-steroids are responsible for depressing macrophage immune function after trauma-hemorrhage. *Am J Physiol* 273: C1335–C1340

35 Luster MI, Pfeifer RW, Tucker AN (1985) Influence of sex hormones on immunoregulation with specific reference to natural and environmental estrogens. In: JA Thomas, KS Korach, JA McLachlan (eds): *Endocrine toxicology*. Raven Press, New York, p. 67–83

36   Roubinian JR, Talal N, Greenspan JS, Goodman JR, Siiteri PK (1979) Delayed andro-
      gen treatment prolongs survival in murine lupus. *Clin Invest* 63: 902–922
37   Viselli SM, Stanziale S, Shults K, Kovacs WJ, Olsen NJ (1995) Castration alters periph-
      eral immune function in normal male mice. *Immunology* 84: 337–342
38   Waynforth H (1980) Orchiedectomy (Castration). In: Anonymous: *Experimental and
      surgical technique in the rat*. Academic Press, London, 160–161
39   Wichmann MW, Zellweger R, DeMaso CM, Ayala A, Chaudry IH (1996) Mechanisms
      of immunosuppression in males following trauma-hemorrhage: critical role of testos-
      terone. *Arch Surg* 131: 1186–1192
40   Angele MK, Wichmann MW, Ayala A, Cioffi WG, Chaudry IH (1997) Testosterone
      receptor blockade after hemorrhage in males: restoration of the depressed immune func-
      tions and improved survival following subsequent sepsis. *Arch Surg* 132: 1207–1214
41   Walker SE, Besch-Williford CL, Keisler DH (1994) Accelerated deaths from systemic
      lupus erythematosus in NZB × NZW F_1 mice treated with the testosterone-blocking
      drug flutamide. *J Lab Clin Med* 124: 401–407
42   Olsen NJ, Kovacs WJ (1996) Gonadal Steroids and Immunity. *Endocrine Reviews* 17:
      369–384
43   Olsen NJ, Kovacs WJ (1995) Case report: Testosterone treatment of systemic lupus ery-
      thematosus in a patient with Klinefelter's syndrome. *Am J Med Sci* 310: 158–160
44   Zellweger R, Wichmann MW, Ayala A, Stein S, DeMaso CM, Chaudry IH (1995)
      Females in proestrus state maintain splenic immune functions and tolerate sepsis better
      than males. *Crit Care Med* 25: 106–110
45   Weinstein Y, Ran S, Segal S (1984) Sex-associated differences in the regulation of
      responses controlled by the MHC of the mouse. *J Immunol* 132: 656–661
46   Calzolari A (1898): Recherches experimentales sur un rapport probable entre la func-
      tion du thymus et celle des testicules. *Arch Ital Biol* 30: 71–77
47   Ansar AS, Penhale WJ, Talal N (1985) Sex hormones, immune responses and autoim-
      mune diseases: Mechanisms of sex hormone action: *Am J Pathol* 121: 531–551
48   Grossmann CJ (1985): Interactions between the gonadal steroids and the immune
      response. *Science* 227: 257–261
49   Grossmann CJ, Roselle GA (1986) The control of immune response by endocrine fac-
      tors and the clinical significance of such regulation. *Proc Clin Biochem Med* 4: 9–56
50   Butterworth MB, McClellan B, Alansmith M (1967) Influence of sex on immunoglobu-
      lin levels. *Nature* 214: 1224–1225
51   Ainbender E, Weisinger R, Hevizy M, et al (1968) Difference in immunoglobulin class
      of polio antibody in the serum of men and women. *J Immunol* 101: 92–98
52   Terres G, Morrison SL, Habicht GS (1968) A quantitative difference in the immune
      response between male and female mice. *Proc Soc Exp Biol Med* 127: 664–667
53   Grossman CJ (1989) Possible underlying mechanisms of sexual dimorphism in the
      immune response, fact and hypothesis. *J Steroid Biochem* 34: 241–251
54   Shen GK, Montgomery DW, Ulrich ED, Mahoney KR, Zukoski CF (1992) Up-regula-

tion of prolactin gene expression and feedback modulation of lymphocyte proliferation during acute allograft rejection. *Surgery* 112: 387–394

55 Gala RR (1991) Prolactin and growth hormone in the regulation of the immune system (Minireview). *Proc Soc Exp Biol Med* 198: 513–527

56 Athreya BH, Pletcher J, Zulian F, et al (1993): Subset-specific effects of sex hormones and pituitary gonadotropins on human lymphocyte proliferation *in vitro*. *Clin Immunol Immunopathol* 66: 201–211

57 Ayala A, Kisala JM, Felt JA, Perrin MM, Chaudry IH (1992) Does endotoxin tolerance prevent the release of inflammatory monokines (IL-1, IL-6, of TNF) during sepsis? *Arch Surg* 127: 191–197

58 Ayala A, Perrin MM, Kisala J, Ertel W, Chaudry IH (1990) Sepsis selectively activates periotoneal but not alveolar macrophage to release inflammatory mediators (IL-1, IL-6 and TNF). *Surg Forum* 41: 117–119

59 Brouwers JRBJ, Assies J, Wiersinga WM, Huizing G, Tytgat GN (1980): Plasma prolactin levels after acute and subchronic oral administration of domperidone and of metoclopramide: A cross-over study in healthy volunteers. *Clin Endocrinol* 12: 435-440

60 Zhu XH, Zellweger R, Wichmann MW, Ayala A, Chaudry IH (1997) Effects of prolactin and metoclopramide on macrophage cytokine gene expression in late sepsis. *Cytokine* 6: 437–446

61 Zellweger R, Zhu XH, Wichmann MW, Ayala A, DeMaso CM, Chaudry I (1996) Prolactin administration following hemorrhagic shock improves macrophage cytokine release capacity and decreases mortality from subsequent sepsis. *J Immunology* 157: 5768–5754

62 De M, Sanford TR, Wood GW (1992) Interleukin-1, interleukin-6, and tumor necrosis factor α are produced in the mouse uterus during the estrous cycle and are induced by estrogen and progesterone. *Dev Biol* 151: 297–305

63 Huet-Hudson YM, Chakraborty C, De SK, Suzuki Y, Andrews GK, Dey SK (1990): Estrogen regulates the synthesis of epidermal growth factor in mouse uterine epithelial cells. *Mol Endocrinol* 4: 510–523

64 De M, Wood GW (1990) Influence of estrogen and progesterone on macrophage distribution in the mouse uterus. *J Endocrinol* 126: 417–424

65 Ahmed SA, Penhale WJ, Talal (1985) Sex hormones, immune responses, and autoimmune diseases. *Am J Pathol* 121: 531–551

66 Baue A (1975) Multiple, progressive, or sequential systems failure: a syndrome of the 1970s. *Arch Surg* 110: 779–781

67 Cerra FB (1989) Multiple organ failure syndrome. In: DJ Bihari, FB Cerra (eds): *Multiple organ failure*. Society of Critical Care Med., Fullerton, CA, 1–24

68 Faist E, Baue AE, Dittmer H (1983) Multiple organ failure in polytrauma patients. *J Trauma* 23: 775–787

69 Barrow RE, Herndon DN (1990) Incidence of mortality in boys and girls after severe thermal burns. *Surgery* 170: 295–298

70 Deitch EA (1990): Multiple organ failure: Summary and overview. In: EA Deitch (ed): *Multiple organ failure*. Thieme Medical Publishers, New York, 285–299

71 Inoue S, Wirman JA, Alexander JW, Trocke O, Cardell RR (1988) *Candida albicans* translocation across the gut mucosa following burn injury. *J Surg Res* 44: 479–492

72 Beutler B, Cerami A (1989) The biology of cachectin/TNF – a primary mediator of the host response. *Ann Rev Immunol* 7: 625–655

73 Rosenstreich DL, Vogel SN, Jacques A, Wahl LM, Scher I, Mergenhagen SE (1978) Differential endotoxin sensitivity of lymphocytes and macrophages from mice with an X-linked defect in B-cell maturation. *J Immunol* 121: 685–690

74 Vogel SN, Hansen CT, Rosenstreich DL (1979) Characterization of a congenitally LPS-resistant, athymic mouse strain. *J Immunol* 122: 619–622

75 Schirmer WJ, Schirmer JM, Fry D (1989) Recombinant human tumor necrosis factor produces hemodynamic changes characteristic of sepsis and endotoxemia. *Arch Surg* 124: 445–448

76 Tracey KJ, Lowry SF, Fahey TJ, Albert JD, Fong Y, Hesse D, Beutler B, Manogue KR, Calvano S, Wei H, Cerami A, Shires GT (1987) Cachetin/tumor necrosis factor induces lethal shock and stress hormone responses in the dog. *Surg Gynecol Obstet* 164: 415–422

77 Chandra RK (1983): Nutrition, immunity, and infection: present knowledge and future directions. *Lancet* i: 688–691

78 Islikar H, Schurch B (eds) (1981) *The impact of malnutrition on immune defense in parasitic infestation*. Hans Huber Verlag, Bern

79 Chandra RK (ed) (1988) *Nutrition and immunology*. Alan R. Liss, New York

80 Chandra RK (1988) Nutrition, immunity, and outcome. Past, present, and future. 11th Gopalan Gold Medal Oration. *Nutr Res* 8: 132–146

81 Chandra RK (1991) Immunocompetence is a sensitive and functional barometer of nutritional status. *Acta Paediatr Scand Suppl* 374: 129–132

82 Chandra RK (1993) Nutrition and the Immune System. *Proc Nutr Soc* 52: 77–84

83 Bendich A, Chandra RK (eds) (1990) *Micronutrient effects on immunologic functions*. New York Academy of Sciences, New York

84 Chandra RK (1984) Excess intake of zinc impairs immune responses. *JAMA* 252: 1443–1446

85 Kelley DS, Branch LB, Iacono JM (1989) Nutritional modulation of human immune system. *Nutr Res* 9: 965–975

86 Kelley DS, Dougherty RM, Branch LB, Taylor PC, Iacono JM (1992) Concentration of dietary *n*-6 polyunsaturated fatty acids and the human immune status. *Clin Immunol Immunopathol* 62: 240–244

87 Meydani SN, Lichtenstein AH, Cornwall S, Dinarello CA, Rasmussen H, Schaefer EJ (1992) Immunological effects of low fat high polyunsaturated fatty acid (NCEP – Step 2) diets on immune response of human. *FASEB J* 6: A1370 (abstr)

88 Barone J, Hebert JR, Reddy MM (1989) Dietary fat and natural-killer-cell activity. *Am J Clin Nutr* 50: 861–7

89 Rasmussen LB, Liens B, Pederson BD, Richer EA (1994) Effect of diet and plasma fatty acid composition on immune status of elderly men. *Am J Clin Nutr* 59: 572–577

90 Endres S, Ghorbani R, Kelley VE, Georgilis K, Lonnemann G, Van der Meer JW, Cannon JG, Rogers TS, Klempner MS, Weber PC, et al (1989) The effect of dietary supplementation with *n*-3 polyunsaturated fatty acids on the synthesis of interleukin-1 and tumor necrosis factor by mononuclear cell. *N Engl J Med* 320: 265–271

91 Endres S, Meydani SN, Ghorbani R, Schindler R, Dinarello CA (1993) Dietary supplementation with *n*-3 fatty acids suppresses interleukin-2 production and mononuclear cell proliferation. *J Leukocyte Biol* 43: 599–603

92 Cerra FB, Lehman S, Konstantinides K, Kostantinides F, Shronts EP, Holman R (1990) Effect of enteral nutrient on *in vitro* tests of immune function in ICU patients: a preliminary report. *Nutrition* 6: 84–87

93 Liebermann MD, Shou J, Torres AS, Weintraub F, Goldfine J, Sigal R, Daly JM (1990) Effects of nutrient substrates on immune function. *Nutrition* 6: 88–91

94 Cerra FB, Lehmann S, Konstantinides N, Dzik J, Fish J, Konstantinides F, LiCari JJ, Holman T (1991) Improvement in immune function in ICU patients by enteral nutrition supplemented with arginine, RNA, and Menhaden oil is independent of nitrogen balance. *Nutrition* 7: 193–199

95 Alexander JW, Gottschlich MM (1990) Nutritional immunomodulation in burn patients. *Crit Care Med* 18: S149–S153

96 Daly JM, Liebermann MD, Goldfine J, Weintraub F, Rosato EF, Lavin P (1992) Enteral nutrition with supplemental arginine, RNA, and omega-3 fatty acids in patients after operation: immunologic, metabolic, and clinical outcome. *Surgery* 112: 56–57

97 Barton RG, Wells CL, Carlson A, Sing R, Sullivan JJ, Cerra FB (1991) Dietary omega-3 fatty acids decrease mortality and Kupffer cell prostaglandin E_2 production in a rat model of chronic sepsis. *J Trauma* 31: 768–773

98 Krammer TR, Schone N, Douglass LW (1991) Increased vitamin E intake restores fish-oil-induced suppressed blastogenesis of mitogen-stimulated T-lymphocytes. *Am J Clin Nutr* 54: 896–902

99 FAO/WHO (1994) *Fats and oils in human nutrition. Report of a joint expert consultation.* Food and Agriculture Organization, Rome

100 National Research Council (1989) *Recommended dietary allowances.* 10th ed. National Academy Press, Washington, DC

101 Peters EM, Goetzshe JM, Grobbelaar B, Noakes DO (1993): Vitamin C supplementation reduces the incidence of postrace symptoms of upper-respiratory-tract infection in ultramarathon runners. *Am J Clin Nutr* 57: 170–174

102 Schwartz J, Weiss ST (1994) Relationship between dietary vitamin C intake and pulmonary function in the First National Health and Nutrition Examination Survey (NHANES 1). *Am J Clin Nutr* 59: 110–114

103 Mobarhan S, Bowen P, Andersen B, Evans M, Stacewicz-Sapuntzakis M, Sugerman S, Simms P, Lucchesi D, Friedman H (1990) Effects of beta-carotene repletion on beta-

carotene absorption, lipid peroxidation, and neutrophil superoxide formation in young men. *Nutr Cancer* 14: 195–206

104 Garewal H, Shamdas GJ (1991) Intervention trials with beta-carotene in precancerous conditions of the upper aerodigestive tract. In: A Bendich, CE Butterworth Jr (eds): *Micronutrients in health and disease prevention*. Marcel Dekker, New York, 127–140

105 Wayne SJ, Rhyne RL, Garry PJ, Goodwin JS (1990) Cell-mediated immunity as a predictor of morbidity and mortality in subjects over 60. *J Gerontol* 45: 45–48

106 Bogden JD, Bendich A, Kemp FW, Bruenings KS, Shurnick JH, Denny T, Baker H, Louria DB (1994) Daily micronutrient supplements enhance delayed-hypersensitivity skin test responses in older people. *Am J Clin Nutr* 60: 437–47

107 Chandra RK (1992) Effect of vitamin and trace-element supplementation on immune responses and infection in elderly subjects. *Lancet* 340: 1124–1127

108 Scrimshaw NS, Taylor CE, Gordon J (1959) Interactions of nutrition and infection. *Am J Med Sci* 237: 367–403

109 Beisel WR (1992) The history of nutritional immunology. *J Nutr Immunol* 1:5–40

110 Roubenoff R, Rall LC (1993) Humoral Mediation of Changing Body Composition During Aging and Chronic Inflammation. *Nutr Review* 51: 1–11

111 Kuczmarski RJ (1989) Need for body composition information in elderly subjects. *Am J Clin Nutr* 50: 1150–1157

112 Borkan GA, Norris AH (1977) Fat redistribution and the changing body dimensions of the adult male. *Human Biol* 49: 495–514

113 Crist DM, Peake GT, Loftfield RB, Kraner JC, Egan PA (1991) Supplemental growth hormone alters body composition, muscle protein metabolism and serum lipids in fit adults: characterization of dose-dependent and response-recovery effects. *Mech Aging Dev* 58: 191–205

114 Weigent DA, Baxter JB, Wear WE, Smith LR, Bost KL, Blalock JE (1988) Production of immunoreactive growth hormone by mononuclear leukocytes. *FASEB J* 2: 2812–2818

115 Rudman D (1985) Growth hormone, body composition, and aging. *J Am Geriatr Soc* 33: 800–807

116 Rudman D, Feller AG, Nagraj HS, Gergans GA, Lalitha PY, Goldberg AF, Schlenker RA, Cohn L, Rudman IW, Mattson DE (1990) Effects of human growth hormone in men over 60 years old. *N Engl J Med* 323: 1–6

117 Rudman D, Kutner MH, Rogers CM, Lubin MF, Fleming GA, Bain RP (1981) Impaired growth hormone secretion in the adult population. *J Clin Invest* 67:1361–1369

118 Marcus R, Butterfield G, Holloway L, Gilliland L, Baylink DJ, Hintz RL, Sherman BM (1990) Effects of short term administration of recombinant human growth hormone to elderly people. *J Clin Endocrinol Metab* 70: 519–527

119 Finkelstein JW, Roffwarg HP, Boyar RM, Kream J, Hellman L (1972) Age-related change in the twenty-four-hour spontaneous secretion of growth hormone. *J Clin Endocrinol Metab* 35: 665–670

120 Steger RW (1981) Age related changes in the control of prolactin secretion in the female rat. *Neurobiol Aging* 2: 119–123

121 Forbes GB, Reina JC (1970) Adult lean body mass declines with age: some longitudinal observations. *Metabolism* 19: 653–663

122 Broughton DL, James OFW, Alberti KGMM, Taylor R (1991) Peripheral and hepatic insulin sensitivity in healthy elderly human subjects. *Eur J Clin Invest* 21:13–21

123 Saposky RM (1992) Do glucocorticoid concentrations rise with age in the rat? *Neurobiol Aging* 13: 171–174

124 Waltman C, Blackman MR, Chrousos GP, Riemann C, Harmann SM (1991) Spontaneous and glucocorticoid-inhibited adrenocorticotropic hormone and cortisol secretion are similar in healthy young and old men. *J Clin Endocr Metab* 73: 495–502

125 Peterson PK, Chao CC, Carson P, Hu S, Nichol K, Janoff EN (1994) Levels of tumor necrosis factor α, Interleukin-6, Interleukin-10, and transforming growth factor β are normal in the serum of the healthy elderly. *Clin Infect Dis* 19: 1158–1159

126 Mooradian AD, Reed RL, Osterweil D, Clements N, Scuderi P (1990) Lack of an association between the presence of tumor necrosis factor or interleukin-1 alpha in the blood and weight loss among elderly subjects. *J Am Geriatr Soc* 38: 397–401

127 Gon Y, Hashimoto S, Hayashi S, Koura T, Matsumoto K, Horie T (1996) Lower serum concentrations of cytokines in elderly patients with pneumonia and the impaired production of cytokines by peripheral blood monocytes in the elderly. *Clin Exp Immunol* 106: 120–126

Genetics: cytokine polymorphisms

Frank Stüber

Klinik und Poliklinik für Anästhesiologie und spezielle Intensivmedizin, Friedrich-Wilhelms-Universität Bonn, Sigmund-Freud-Str. 25, D-53105 Bonn, Germany

Introduction

New anti-mediator strategies and their application in clinical trials of severe sepsis and septic shock [1, 3] have not changed the fact that severe systemic inflammation remains a major cause of death even in modern intensive care units. Cytokines play an important role as endogenous mediators of infectious, as well as non-infectious, causes of multiple organ dysfunction which represents an end stage of systemic inflammatory disease. The recent failure of immunomodulatory approaches in sepsis therapy may question the concept of anti-mediator strategies. Even more important, it uncovers the diagnostic dilemma physicians face when an immunomodulatory drug is to be given to the right patient at the right point in time. We simply do not know when to antagonize tumor necrosis factor (TNF), a major proinflammatory cytokine, or, on the other hand, when to increase performance of the macrophage system by γ-interferon. The first may inactivate a potent agent against invading pathogens, whereas the latter may induce an over-abundant release of systemic proinflammatory cytokines.

The immune response to infectious and non-infectious challenges involves a complex pattern of primary, secondary and tertiary humoral and cellular responses. In this view, the role of the genetic background in cytokine responses is influenced by genetic variabilities of cytokines which constitute the pathways of systemic inflammation.

Primary responses to infectious challenges are mediated by proinflammatory cytokines such as tumor necrosis factor (TNF) and interleukin-1 (IL-1) [4]. Secondary proinflammatory mediators like interleukin-6 (IL-6) and interleukin-8 (IL-8) are induced by TNF and IL-1 [4]. Tertiary mediators comprise factors of different, even non-cytokine origin such as proteases, coagulation factors, kinins, eicosanoids, nitric oxide and others which take effect in the distal part of mediator cascades [5].

Recent evidence suggests that not only proinflammatory mechanisms contribute to organ failure and death induced by severe systemic inflammation but that anti-

Cytokines in Severe Sepsis and Septic Shock, edited by H. Redl and G. Schlag[†]
© 1999 Birkhäuser Verlag Basel/Switzerland

inflammatory mediators have important effects on the host's immune system as well [6]. Anti-inflammatory mediators induce a state of immunosuppression in sepsis which has been named "immunoparalysis" [7]. This state of decreased immunoreactivity is accompanied by high levels of anti-inflammatory cytokines such as interleukin-10 (IL-10) and interleukin-1 receptor antagonist (IL-1ra) [8]. Symptoms of immunosuppression comprise a decreased number of circulating monocytes expressing surface HLA class II molecules and impaired *ex vivo* responses of macrophages and lymphocytes to lipopolysaccharide (LPS) [9].

Pro- and anti-inflammatory responses at the same time contribute to the outcome of severe sepsis and septic shock. Therefore, all genes encoding proteins involved in inflammatory responses are candidate genes for determining the human genetic background which is responsible for inter-individual differences in the extent and sequelae of systemic inflammation.

The genetically-determined capacity of cytokine production and release and expression of other genes involved in inflammation may contribute to a wide range of clinical manifestations in inflammatory disease states. A patient with peritonitis, e.g. may present without symptoms of sepsis and recover within days or may suffer from fulminant septic shock resulting in death within hours.

As well as the basic scientific interest concerning the role and interaction of mediators, there are several very practical and clinical considerations: Which group of patients carries the greatest risk of developing severe sepsis and multiple organ dysfunction caused by systemic inflammation? Is it possible to identify a high risk group for non-survival? Will certain patients benefit more than others from anti-mediator strategies because of their genetic determination enabling high cytokine release in systemic inflammation?

One task in determining the role of genetic factors influencing incidence and/or outcome of severe sepsis and septic shock is to identify genomic markers suitable for clinical use and risk stratification of patients. Another goal is to understand the influence of genomic variations on gene regulation and protein expression.

Genomic polymorphisms of proinflammatory cytokines

Primary proinflammatory cytokines such as TNF and IL-1 induce secondary pro- and anti-inflammatory mediators like IL-6 and IL-10. They have been shown to contribute substantially to the host's primary inflammatory response. Both TNF and IL-1 are capable of inducing the same symptoms and the same severity of septic shock and organ dysfunction as an endotoxin challenge in experimental settings and in humans [10]. Genetic variations in the TNF and IL-1 genes are of major interest concerning genetically-determined differences in the response to endotoxin.

Tumor necrosis factor

TNF is considered as one of the most important mediators of endotoxin-induced effects. Inter-individual differences of TNF release have been described [11, 12].

The TNF locus consists of three functional genes. TNF is positioned between lymphotoxin α (LTα) in the upstream direction and lymphotoxin β (LTβ) in the downstream direction (Fig. 1). Genomic polymorphisms within the TNF locus have been under intense investigation. Genetic variation within the TNF locus, particularly the coding region, is rare as the TNF gene is well conserved throughout evolution [13].

The main interest has been focused on the genomic variations of the TNF locus depicted in Figure 1. Two allele polymorphisms defined by restriction enzymes (NcoI, AspHI) or single base changes (-308, -238) as well as multiallelic microsatellites (TNFa-e) have been investigated in experimental studies and also in various diseases in which TNF has a pathogenetic role. Functional importance in the regulation of the TNF gene has been suggested for two polymorphisms within the TNF promoter region. Single base changes have been detected at position -308 and position -238 [14, 15].

A G to A transition at position -308 has been associated with susceptibility to cerebral malaria [16]. The rare allele TNF2 (A at position -308) was supposed to be linked to high TNF promoter activity [16]. Autoimmune diseases like diabetes mellitus or lupus erythematosus did not, however, show differences in allele frequencies or genotype distribution between patients and controls [17, 18]. In addition, patients with severe sepsis and a high proportion of Gram-negative bacteria also did not display altered allele frequencies concerning the biallelic promoter polymorphism (position -308) [19]. Analysis of the TNF promoter by means of reporter gene constructs revealed contradictory results. The first report found that there was a functional importance of the -308 G to A transition [16]. Two investigations could not confirm differences in the TNF promoter activity in relation to the -308 polymorphism [19, 20]. A recent study reports on a possible influence on TNF promoter activity by the -308 G to A transition in a B cell line [21]. Genotyping of this polymorphism in patients with severe sepsis does not contribute to risk assessment. The -308 polymorphism is neither a marker for susceptibility to, nor for outcome of severe sepsis caused by a Gram-negative infection [19].

In contrast to genomic variations located in the promoter region, intronic polymorphisms are more difficult to associate with a possible functional relevance. Two biallelic polymorphisms located within intron two of LTα have been studied in autoimmune disease [22, 23]. One polymorphism is characterized by the absence or presence of a NcoI restriction site. First reports demonstrated genomic blots revealing characteristic 5.5 or 10.5 kbp bands, after genomic NcoI digest, which hybridize to TNF-specific probes [24]. These bands correspond to the presence and absence, respectively, of a NcoI restriction site within intron one of LTα.

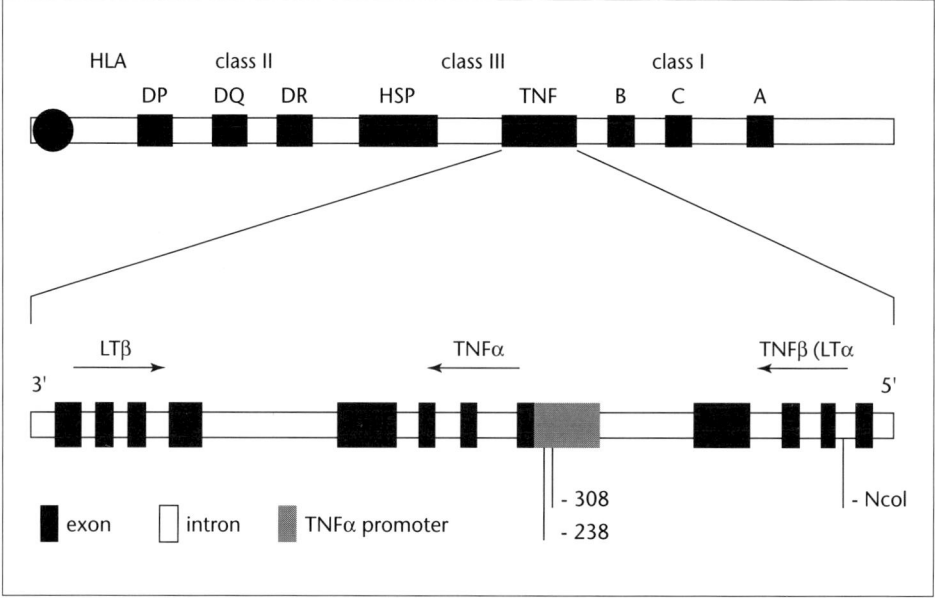

Figure 1
Genomic polymorphisms located within the tumor necrosis factor (TNF) locus on the short arm of chromosome six.

The allele TNFB2 of this NcoI polymorphism (10.5 kbp band) is associated with high TNFα release *ex vivo* [25]. One study showed no differences between genotypes in *ex vivo* TNF induction [12], while another study suggests an increased LTα response in TNFB2 homozygotes [25]. The question as to which genotype is clearly associated with a high proinflammatory response in the clinical situation of severe sepsis and septic shock cannot yet be answered by *ex vivo* studies. Our own results show increased TNF mRNA levels induced by LPS *ex vivo* in whole blood drawn from healthy volunteers typed TNFB2 homozygous (Fig. 2), while TNFB2 homozygous patients with severe sepsis display high initial TNF values [26].

Different conditions of cell culture and cytokine induction contribute to differing results. In addition, the genomic NcoI polymorphism within intron one of the LTα gene may represent a genomic marker without evidence for functional importance in gene regulation. This genomic marker may coincide with as yet undetected genomic variations which are responsible for genetic determination of a high proinflammatory response to infection.

Several studies in chronic inflammatory autoimmune diseases suggest an association between TNFB2 and incidence or severity and outcome of the disease [22, 23, 27]. Studies in acute inflammatory diseases like severe sepsis in patients on surgical

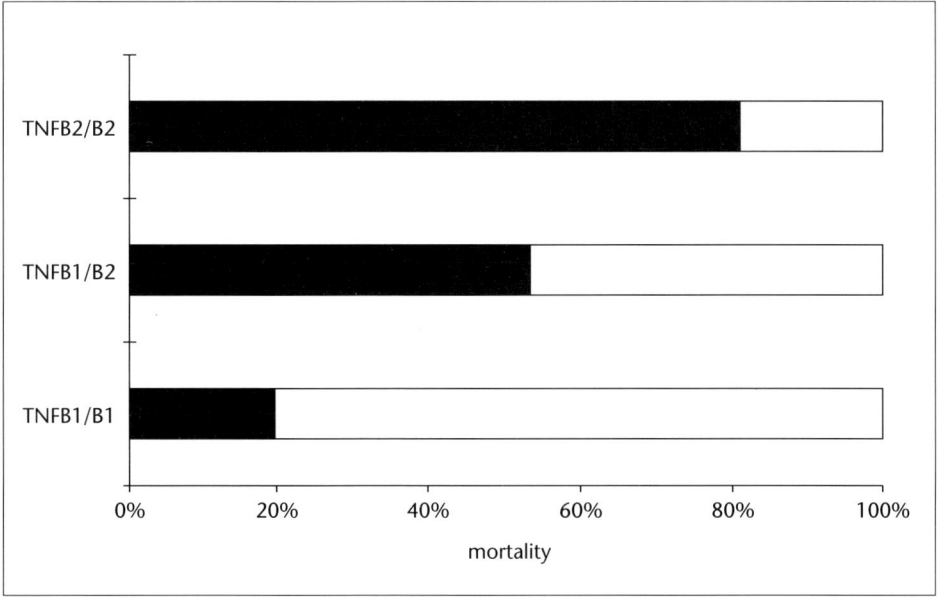

Figure 2
Mortality of patients with severe sepsis (n = 105). Patients are grouped according to three genotypes of the TNFβ Ncol polymorphism.

intensive care units showed a correlation between TNFB2 homozygosity and mortality (Fig. 2). TNFB2 homozygotes display a relative risk of death from severe sepsis of 2.9 when compared to corresponding genotypes.

Interleukin-1

IL-1 is a proinflammatory cytokine released by macrophages in response to endotoxin. This potent cytokine is capable of inducing the symptoms of septic shock and organ failure in animal models and is regarded as a primary mediator of the systemic inflammatory response. Antagonizing IL-1 in endotoxin-challenged animals including primates abrogates the lethal effects of endotoxin [28]. IL-1β, the secreted cytokine, is regarded as being more important than the membrane bound protein IL-1α. A biallelic TaqI polymorphism has been described within the coding region (exon 5) of IL-1β [29, 30]. Despite the finding that a homozygous TaqI genotype correlates with high IL-1β secretion [29], genotyping of patients with severe sepsis did not reveal any association with incidence or outcome of the disease (data not shown).

Interleukin-6

IL-6 is a secondary mediator with important immunological functions such as enhancement of B lymphocyte proliferation. It is released by macrophages and endothelial cells. Although direct toxic effects mediated by IL-6 in severe sepsis and septic shock have not been demonstrated yet, the proinflammatory activity is obvious. The signaling of IL-6 through the IL-6 receptor also exerts some anti-inflammatory effects mediated by the gp130 protein.

IL-6 gains importance as a new clinical parameter for monitoring the inflammatory activity in the course of acute inflammatory diseases. A study testing the anti-TNF monoclonal antibody approach in the treatment of severe sepsis used IL-6 levels as a criterion of hyperinflammation. Only patients with IL-6 plasma levels of more than 1 ng/ml at study entry were enrolled [31].

Genomic polymorphisms of the IL-6 gene have been described in the 3' flanking region [32]. In addition, two single base changes have been reported for a MspI and a BcgII restriction site [33, 34]. Functional studies of these genomic variations concerning influences on gene transcription or mRNA stability do not exist. Another study of allele frequencies and genotype distributions of the BcgII biallelic polymorphism in patients with rheumatoid arthritis did not reveal differences when compared to normal controls [27]. As for the second biallelic polymorphism characterized by the presence or absence of the MspI site, the functional relevance of this polymorphism is unknown.

Currently, there are no data available in the field of acute systemic inflammatory disease. Neither *ex vivo* data concerning the relationship between genomic variations and the quantity of IL-6 release exist, nor have associations of the IL-6 polymorphisms with incidence or outcome of severe sepsis been studied. Therefore, the contribution of IL-6 gene polymorphisms to the genetic background of systemic inflammation remains obscure.

Interleukin 8

IL-8 is, like IL-6, another secondary proinflammatory cytokine with important chemotactic properties in systemic inflammation [35]. IL-8 has been associated with inflammatory processes in lung dysfunction. This cytokine is present in bronchoalveolar lavage fluids of patients with acute respiratory distress syndrome (ARDS) as part of the multiple organ dysfunction syndrome, where it acts as a chemoattractant for neutrophils [36]. Serum levels of IL-8 correlated with the course of severe sepsis, especially with lactacidemia [37]. Antibodies to IL-8 increase survival in rabbits challenged by endotoxin [38]. Only one genomic polymorphism of the IL-8 gene has been described so far [39]. A biallelic Hind III polymorphism is detectable by a IL-8 cDNA probe on the long arm of chromosome four. Up to date, no data are available on the functional impact of this polymorphism on IL-8 expression. In addition, no data exist with regard to allele frequencies or genotype distributions in patients with severe sepsis or septic shock.

Genomic polymorphisms of anti-inflammatory cytokines

Interleukin-1 receptor antagonist

Proinflammatory mediators comprise the hyperinflammatory side of systemic inflammation. At the same time, anti-inflammatory mediators are induced by proinflammatory cytokines and function to counterbalance the overshoot of inflammatory activity. This physiological process of limiting the extent of inflammation by release of anti-inflammatory proteins may escape physiological boundaries of local and systemic concentrations of these mediators. Proteins like IL-4, IL-10, IL-11 or IL-13 or IL-1ra contribute to a very powerful downregulation of soluble and cellular proinflammatory activities. This downregulation results in decreased expression of class II molecules in antigen presenting cells as well as reduced *ex vivo* responses of immunocompetent cells to inflammatory stimuli. This state of imunosuppression has also been termed "immunoparalysis" [7]. It results in a state of deactivation and diminished capacity to eliminate microbial pathogens. A new term for this anti-inflammatory state has recently been created: the compensatory anti-inflammatory response syndrome (CARS) [40]. The outcome of patients with severe sepsis is not only influenced by hyperinflammation with progressive organ dysfunction but may also be affected by immunosuppression and lack of restoration of immune function. In this view, innate interindividual differences in the release of anti-inflammatory mediators contribute to the human inflammatory response.

A genomic polymorphism of the anti-inflammatory cytokine IL-1ra is located within intron two and consists of variable numbers of a tandem repeat (VNTR) of a 86 bp motif (Fig. 3). This 86 base pair motif contains at least three known binding sites for DNA binding proteins [41]. *Ex vivo* experiments suggest higher IL-1ra responses combined with alleles containing low numbers of the 86 bp repeat. *Ex vivo* studies also demonstrate a higher level of IL-1ra protein expression and protein release of A2 homozygous individuals compared to heterozygotes following stimulation with lipopolysaccharide [42]. In LPS-stimulated whole blood cultures, A2 homozygotes also express higher levels of IL-1ra mRNA and protein (data not shown).

The allele A2 has been associated with an increased incidence of autoimmune diseases like lupus erythematosus and insulin dependent diabetes mellitus [43, 44]. In acute systemic inflammation, there is no difference between surviving or non-surviving patients with severe sepsis. This finding is in contrast to the results concerning the biallelic NcoI polymorphism within intron one of LTα: Homozygotes for the TNFB2 genotype revealed a high mortality when compared to heterozygotes and

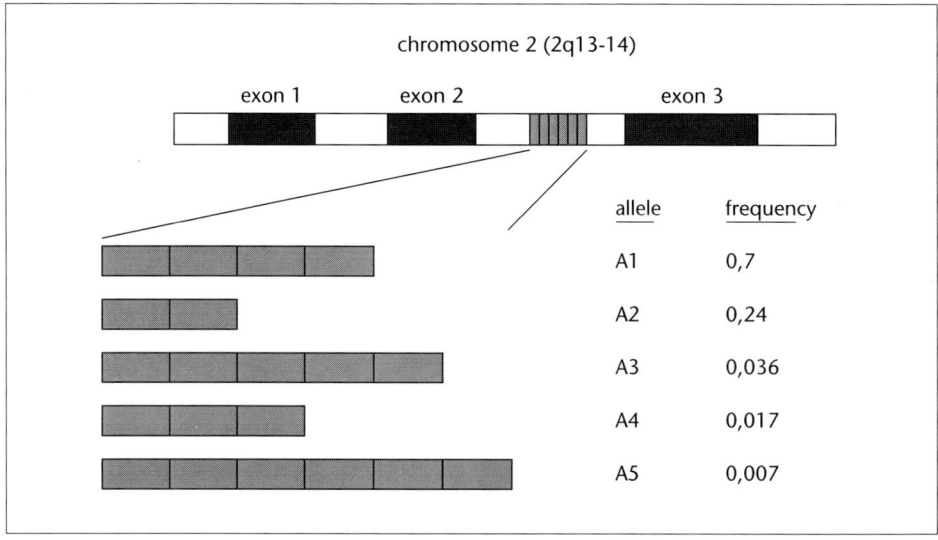

Figure 3
A genomic polymorphism of a variable number of tandem repeats (VNTR) is located within the second intron of the Interleukin-1 receptor antagonist (IL-1ra) gene.

TNFB1 homozygotes. The overall group of patients with severe sepsis did not show an increase in the TNFB2 allele frequency. For the IL-1ra polymorphism, however, an increase of the allele A2 in the patients with severe sepsis was detected (Fig. 4). Patients carrying the TNFB2 homozygous and A2 homozygous haplotype did not survive in this study.

Interleukin-4

IL-4 is a cytokine, predominantly released by TH2 lymphocytes, with anti-inflammatory properties which contributes to the anti-inflammatory response evoked by systemic inflammation [45]. An overwhelming release of IL-4 may contribute to states of immunosuppression or the compensatory anti-inflammatory response syndrome [40]. Genomic polymorphisms of the IL-4 gene consist of repeat polymorphisms [46] as well as polymorphisms in the promoter region which regulates transcription [47]. Studies of IL-4 polymorphisms have been conducted in asthma patients [47] and patients with multiple sclerosis [48]. Data on severe sepsis/septic shock or IL-4 expression with regard to genomic polymorphisms have not been published.

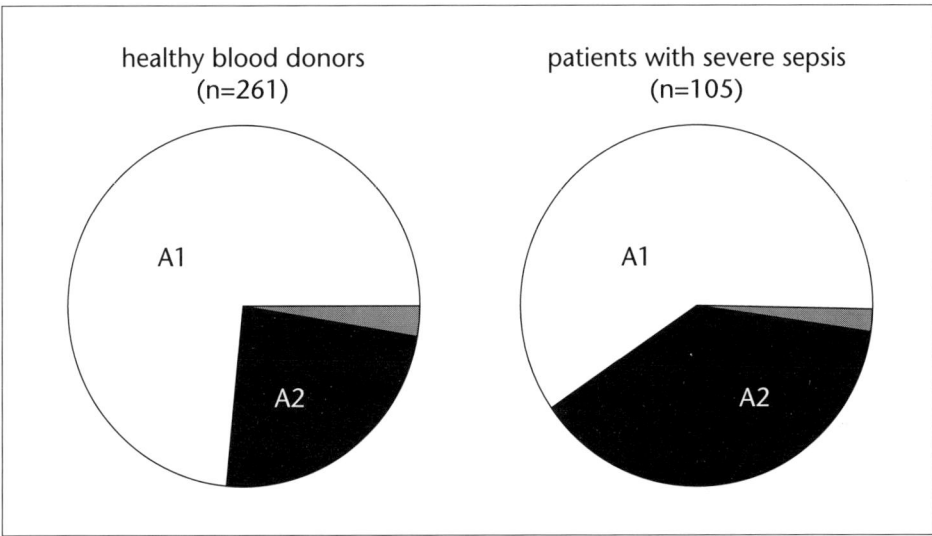

Figure 4
Frequency of the allele A2 of the IL-1ra VNTR polymorphism is significantly higher in patients with severe sepsis compared to healthy controls (p < 0.05, χ²test).

Interleukin-10

Recent work suggests that the ant-inflammatory cytokine Interleukin-10 (IL-10) contributes significantly to the counterregulation of the proinflammatory response evoked by LPS in human sepsis [7]. In a murine model of peritonitis, therapeutic intervention using IL-10 attenuated the rise in proinflammatory serum cytokines [49]. The genomic structure of the IL-10 gene reveals nucleotide variations in the regulatory promoter region of the IL-10 gene. Biallelic polymorphisms (RsaI and MaeIII restriction sites) as well as dinucleotide repeats with sixteen different alleles have been described [50, 51]. Associations between IL-10 genotype and the individual's capacity for IL-10 secretion have been demonstrated. Innate, low IL-10 secretion was correlated to a high rejection rate in organ transplant recipients [52]. Another study reported a correlation between certain IL-10 microsatellite alleles and autoantibody production in lupus erythematosus [53]. Data linking the capacity of IL-10 secretion to genomic variations of the IL-10 gene are rare. Also, no data are available on allele frequencies and genotype distribution in sepsis. The importance of the IL-10 molecule in regulating inflammation warrants further investigation of the genetic background of IL-10 expression.

Conclusion

Understanding the contribution of genomic variations in cytokine genes to the individual systemic inflammatory response which contains the risk of evoking severe sepsis, septic shock, and finally death, is a major task. Currently, there is a lack of understanding in the regulation of systemic inflammatory responses, a lack of diagnostic tools identifying individuals at risk of developing or dying from severe sepsis, and a lack of knowledge about which patients to treat with immunomodulatory agents. Evaluation of this genetic background has just started. Genomic markers will need to be studied in the context of extended haplotypes which will characterize an individual patient's genetic background of cytokine responses in systemic inflammation.

References

1   Opal SM, Fisher CJ, Jr., Dhainaut JF, Vincent JL, Brase R, Lowry SF, Sadoff JC, Slotman GJ, Levy H, Balk RA et al (1997) Confirmatory interleukin-1 receptor antagonist trial in severe sepsis: a phase III, randomized, double-blind, placebo-controlled, multicenter trial. The Interleukin-1 Receptor Antagonist Sepsis Investigator Group. *Crit Care Med* 25: 1115–1124

2   Fisher CJ, Jr., Agosti JM, Opal SM, Lowry SF, Balk RA, Sadoff JC, Abraham E, Schein RM, Benjamin E (1996) Treatment of septic shock with the tumor necrosis factor receptor:Fc fusion protein. The Soluble TNF Receptor Sepsis Study Group. *N Engl J Med* 334: 1697–1702

3   Abraham E, Glauser MP, Butler T, Garbino J, Gelmont D, Laterre PF, Kudsk K, Bruining HA, Otto C, Tobin E et al (1997) p55 Tumor necrosis factor receptor fusion protein in the treatment of patients with severe sepsis and septic shock. A randomized controlled multicenter trial. Ro 45-2081 Study Group. *JAMA* 277: 1531–1538

4   Blackwell TS, Christman JW (1996) Sepsis and cytokines: current status. *Br J Anaesth* 77: 110–117

5   Bernard GR, Wheeler AP, Russell JA, Schein R, Summer WR, Steinberg KP, Fulkerson WJ, Wright PE, Christman BW, Dupont WD et al (1997) The effects of ibuprofen on the physiology and survival of patients with sepsis. The Ibuprofen in Sepsis Study Group. *N Engl J Med* 336: 912–918

6   van der Poll T, de Waal Malefyt R, Coyle SM, Lowry SF (1997) Antiinflammatory cytokine responses during clinical sepsis and experimental endotoxemia: sequential measurements of plasma soluble interleukin (IL)-1 receptor type II, IL-10, and IL-13. *J Infect Dis* 175: 118–122

7   Volk HD, Reinke P, Krausch D, Zuckermann H, Asadullah K, Muller JM, Docke WD, Kox WJ (1996) Monocyte deactivation – rationale for a new therapeutic strategy in sepsis. *Intensive Care Med* 22 Suppl 4: S474-481

8   Fisher CJ, Jr., Slotman GJ, Opal SM, Pribble JP, Bone RC, Emmanuel G, Ng D, Bloedow DC, Catalano MA (1994) Initial evaluation of human recombinant interleukin-1 receptor antagonist in the treatment of sepsis syndrome: a randomized, open- label, placebo-controlled multicenter trial. The IL-1RA Sepsis Syndrome Study Group. *Crit Care Med* 22: 12–21

9   Docke WD, Randow F, Syrbe U, Krausch D, Asadullah K, Reinke P, Volk HD, Kox W (1997) Monocyte deactivation in septic patients: restoration by IFN-gamma treatment. *Nat Med* 3: 678–681

10 Weinberg JR, Boyle P, Meager A, Guz A (1992) Lipopolysaccharide, tumor necrosis factor, and interleukin-1 interact to cause hypotension. *J Lab Clin Med* 120: 205–211

11 Westendorp RG, Langermans JA, Huizinga TW, Elouali AH, Verweij CL, Boomsma DI, Vandenbrouke JP (1997) Genetic influence on cytokine production and fatal meningococcal disease. *Lancet* 349: 170–173

12 Whichelow CE, Hitman GA, Raafat I, Bottazzo GF, Sachs JA (1996) The effect of TNF*B gene polymorphism on TNF-alpha and -beta secretion levels in patients with insulin-dependent diabetes mellitus and healthy controls. *Eur J Immunogenet* 23: 425–435

13 Gray PW, Aggarwal BB, Benton CV, Bringman TS, Henzel WJ, Jarrett JA, Leung DW, Moffat B, Ng P, Svedersky LP et al (1984) Cloning and expression of cDNA for human lymphotoxin, a lymphokine with tumour necrosis activity. *Nature* 312: 721–724

14 Wilson AG, di Giovine FS, Blakemore AI, Duff GW (1992) Single base polymorphism in the human tumour necrosis factor alpha (TNF alpha) gene detectable by NcoI restriction of PCR product. *Hum Mol Genet* 1: 353

15 Brinkman BM, Huizinga TW, Kurban SS, van der Velde EA, Schreuder GM, Hazes JM, Breedveld FC, Verweij CL (1997) Tumour necrosis factor alpha gene polymorphisms in rheumatoid arthritis: association with susceptibility to, or severity of, disease? *Br J Rheumatol* 36: 516–521

16 McGuire W, Hill AV, Allsopp CE, Greenwood BM, Kwiatkowski D (1994) Variation in the TNF-alpha promoter region associated with susceptibility to cerebral malaria. *Nature* 371: 508–510

17 Pociot F, Wilson AG, Nerup J, Duff GW (1993) No independent association between a tumor necrosis factor-alpha promotor region polymorphism and insulin-dependent diabetes mellitus. *Eur J Immunol* 23: 3050–3053

18 Wilson AG, Gordon C, di Giovine FS, de Vries N, van de Putte LB, Emery P, Duff GW (1994) A genetic association between systemic lupus erythematosus and tumor necrosis factor alpha. *Eur J Immunol* 24: 191–195

19 Stüber F, Udalova IA, Book M, Drutskaya LN, Kuprash DV, Turetskaya RL, Schade FU, Nedospasov SA (1995) -308 tumor necrosis factor (TNF) polymorphism is not associated with survival in severe sepsis and is unrelated to lipopolysaccharide inducibility of the human TNF promoter. *J Inflamm* 46: 42–50

20 Brinkman BM, Zuijdeest D, Kaijzel EL, Breedveld FC, Verweij CL (1995) Relevance of

the tumor necrosis factor alpha (TNF alpha) -308 promoter polymorphism in TNF alpha gene regulation. *J Inflamm* 46: 32–41

21   Wilson AG, Symons JA, McDowell TL, McDevitt HO, Duff GW (1997) Effects of a polymorphism in the human tumor necrosis factor alpha promoter on transcriptional activation. *Proc Natl Acad Sci USA* 94: 3195–3199

22   Pociot F, Molvig J, Wogensen L, Worsaae H, Dalboge H, Baek L, Nerup J (1991) A tumour necrosis factor beta gene polymorphism in relation to monokine secretion and insulin-dependent diabetes mellitus. *Scand J Immunol* 33: 37–49

23   Bettinotti MP, Hartung K, Deicher H, Messer G, Keller E, Weiss EH, Albert ED (1993) Polymorphism of the tumor necrosis factor beta gene in systemic lupus erythematosus: TNFB-MHC haplotypes. *Immunogenetics* 37: 449–454

24   Badenhoop K, Schwarz G, Trowsdale J, Lewis V, Usadel KH, Gale EA, Bottazzo GF (1989) TNF-alpha gene polymorphisms in type 1 (insulin-dependent) diabetes mellitus. *Diabetologia* 32: 445–448

25   Pociot F, Briant L, Jongeneel CV, Molvig J, Worsaae H, Abbal M, Thomsen M, Nerup J, Cambon-Thomsen A (1993) Association of tumor necrosis factor (TNF) and class II major histocompatibility complex alleles with the secretion of TNF-alpha and TNF-beta by human mononuclear cells: a possible link to insulin-dependent diabetes mellitus. *Eur J Immunol* 23: 224–231

26   Stüber F, Petersen M, Bokelmann F, Schade U (1996) A genomic polymorphism within the tumor necrosis factor locus influences plasma tumor necrosis factor-alpha concentrations and outcome of patients with severe sepsis. *Crit Care Med* 24: 381–384

27   Vinasco J, Beraun Y, Nieto A, Fraile A, Mataran L, Pareja E, Martin J (1997) Polymorphism at the TNF loci in rheumatoid arthritis. *Tissue Antigens* 49: 74–78

28   Boermeester MA, Van Leeuwen PA, Coyle SM, Wolbink GJ, Hack CE, Lowry SF (1995) Interleukin-1 blockade attenuates mediator release and dysregulation of the hemostatic mechanism during human sepsis. *Arch Surg* 130: 739–748

29   Pociot F, Molvig J, Wogensen L, Worsaae H, Nerup J (1992) A TaqI polymorphism in the human interleukin-1 beta (IL-1 beta) gene correlates with IL-1 beta secretion *in vitro*. *Eur J Clin Invest* 22: 396–402

30   Guasch JF, Bertina RM, Reitsma PH (1996) Five novel intragenic dimorphisms in the human interleukin-1 genes combine to high informativity. *Cytokine* 8: 598–602

31   Reinhart K, Wiegand-Lohnert C, Grimminger F, Kaul M, Withington S, Treacher D, Eckart J, Willatts S, Bouza C, Krausch D et al (1996) Assessment of the safety and efficacy of the monoclonal anti-tumor necrosis factor antibody-fragment, MAK 195F, in patients with sepsis and septic shock: a multicenter, randomized, placebo-controlled, dose- ranging study. *Crit Care Med* 24: 733–742

32   Bowcock AM, Ray A, Erlich H, Sehgal PB (1989) Rapid detection and sequencing of alleles in the 3' flanking region of the interleukin-6 gene. *Nucleic Acids Res* 17: 6855–6864

33   Fugger L, Morling N, Bendtzen K, Ryder LP, Svejgaard A (1989) BglII polymorphism in the human interleukin 6 (IL 6) gene. *Nucleic Acids Res* 17: 7548

34 Fugger L, Morling N, Bendtzen K, Ryder L, Odum N, Georgsen J, Svejgaard A (1989) MspI polymorphism in the human interleukin 6 (IL 6) gene. *Nucleic Acids Res* 17: 4419

35 Solomkin JS, Bass RC, Bjornson HS, Tindal CJ, Babcock GF (1994) Alterations of neutrophil responses to tumor necrosis factor alpha and interleukin-8 following human endotoxemia. *Infect Immun* 62: 943-947

36 Miller EJ, Cohen AB, Matthay MA (1996) Increased interleukin-8 concentrations in the pulmonary edema fluid of patients with acute respiratory distress syndrome from sepsis. *Crit Care Med* 24: 1448-1454

37 Biron C, Bengler C, Gris JC, Schved JF (1997) Acquired isolated factor VII deficiency during sepsis. *Haemostasis* 27: 51-56

38 Carvalho GL, Wakabayashi G, Shimazu M, Karahashi T, Yoshida M, Yamamoto S, Matsushima K, Mukaida N, Clark BD, Takabayashi T et al (1997) Anti-interleukin-8 monoclonal antibody reduces free radical production and improves hemodynamics and survival rate in endotoxic shock in rabbits. *Surgery* 122: 60-68

39 Fey MF, Tobler A (1993) An interleukin-8 (IL-8) cDNA clone identifies a frequent HindIII polymorphism. *Hum Genet* 91: 298

40 Bone RC (1996) Sir Isaac Newton, sepsis, SIRS, and CARS. *Crit Care Med* 24: 1125–1128

41 Tarlow JK, Blakemore AI, Lennard A, Solari R, Hughes HN, Steinkasserer A, Duff GW (1993) Polymorphism in human IL-1 receptor antagonist gene intron 2 is caused by variable numbers of an 86-bp tandem repeat. *Hum Genet* 91: 403–404

42 Danis VA, Millington M, Hyland VJ, Grennan D (1995) Cytokine production by normal human monocytes: inter-subject variation and relationship to an IL-1 receptor antagonist (IL-1Ra) gene polymorphism. *Clin Exp Immunol* 99: 303–310

43 Blakemore AI, Tarlow JK, Cork MJ, Gordon C, Emery P, Duff GW (1994) Interleukin-1 receptor antagonist gene polymorphism as a disease severity factor in systemic lupus erythematosus. *Arthritis Rheum* 37: 1380–1385

44 Metcalfe KA, Hitman GA, Pociot F, Bergholdt R, Tuomilehto-Wolf E, Tuomilehto J, Viswanathan M, Ramachandran A, Nerup J (1996) An association between type 1 diabetes and the interleukin-1 receptor type 1 gene. The DiMe Study Group. Childhood Diabetes in Finland. *Hum Immunol* 51: 41–48

45 Bone RC (1991) The pathogenesis of sepsis. *Ann Intern Med* 115: 457–469

46 Mout R, Willemze R, Landegent JE (1991) Repeat polymorphisms in the interleukin-4 gene (IL4). *Nucleic Acids Res* 19: 3763

47 Rosenwasser LJ, Borish L (1997) Genetics of atopy and asthma: the rationale behind promoter-based candidate gene studies (IL-4 and IL-10). *Am J Respir Crit Care Med* 156: S152–5

48 Vandenbroeck K, Martino G, Marrosu M, Consiglio A, Zaffaroni M, Vaccargiu S, Franciotta D, Ruggeri M, Comi G, Grimaldi LM (1997) Occurrence and clinical relevance of an interleukin-4 gene polymorphism in patients with multiple sclerosis. *J Neuroimmunol* 76: 189–192

49 Rongione AJ, Kusske AM, Ashley SW, Reber HA, McFadden DW (1997) Interleukin-10

prevents early cytokine release in severe intraabdominal infection and sepsis. *J Surg Res* 70: 107–112

50 Eskdale J, Kube D, Tesch H, Gallagher G (1997) Mapping of the human IL10 gene and further characterization of the 5' flanking sequence. *Immunogenetics* 46: 120–128

51 Eskdale J, Kube D, Gallagher G (1996) A second polymorphic dinucleotide repeat in the 5' flanking region of the human IL10 gene. *Immunogenetics* 45: 82–83

52 Turner D, Grant SC, Yonan N, Sheldon S, Dyer PA, Sinnott PJ, Hutchinson IV (1997) Cytokine gene polymorphism and heart transplant rejection. *Transplantation* 64: 776–779

53 Eskdale J, Wordsworth P, Bowman S, Field M, Gallagher G (1997) Association between polymorphisms at the human IL-10 locus and systemic lupus erythematosus. *Tissue Antigens* 49: 635–639

Diagnostic

Possibilities and problems of cytokine measurements

Jean-Marc Cavaillon

Unité d'Immuno-Allergie, Institut Pasteur, 28 rue du Dr. Roux, F-75015 Paris, France

Sepsis is associated with an exacerbated production of cytokines

The appearance of detectable pro- as well as anti-inflammatory cytokines in the blood-stream during sepsis is indicative of their exacerbated production. The interaction of micro-organisms and their derived products with host cells rapidly leads to the production of many inflammatory mediators including cytokines. Two major features characterize the production of these factors: cascade and regulatory loops. This means that, once produced, a given cytokine can induce the production of others which can further induce cytokine release or, on the contrary, down-regulate the upstream synthesis. Usually absent from the plasma at homeostasis, many cytokines are produced in such large amounts during sepsis that they can be detected in the circulation of the patients. Due to limitation of space, this review will attempt to focus on human sepsis, while mentioning animal models when necessary.

Interleukin-1 (IL-1)

The cascade of inflammatory events is orchestrated by two cytokines, namely interleukin-1 (IL-1) and tumor necrosis factor (TNF). IL-1β has been regularly reported in the plasma of sepsis patients whereas IL-1α has never been observed when investigated [1, 2]. However, measurements of plasma IL-1β led to technical difficulties: in the early time, circulating IL-1β was found in healthy controls [1, 3] while it was not detected in sepsis [4]! Indeed, IL-1β is probably the most delicate cytokine to measure in plasma [5]. While plasma chloroform extraction was recommended [1] and performed in some studies [2, 6], it is not used anymore. Furthermore, the use of either radioimmunoassays (RIA), bioassays, or enzyme-linked immunoassays (ELISA) contributed to the great heterogeneity in the various reports. While most authors now agree that there is no detectable circulating IL-1β at homeostasis, this cytokine was demonstrated in 0 to 90% of septic patients depending on the studies, the nature of the sepsis, and most probably on the nature of the technique used to assess its presence. The highest frequency of detectable levels of IL-1β was observed among patients with meningococcal sepsis [7, 8] and high levels of IL-1β correlate with the severity of meningococcemia, the presence of shock, high acute physiology and chronic health evaluation (APACHE II) scores and rapid fatal outcome [7–10]. Such correlations were not observed in other sepsis patients [2, 11]. In a few studies, IL-1β was monitored over a period of time and either high levels at admission, followed by a decrease, or sustained levels were reported [2, 8, 12].

Tumor necrosis factor (TNF)

In 1986, tumor necrosis factor was the first cytokine to be described in the serum of patients with septicemia [13], and later in patients with meningococcal sepsis [9, 14]. Like IL-1β, TNF was investigated using either a bioassay, RIA or ELISA. Accordingly, the frequency of positive samples was influenced by the technique used and the low numbers of positive samples (17–23%) were reported by authors employing bioassays [11, 13], whereas other techniques allowed a frequency as high as over 80% [2, 8, 9, 12, 15, 16]. It is worth noting that the levels of TNF usually never exceed a few hundred picograms per mL. However, higher amounts can be reached as illustrated by the 14, 630 pg/mL value observed in a patient, 3.6 h following self-administration of 3750 times the amount of lipopolysaccharide (LPS) administered to human volunteers [17]. There is disagreement as to whether a correlation exists between high levels of measured circulating TNF and fatal outcome. While this seems to be the case in meningococcal sepsis [9, 14], in other sepsis some authors did observe such a correlation [12, 18], and others did not [2, 11, 15]. Different authors have followed up the kinetics of plasma TNF and observed either an increase, a decrease or sustained levels [2, 4, 12, 18, 19]. Indeed, as first shown by Baud et al. [15], and confirmed by Pinsky et al. [20], it seems that it is the persistence of detectable TNF rather than its peak level which is associated with the fatal outcome. When addressed, the TNF levels correlate with the severity of illness and APACHE II scores [1, 8, 15], with IL-6 levels [7, 11, 21] and with nitrate [22]. It is worth noting that in intraperitoneal sepsis, on the contrary, high levels of circulating TNF are associated with a good prognosis while low levels are correlated with fatal outcome [23, 24]. Some authors reported that the TNF levels were higher in Gram-negative than in Gram-positive sepsis [16, 25] although this was not observed in all studies [2, 26]. In meningococcal sepsis levels of TNF are higher in cerebrospinal fluids than in plasma [27] and not detected in CSF of non-bacterial meningitis [28]. Injection of LPS in human volunteers and in animal models leads to a plasma peak of TNF at 90 min, and its levels may be up-regulated by administration of ibuprofen [29] or granulocyte CSF (G-CSF) [30], and down-regulated by epinephrine [31].

Lymphotoxin-α (Ltα)

Lymphotoxin-α is a rare cytokine which is produced by a limited number of cells, essentially activated T-lymphocytes. It shares with TNFα the same receptors and thus most of its activities. Ltα should be essentially expected in Gram-positive sepsis since Gram-positive bacteria release various T cell activators known as superantigens. While the use of neutralizing antibodies could suggest that *Pseudomonas aeruginosa* infusion led to the appearance of TNFα and Ltα in the circulation of pigs [32], Ltα has never been reported so far in human Gram-negative sepsis [10]. On the contrary, in patients with streptococcal toxic shock syndrome, circulating Ltα was found to parallel the levels of circulating superantigen [33].

Interleukin-2 (IL-2)

IL-2 is another cytokine which reflects T cell activation. While rarely reported in humans [10, 20], IL-2 was found in the circulation within two hours following injection of bacterial superantigens in mice [34] and baboons [35].

Interleukin-6 (IL-6)

Although IL-6 is often considered as an inflammatory cytokine, most of its activities are probably associated with a negative control of inflammation thanks to its potent capacity to induce the production of acute phase proteins by the liver as well as the release of IL-1 receptor antagonist (IL-1ra) and soluble TNF receptors (sTNFR) [36]. Its presence in plasma of sepsis patients was first reported in 1989 [10, 37, 38]. Until 1992, plasma IL-6 was evaluated by bioassays using the growth of a hybridoma B cell line (B9 or 7TD1) or the protein synthesis by a hepatoma cell line (Hep3B). Since then, RIA and mainly ELISA have confirmed the first observations. Plasma IL-6 has been observed in 64% to 100% of the studied patients. Most investigators have demonstrated that levels of circulating IL-6 correlate with severity of sepsis and may predict outcome [2, 10, 11, 21, 37] as illustrated by the correlation between IL-6 levels and APACHE II scores [4, 8, 11]. Numerous correlations between IL-6 levels and other markers have been reported including C3a, lactate [37], circulating endotoxin [7], C-reactive protein (CRP) [4], and TNF [7, 10, 11, 21]. IL-6 levels are similar in Gram-positive or Gram-negative sepsis [2, 16].

Injection of endotoxin in human volunteers revealed that the peak levels were reached 2 h after injection [39].

Leukemia inhibitory factor (LIF), oncostatin M (OSM), ciliary neurotrophic factor (CNTF) and interleukin-11 (IL-11)

LIF, OSM, CNTF and IL-11 belong to the IL-6 superfamily, sharing the gp130 chain of the receptor. However, while IL-6 and IL-11 possess certain anti-inflammatory properties and may protect against sepsis [40, 41], LIF [42] and OSM [43] are involved in the pathogenesis of inflammation. First reported in 1992, detectable levels of LIF were occasionally found in the plasma of 9 to 40% of septic patients [16, 44–46]. Levels of circulating LIF correlate with shock, temperature, creatinine and IL-6 [45]. The correlation of LIF with IL-6 has been confirmed in a baboon model of sepsis [47]. Levels of plasma CNTF and OSM are elevated in 60% and 100% of septic patients, respectively [46]. Divergent reports concern IL-11, which was detected in 67% of patients with disseminated intravascular coagulation complicated by sepsis [48], but not in patients suffering from septic shock [46].

Interleukin-8 (IL-8) and chemokines

Sepsis is often associated with organ dysfunction. It reflects the inflammatory process occurring in the tissues. One of the major features of this phenomenon is the recruitment of inflammatory leukocytes, following their adherence to the endothelium and their response to the locally-produced chemokines. These chemokines contribute to the inflammatory cell infiltrate favoring the damage of tissue integrity. For example, it was reported that neutralization of IL-8 profoundly inhibited neutrophil recruitment in an endotoxin-induced rabbit model of pleurisy, indicating that IL-8 is a major chemotactic factor in this model of acute inflammation [49]. However, this first encounter of neutrophils with IL-8 may lead to their desensitization to further signals delivered locally by IL-8 and some cross-reacting chemokines. So, the presence of IL-8 in the intravascular space may well be a mechanism to suppress neutrophil accumulation at extracellular sites as illustrated by the defect in neutrophil migration during sepsis or endotoxemia [50, 51]. Similarly, while monocyte-chemoattractant protein-1 (MCP-1) contributes to the recruitment of inflammatory macrophages within the tissues, neutralization of MCP-1 by specific antibodies before LPS administration resulted in a striking increase in mortality, and injection of MCP-1 was protective [52]. As first reported in 1992, a great amount of IL-8 is detectable within the blood compartment during sepsis [53, 54], in bronchoalveolar lavages (BAL), and edema fluids of acute respiratory distress syndrome (ARDS)-associated to sepsis [55]. In the later study, patients with high levels of BAL IL-8 had a high mortality rate. Similarly, high levels of plasma IL-8 correlate with poor outcome in many studies [53, 54, 56]. No difference in IL-8 plasma levels were found between Gram-negative and Gram-positive infection [54] while in bacteremic pneumonia the type of pathogen influenced the measurable levels of IL-8 [16]. Furthermore, IL-8 levels in septic shock were higher than in septic patients without shock [57] and higher in patients with septic multiple organ failure (MOF) than in nonseptic MOF [56]. In this later comparison, IL-6 could not discriminate between both types of MOF. IL-8 levels also correlate with various markers including IL-6 [7, 11, 54, 56], C3a, α1-anti-trypsin, lactate [54], IL-10, IL-1ra and soluble TNF receptors (sTNF R) [7]. Correlation with plasma TNF led to controversial results [7, 11]. More interestingly, local levels of IL-8 often correlate with the number of recruited neutrophils [55] and plasma levels are associated with granulocyte activation as evidenced by massive release of elastase, detectable in the circulation of bacteremic baboons [58], and by correlation between elastase and IL-8 in human sepsis [57].

While chemokines represent a family of more than 40 members, very little is known about the contribution and the presence of other molecules in sepsis, except for MCP-1 and MCP-2 which have been found in plasma of sepsis patients [59]. MCP-1 levels were higher in patients with the more severe forms of sepsis (i.e. those with shock or a lethal outcome).

Interferon-γ (IFNγ)

Gamma-interferon is an efficient amplificatory cytokine produced by T-lymphocytes in response either to IL-12, produced by monocytes/macrophages activated by microbial products, or directly to superantigens or viruses. Its synergy with the detrimental activities of LPS has been clearly established: IFNγ enhanced LPS-induced circulating TNFα as well as LPS- and TNF-induced mortality [60, 61], and anti-IFNγ antibodies protected against LPS- and *E. coli*-induced mortality [60, 62]. As a consequence, a clinically silent viral infection may induce hypersensitivity to Gram-negative bacterial endotoxin through T cell activation and subsequent IFNγ production, leading to a hyperproduction of TNFα [63]. On the other hand, IFNγ may be considered as a useful cytokine for restoring immune responsiveness which is often suppressed during sepsis [64]. The study of circulating IFNγ in human sepsis led to contradictory results. While in sepsis and purpura fulminans IFNγ was found in patients with the most severe disease [9], no correlation was reported with outcome in other studies on sepsis and septic shock [12, 20], and no detectable IFNγ was reported in meningococcal septic shock [10] or in human volunteers receiving systemic endotoxin [65]. In a baboon septic shock model, the IFNγ level was threefold higher in lethally-challenged animals than in those receiving sublethal doses [66]. These data suggest that in human studies the IFNγ level may often be below the detection limits of measurement.

Interleukin-12 (IL-12)

IL-12 is a heterodimeric cytokine consisting of p40 and p70 subunits. The measurement of p70 is correlated with IL-12 bioactivity. As mentioned previously, IL-12 is a potent inducer of IFNγ. In a bacille Calmette Guérin (BCG)-primed model of LPS-induced shock and lethality in mice, anti-IL-12 antibodies were associated with decreased IFNγ and protection [67]. An intravenous bolus of *Escherichia coli* LPS in human volunteers did not lead to changes in the plasma levels of IL-12 [65] whereas unexpected results were obtained in baboons: higher levels of IL-12 were detectable in the plasma of animals injected with sublethal doses of *E. coli* than in animals challenged with lethal doses [66].

Colony stimulating factors (CSF)

Among hematopoietic factors, macrophage-CSF (M-CSF) and G-CSF are two cytokines mainly involved in helping the immune system to fight the infectious process. This is also true for IL-3 and GM-CSF which, in addition, favor IL-1 and TNFα production and thus behave as pro-inflammatory cytokines. This is illustrated by GM-CSF-deficient mice in which LPS-induced hypothermia and loss in body weight were markedly attenuated when compared to normal mice; levels of circulating IFNγ, IL-1α, and IL-6 were lower and survival of a LD100 of LPS was 42% [68]. In humans, M-CSF is present at homeostasis in the circulation and its level is increased in patients with sepsis and higher in patients with hemophagocytosis associated with sepsis [69]. G-CSF is also increased in sepsis and reaches higher levels during severe sepsis when compared to sepsis or bacteremia [16, 70]. Enhanced levels of circulating G-CSF have been particularly associated with infection and sepsis in neonates [71, 72]. In meningococcemia, plasma GM-CSF concentrations were briefly present in subjects with life-threatening septic shock and were strongly associated with fulminant disease [70].

Macrophage migration inhibitory factor (MIF)

MIF was first discovered in 1966 as a T cell product released during delayed-type hypersensitivity and rediscovered in 1993 as a pituitary-derived cytokine that potentiates lethal endotoxemia [73] as well as a macrophage product induced by the action of glucocorticoids [74]. Bernhagen et al. [73] reported that injection of MIF together with one LD40 of LPS greatly potentiated lethality and that anti-MIF antibodies fully protected against a LD50 of LPS. Interestingly, it was recently shown that MIF is expressed constitutively in many tissues including lung, liver, kidney, spleen, adrenal gland, and skin. MIF exists as a preformed cytokine which is rapidly released following LPS injection [75].

IL-10 and anti-inflammatory cytokines

Sepsis is not associated with a deficient anti-inflammatory response. On the contrary, specific cytokine inhibitors such as the soluble TNF receptors (sTNFRI & sTNFRII) [76, 77], soluble IL-1 receptors (sIL-1RI & sIL-1RII) [78], cytokine receptor antagonists (IL-1ra) [8], and anti-inflammatory cytokines, particularly IL-10 [79, 80], are detected in great amounts in the circulation of septic patients. Most frequently the highest plasma levels of these regulatory molecules are detected in the most severe cases, leading to the concept of "compensatory anti-inflammatory response syndrome" (CARS) [81]. However, local production may lead to different patterns. In this context, it is interesting to recall the observation by Donnelly et al. [82] showing that a poor prognosis in patients with adult respiratory distress syndrome was significantly associated with the lowest levels of IL-10 and IL-1ra.

In addition to IL-10, TGFβ, IL-4, IL-13 and interferon-α also possess strong anti-inflammatory activities and a potent capacity for inhibiting the synthesis of the pro-inflammatory cytokines. Each individual anti-inflammatory cytokine has been demonstrated to be capable of reducing mortality in various endotoxic or septic shock models. Circulating IL-4, IL-13, or interferon-α have been rarely studied in sepsis, and absence of detectable levels [65], no modified levels [9], or rare positive cases [83] have been reported. Results concerning TGFβ are controversial, most probably because of the difficulty in measuring it and the fact that a latent and an active form already exist at homeostasis. Furthermore, since platelets are an important source of TGFβ, measurements in plasma, platelet-poor plasma, or sera may explain the discrepancy in the literature. Karres et al. [84] and Astiz et al. [85] reported a reduced level in sera from septic patients. The mean levels of serum TGFβ1 in healthy controls were in the range of ng/mL in one study and pg/mL in the other, illustrating the difficulty linked to the measurements. On the other hand, we found enhanced levels in plasma and platelet-poor plasma in patients with sepsis [86]. In a baboon septic model, Junger et al. [87] reported that active TGFβ1 levels increased while total TGFβ1 decreased.

Interleukin-1 receptor antagonist (IL-1ra), a natural IL-1 inhibitor, is also present in plasma at homeostasis. Enhanced levels of IL-1ra have been regularly reported in critically ill patients, septic adult, and new born patients [8, 88]. It may correlate with the APACHE II score [8]. As an antagonist, its concentration has to be at least 100 fold higher than that of IL-1 to efficiently block the effects of IL-1. Indeed 2,000 fold higher concentration have been noted in patients with septic shock [8]. In two patients who died within 3 h to 8 h after admission with a *Streptococcus* group A or *Neisseria meningitidis* septicemia we found a 3,400 and 61,000 fold higher concentration of IL-1ra than IL-1β, respectively [89, 90]. These observations suggest that the balance between pro- and anti-inflammatory cytokines seems adequate in limiting the effects of pro-inflammatory cytokines.

Where to measure cytokines?

Biological fluids

Since sepsis is a systemic inflammatory response syndrome, plasma levels of cytokines have been particularly investigated (see above). However, other biological fluids can reflect either a local production or exchange with plasma proteins following an enhanced vascular permeability. The local production is illustrated with the measurements performed in cerebrospinal fluid (CSF) during meningitis. During this severe infection, levels of TNF in CSF correlate with outcome [27]. In the CSF, cytokine levels are more frequently detected and in higher concentrations than in serum [91]. Local production and exchange between plasma and other milieu are also illustrated by the measurement performed in the peritoneal exudate [92] or in pleural effusion [93]. In the latter study we did not observe any differences between septic and non-septic patients suggesting that, in some instances, inflammatory stress can lead to similar cytokine patterns as infectious insult. Other biological fluids may not be relevant to sepsis (e.g. gingival fluid, synovial fluid, tears, saliva, sputum) but have been widely investigated in the study of locally-associated inflammatory diseases. Except in the case of urinary infections, urine has been poorly studied even though it might provide some interesting information [94].

Lavages

When fluids are absent, lavages can be performed to further analyze cytokines as in the case of bronchoalveolar lavages (BAL). While divergent results were reported on using the levels of plasma TNF to predict at risk-patients for developing acute adult respiratory distress syndrome (ARDS) [26, 95], measurement of TNF within BAL showed high levels in early severe ARDS when compared with early mild ARDS and late ARDS [96]. Other BAL cytokines like IL-8 may correlate with severity [55].

Cell-associated cytokines

Circulating cytokines represent the tip of the iceberg [97] (Fig. 1). Once produced, cytokines are present in a cellular environment and consequently can be trapped by surrounding cells which possess specific receptors. If one considers the blood com-

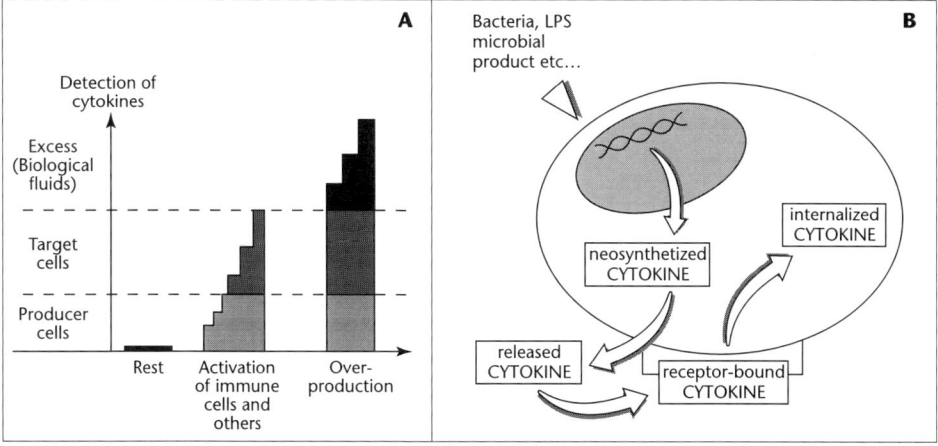

Figure 1

(A) The detection of a given cytokine in a biological fluid is possible once, following activation of producing cells, the released cytokine which can be efficiently trapped by the environmental cells has been produced in sufficient excess to allow its presence as a free molecule [97].

(B) Thus, the earlier levels of detection are the environmental cells. Cell-associated cytokine can represent the neosynthetized form, if the cell is the producing one, and can been found bound to the receptor or following its internalization by the target cell.

partment, it is obviously not possible to analyze endothelial cells, but circulating cells may be considered as useful tools. Indeed, we showed that IL-1α, IL-1β and TNF could be found associated with monocytes. Surprisingly, while IL-1 is a cytokine which can be found accumulated within the monocytes following *in vitro* activation, TNF was the most frequently found [2] (Tab. 1). Interestingly, at the end of the follow up of the patients, while most survivors did not have any more detectable circulating TNF, a majority had still detectable cell-associated TNF. More recently we investigated cell-associated IL-8. While Darbonne et al. [98] had coined the phrase that "red cells were a sink for IL-8", this statement referred to experiments performed in the absence of leukocytes. Indeed, while red cells can trap IL-8 via their Duffy antigen, we showed that their contribution remains lower than that of both polymorphonuclear cells and peripheral blood mononuclear cells [99]. In septic patients a tremendous amount of cell-associated IL-8 has been detected. Such measurements may offer more precise information in terms of follow-up and possible association with infection [100]. The presence of cell-associated cytokine should

Table 1a - Monocyte-associated cytokines in septic patients

	Measurements performed at admission in ICU		Maximum levels during the follow-up of the patients	
	% positive patients	range or mean ± SEM (pg/10^6 monocytes)	% positive patients	range or mean ± SEM (pg/10^6 monocytes)
IL-1α	6%	< 15 – 25	25%	< 15 – 90
IL-1β	25%	< 70 – 190	50%	153 ± 60
TNFα	81%	275 ± 58	88%	410 ± 65

Table 1b - Mean values of circulating TNFα and monocyte-associated TNFα at the end of the longitudinal study among septic patients

		surviving	non surviving
Day of the last measurement ± SEM		14 ± 2	10 ± 3
Plasma TNFα	% positive patients	17%	67%
	(range or mean ± SEM; pg/ml)	(< 70 – 150)	(125 ± 53)
Monocyte-associated TNFα			
	% positive patients	67%	100%
	(mean ± SEM; pg/10^6 monocytes)	(233 ± 67)	(372 ± 90)

adapted from [2]

not be always interpreted as an indication of the cellular source of a given cytokine since internalization of receptor-bound environmental cytokine could also take place. In addition to circulating leukocytes, cells recovered from various fluids or broncho-alveolar lavages can also be analyzed and may provide useful information. We have particularly analyzed cell lysates and measured cytokines by ELISA but flow cytometry is another useful tool for performing such analyses. Indeed, flow cytometric values for IL-1β and TNF were shown to correlate with the immunoreactive cytokine [101]. Using for the first time such a technique in ICU patients, Yentis et al. [102] described the presence of IL-1β positive cells among circulating leukocytes. Analysis of T-lymphocyte-associated cytokines has been particularly studied by flow cytometry and the usefulness and limitations of various currently available cytokine products have been recently reported [103]. However, flow cytometry may not be appropriate for studying all cells and all cytokines. For example, we showed that the permeabilization technique required for such an analysis led to the linking of all intracellular IL-8 measured in neutrophils by ELISA (C. Marie, unpublished observation). Immunocytochemistry has also been employed to detect cell-associated cytokine and concomitant analysis of many different cytokines can be performed as demonstrated with human tonsil tissues [104] and computerized assessment has been now rendered possible [105]. In human sepsis and sepsis-related pathologies, few investigations have employed immunocytochemistry analysis. In ARDS patients the presence of numerous IL-8 positive alveolar macrophages has confirmed the putative detrimental role of IL-8 in the development of that syndrome [106]. In animal models of sepsis or endotoxic shock, immunocytochemical analysis of tissues may be easier. For example, immunostaining of IL-1α in rat glomeruli [107], IL-1β in rat pituitary [108], and TNF in rat liver [109], mouse bone marrow cells [110] and diaphragm muscle [111] has been demonstrated after endotoxin administration.

What and how to measure?

Sampling

Blood sampling and storage may be sources of artifactual results. These may be the consequence of either *in vitro* activation which may lead to false positive results or cytokine degradation or trapping by environmental leukocytes which lead to underestimated values. While endotoxin-free heparin-containing tubes are now available [112], this has not always been the case and endotoxin-contaminated heparin has led to *in vitro* activation of leukocytes and false positive results [113]. As a consequence ethylene diamine tetraacetate (EDTA), which prevents cytokine production, has been recommended as an anticoagulant for cytokine measurements by immuno-assays. Of course, EDTA is not appropriate for bioassays and for *in vitro* cell-culture and the use of citrate has been suggested [114]. Storage of blood may be another source of artifacts. Proteolysis has been postulated to occur but the use of protease inhibitors such as aprotinin is no longer recommended [115]. At room temperature, cytokines in plasma can be taken up by environmental leukocytes and storage at 4° C would limit the decrease in plasma value noticed, for example, when studying TNF [116]. However, such low temperature storage will limit the reactivity of leukocytes if analyzed later on for their capacity to release cytokines upon *in vitro* activation [117]. Once collected, plasma should be aliquoted to avoid freezing-thawing of the samples. Indeed, some cytokines such as TNF and IL-10 are extremely sensitive to repeated freezing-thawings.

Bio-activity

To assess the presence of cytokines, bioassays have been used particularly during the early time of cytokine measurements. They usually require a cell line the growth of which is cytokine-dependent (e.g. CTLL-2 for IL-2, B9 or 7TD1 for IL-6) or which is killed by a given cytokine (e.g. L929 or WEHI-164 for TNF; MuLv1 for TGFβ). Since these measurements depend on the interaction of the cytokine with its high affinity receptor, they are usually highly sensitive (detection limit in the range of 1 to 5 pg/mL), and allow the detection of a bioactive cytokine. They are rather cheap although perpetuating the cell line may require recombinant cytokines. However, they are not totally specific and the use of antibodies is often necessary in assessing the real contribution of the analyzed cytokine (e.g. CTLL-2 also proliferates in the presence of IL-4, IL-15 and TGFβ). Furthermore, they are influenced by cytokine ligands such as soluble receptors which may amplify (e.g. sIL-6R) or inhibit (e.g. sTNFR) the bioactivity. For example, we have shown that in pleural effusions from septic or non-septic patients containing similar levels of IL-6 as judged by ELISA, the IL-6 bioactivity was significantly affected by the different levels of soluble IL-6 receptors [93]. However, the presence of soluble gp130 in these biological fluids may play an inhibiting role. To be detected by bioassays, TNF levels must be higher than those of its inhibitors. This is probably rarely the case for TNF in septic patients since circulating soluble TNF receptors, already present at homeostasis, are found in great amounts during sepsis. This may explain why the frequency of sepsis patients with detectable TNF was low when the cytokine was analyzed by bioassays [11, 14]. As a consequence, measurement of circulating soluble receptors is another important parameter to monitor. However, one should avoid overinterpretating the meaning of the ratio [cytokine] : [soluble cytokine receptor]. As previously mentioned, the measurements of free cytokines represent only a part of the total level of all released. On the other hand, the levels of soluble receptor are a true reflection of the vast majority of this product once released or shed by the cells.

Immunoreactive cytokines

Initially with radio-immunoassays and now with ELISA, cytokines are easily measured in any fluid. While many other techniques can assess the presence of cytokines, ELISA is the most frequently employed technique although its use is associated with various difficulties and problems. In the early 90's, it became evident that the use of various available commercial kits were in part responsible for the discrepancies observed from one study to another [95, 118]. For example, the influence of soluble TNFR was noticed with the first marketed ELISAs for TNF [119]. In 1993, Dinarello and Cannon wrote in an editorial: "The clinical study is in disarray because of the proliferation of commercial assay kits that are poorly characterized by the manufacturers and are used indiscriminately by researchers" [120]. To further compare commercial ELISA kits, we attempted to obtain more uniform measurements using international cytokine standards [121].

Despite our efforts, none of the kits gave similar values for individual plasma samples from septic patients. Most probably, numerous events may or may not interfere with the measurement as a reflection of the different monoclonal antibodies used in the various ELISA kits: (i) denaturation of the recognized epitope within the natural cytokine, (ii) fragmentation of the cytokine following enzymatic cleavage, (iii) depolymerization or polymerization, (iv) variable glycosylation of the natural cytokines, (v) recognition of precursor forms, (vi) binding of cytokines to undefined ligands. However, for the latter hypothesis, we showed that neither soluble cytokine receptors nor α2-macroglobulin interfered with the kits studied.

mRNA

Cytokines can remain below detection in the fluid under study while they are still being produced and may be trapped by environmental cells. The presence of their specific mRNA may reflect their local production, although the transcription of mRNA may not be associated with an effective translation. Analysis of mRNA may help to identify the source of the cytokine. This is obviously not easy in humans where most studied cells are leukocytes isolated from biological fluids. In sepsis, leukocytes may not be the major sources of the circulating cytokines as assessed by the presence of high levels of cytokines in plasma of neutropenic patients in the same range as that of non-neutropenic septic patients [122, 123]. TNF mRNA expression has been reported by *in situ* hybridization in cerebrospinal fluid cells from patients with bacterial meningitis [124] and in alveolar macrophages from bronchoalveolar lavages performed in ARDS patients [125]. Reverse transcriptase polymerase chain reaction (RT-PCR) revealed the presence of mRNA-positive blood and CSF cells for TNF, lymphotoxin-α, IL-1, IL-6, IFNγ and TGFβ in multiple sclerosis patients with acute bacterial meningitis [126]. However, a study using *in situ* hybridization suggests that IL-4, IL-6, IL-10, IFNγ, and TGFβ may be occasionally found in peripheral mononuclear cells from healthy individuals [127]. Altogether these data suggest that caution should be taken when analyzing cytokine mRNA and more studies are necessary in this area. Animal models of endotoxemia or sepsis can address the cytokine mRNA expression in tissues. In 1992, Giroir et al. [128] published a provocative observation: using the chloramphenicol acetyltransferase reporter gene, they demonstrated that tissues such as kidney, heart, islet of Langerhans, lungs, uterus, and fallopian tubes could transcribe the TNF gene following LPS injection. Since this study, many other tissues have been shown to contribute to cytokine mRNA production. Spleen makes TNF, lymphotoxin-α, IL-2, and IFNγ in response to bacterial superantigens [34] and IL-1α, IL-1β, and IL-1ra in response to LPS as do liver and bowel [129], which also synthetize IL-6 mRNA [130] and TNF mRNA [131].

Cell culture

The analysis of circulating cells of sepsis patients as to their ability to further produce cytokine upon *ex vivo* stimulation led to the discovery that these cells are hyporesponsive compared to leukocytes from healthy patients. All T cell, monocyte and neutrophil-derived cytokines studied so far are produced in lower amounts than those obtained with leukocytes from healthy controls, except IL-1ra in whole blood assay (Tab. 2). This hyporesponsiveness is not specific to sepsis patients and such observations have also been reported in numerous stressful situations. It is worth noting that this peripheral hyporesponsiveness may or may not be observed in tissues.

Table 2 - Decreased ex vivo *cytokine production in human sepsis*

Monocytes

Cytokines	Assays	Activators	References
IL-1	Monocytes	Silica	Luger et al (1986) *Crit Care Med* 14: 458
	P.B.M.C.	LPS	Helminen et al (1990) *Scand J Infect* 22: 105
IL-1α, IL-β		LPS	Muñoz et al (1991) *J Clin Invest* 88: 1747
IL-6, TNFα	Monocytes	Streptococcus	Cavaillon et al (1993) *Endot Res Series* 2: 275
		SEB	Astiz et al (1996) *J Lab Clin Med* 128: 594
TNFα	Alveolar MØ	LPS	Simpson et al (1991) *Crit Care Med* 19: 1060
IL-1β, IL-6			Sekatrian et al (1994) *Arch Surg* 129: 187
TNFα	Whole blood	LPS	van Deuren et al (1994) *J Infect Dis* 69: 157
but not IL-1ra			Marchant et al (1995) *J Clin Immunol* 15: 266
			Ertel et al (1995) *Blood* 85: 1341
IL-10	Whole blood	LPS	Marchant et al (1995) *J Clin Immunol* 15: 266
	PMBC HLA DR+ low		Randow et al (1995) *J Exp Med* 181: 1887
IL-12	Whole blood	LPS & SAC ± IFNγ	Ertel et al (1997) *Blood* 89: 1612

Peripheral blood mononuclear cells

Cytokines	Activators	References
IL-2	PHA	Wood et al (1984) *Ann Surg* 200: 311
IFNγ	LPS + IL-12	Ertel et al (1997) *Blood* 89: 1612
IL-2, IL-5	ConA but neither PHA	Muret et al (1998) *submitted*
IL-10	nor anti-CD3	

Neutrophils

IL-1β	LPS but not staphylococcus	McCall et al (1993) *J Clin Invest* 91: 853
IL-8	LPS and streptococcus	Marie et al (1998) *Blood* 91: 3439
IL-1ra	LPS and streptococcus	Marie et al (1999) *submitted*

PHA, phytohaemagglutinin; SAC, Staphylococcus aureus Cowan; PBMC, peripheral blood mononuclear cells

Are cytokine measurements useful at bedside?

This question often occurs and the answer may vary depending on whether you are in charge of the hospital budget or of sales in a company that makes measurement kits! May we expect from cytokine measurements to have a prognostic, a diagnostic or a predictive value? As a prognostic factor, we have mentioned above many reports dealing with various cytokines where correlations with severity or outcome were described. However, a follow-up of circulating cytokines may be necessary and more appropriate for establishing a good correlation than a unique measurement. Furthermore, many other biological markers and clinical scores lead to the same correlations. Thus, one may question the usefulness of such expensive measurements on a routine basis as long as no specific treatments may be initiated depending on the amounts of a given detectable cytokine. So far, cytokine measurements have not helped the physician to diagnose a given pathology or to orient his therapeutic approach. As a predictive factor, cytokine measurements could be interesting in patients who may develop sepsis. For example, IL-6 is a very early marker which appears before CRP and may therefore be useful in the monitoring of patients with a high risk of developing infection. Indeed, there is good evidence that IL-6 analysis obtained within twelve hours after birth appears to be ideal for detecting early-onset neonatal infection with a high degree of sensitivity and specificity [132]. In neutropenic patients, IL-8 plasma levels, in contrast to IL-6, IL-1, TNF, and IL-1ra, were significantly higher in patients who subsequently developed major infection [133]. One may speculate that T cell derived cytokines could be indicators of Gram-positive infection. Rapid detection would be then recommended. Some are already available like the chemiluminescent immunoassays. The measurement of cell-associated cytokines could be an alternative and useful indicator. As long as we do not have an alternative therapy to offer that depends on a defined inflammatory profile, routine measurement will be of little benefit whereas cytokine analysis will remain essential to further understanding the interplay of cytokines during sepsis.

Acknowledgements
The author acknowledges the most valuable contributions of Catherine Fitting and Dr. Christelle Marie. The authors thanks Dr. Carlos Muñoz who initiated this topic in his group and Dr. Jean Carlet and Prof. Didier Payen without whom no study would have been possible.

References

1   Cannon JG, Tompkins RG, Gelfand JA (1990) Circulating interleukin 1 and tumor necrosis factor in septic shock and experimental endotoxin fever. *J Infect Dis* 161: 79–84

2   Muñoz C, Misset B, Fitting C, Bleriot JP, Carlet J, Cavaillon J-M (1991) Dissociation between plasma and monocyte-associated cytokines during sepsis. *Eur J Immunol* 21: 2177–2184

3   Michie H, Manogue K, Spriggs D, Revhaug A, O'Dwyer S, Dinarello C, Cerami A, Wolf S (1988) Detection of circulating TNF after endotoxin administration. *N Engl J Med* 318: 1481–1486

4   Damas P, Ledoux D, Nys M, Vrindts Y, De Groote D, Franchimont P, Lamy M (1992) Cytokine serum level during severe sepsis in human IL-6 as a marker of severity. *Ann Surgery* 215: 356–362

5   Herzyk DJ, Wewers MD (1993) ELISA detection of IL-1β in human sera needs independent confirmation. False positives in hospitalized patients. *Am Rev Respir Dis* 147: 139–142

6   Granowitz EV, Santos AA, Poutsiaka DD, Cannon JG, Wilmore DW, Wolff SM, Dinarello CA (1991) Production of IL-1ra during experimental endotoxaemia. *Lancet* 338: 1423–1424

7   Van Deuren M, Van Der Ven-Jongekrijg H, Baterlink AKN, Van Dalen R, Sauerwein RW, van Der Meer JWM (1995) Correlation between proinflammatory cytokines and antiinflammatory mediators and the severity of disease in meningococcal infections. *J Infect Dis* 172: 433–439

8   Gardlund B, Sjölin J, Nilsson A, Roll M, Wickerts CJ, Wretlind B (1995) Plasma levels of cytokines in primary septic shock in humans: correlation with disease severity. *J Infect Dis* 172: 296–301

9   Girardin E, Grau G, Dayer J, Roux-Lombard P, Group TJ, Lambert P (1988) TNF and IL-1 in the serum of children with severe infectious purpura. *N Engl J Med* 319: 397–400

10   Waage A, Brandtzaeg P, Halstensen A, Kierulf P, Espevik T (1989) The complex pattern of cytokines in serum from patients with meningococcal septic shock. Association between interleukin-6, interleukin-1, and fatal outcome. *J Exp Med* 169: 333–338

11   Friedland JS, Porter JC, Daryanani S, Bland JM, Screaton NJ, Vesely MJJ, Griffin GE, Bennett ED, Remick DG (1996) Plasma proinflammatory cytokine concentrations, acute physiology and chronic health evaluation (APACHE) III scores and survival in patients in an intensive care unit. *Crit Care Med* 24: 1775–1781

12   Calandra T, Baumgartner JD, Grau GE, WU MM, Lambert PH, Schellekens J, Verhoef J, Glauser MP (1990) Prognostic values of tumor necrosis factor/cachectin, interleukin-1, interferon-α, and interferon-γ in the serum of patients with septic shock. *J Infect Dis* 161: 982–987

13   Waage A, Espevik T, Lamvik J (1986) Detection of TNF-like cytotoxicity in serum from patients with septicemia but not from untreated cancer patients. *Scand J Immunol* 24: 739–743

14   Waage A, Halstensen A, Espevik T (1987) Association between tumor necrosis factor in serum and fatal outome in patients with meningococal disease. *Lancet* i: 355–357

15 Baud L, Cadranel J, Offenstadt G, Luquel L, Guidet B, Amstutz P (1990) Tumor necrosis factor and septic shock. *Crit Care Med* 18: 349–350

16 Kragsbjerg P, Holmberg H, Vikerfors T (1996) Dynamics of blood cytokine concentrations in patients with bacteremic infections. *Scand J Infect Dis* 28: 391–398

17 Taveira da Silva AM, Kaulbach HC, Chuidian FS, Lambert DR, Suffredini AF, Danner RL (1993) Shock and multiple-organ dysfunction after self-administration of Salmonella endotoxin. *N Engl J Med* 328: 1457–1460

18 Marano MA, Fong Y, Moldawer LL, Wei H, Calvano SE, Tracey KJ, Barie PS, Manogue K, Cerami A, Shires GT, et al. (1990) Serum cachectin/tumor necrosis factor in critically ill patients with burns correlates with infection and mortality. *Surg Gynecol Obstet* 170: 32–38

19 Leroux-Roels G, Offner F (1990) Tumor necrosis factor in sepsis. *JAMA* 263: 1494–1495

20 Pinsky MR, Vincent JL, Deviere J, Alegre M, Kahn RJ, Dupont E (1993) Serum cytokine levels in human septic shock. Relation to MOF and mortality. Chest 103: 565–575

21 Calandra T, Gerain J, Heumann D, Baumgartner JD, Glauser MP (1991) High circulating levels of IL-6 in patients with septic shock: evolution during sepsis, prognostic value, and interplay with other cytokines. The Swiss-Dutch J5 Immunoglobulin Study Group. *Am J Med* 91: 23–29

22 Groeneveld PHP, Kwappenberg KMC, Langermans JAM, Nibbering PH, Curtis L (1997) Relation between pro- and anti-inflammatory cytokines and the production of nitric oxide in sever sepsis. *Cytokine* 9: 138–142

23 Hamilton GH, Hofbauer S, Hamilton B (1992) Endotoxin, TNF-alpha, IL-6 and parameters of the cellular immune system in patients with intraabdominal sepsis. *Scand J Infect Dis* 24: 361–368

24 Riche F, Panis Y, Laisne MJ, Briard C, Cholley B, Bernard-Poenaru O, Graulet AM, Gueris J, Valleur P (1996) High tumor necrosis factor serum level is associated with increased survival in patients with abdominal septic shock: a prospective study in 59 patients. *Surgery* 120: 801–807

25 Paramo JA, Perez JL, Serrano M, Rocha E (1990) Types 1 and 2 plasminogen activator inhibitor and tumor necrosis factor alpha in patients with sepsis. *Thromb Haemost* 64: 3–6

26 Marks JD, Marks CB, Luce JM, Montgomery AB, Turner J, Metz CA, Murray JF (1990) Plasma tumor necrosis factor in patients with septic shock. Mortality rate, incidence of ARDS and effects of methylprednisolone administration? *Am Rev Respir Dis* 141: 94–97

27 Arditi M, Manogue KR, Caplan M, Yogev R (1990) Cerebrospinal fluid TNF-α and PAF concentrations and severity of bacterial meningitis in children. *J Infect Dis* 162: 139–147

28 Dulkerian SJ, Kilpatrick L, Costarino AT, McCawley L, Fein J, Corcoran L, Zirin S, Harris MC (1995) Cytokine elevations in infants with bacterial and aseptic meningitis. *J Pediatr* 126: 872–876

29   Engelhardt R, Mackensen A, Galanos C, Andreesen R (1990) Biological response to intravenously administered endotoxin in patients with advanced cancer. *J Biol Resp Mod* 9: 480–491

30   Pollmächer T, Korth C, Mullington J, Schreiber W, Sauer J, Vedder H, Galanos C, Holsboer F (1996) Effects of G-CSF on plasma cytokine and cytokine receptor levels and on the *in vivo* host response to endotoxin in healthy men. *Blood* 87: 900–905

31   van der Poll T, Coyle SM, Barbosa K, Braxton CC, Lowry SF (1996) Epinephrine inhibits tumor necrosis factor-alpha and potentiates interleukin-10 production during human endotoxemia. *J Clin Invest* 97: 713–719

32   Leeper-Woodford SK, Carey PD, Byrne K, Jenkins JK, Fisher BJ, Blocher C, Sugerman HJ, Fowler III AA (1991) Tumor necrosis factor alpha and beta subtypes appear in circulation during onset of sepsis-induced lung injury. *Am Rev Respir Dis* 143: 1076–1082

33   Sriskandan S, Moyes D, Cohen J (1996) Detection of circulating bacterial superantigen and lymphotoxin-alpha in patients with streptococcal toxic-shock syndrome. *Lancet* 348: 1315–1316

34   Bette M, Schafer MK, van Rooijen N, Weihe E, Fleischer B (1993) Distribution and kinetics of superantigen-induced cytokine gene expression in mouse spleen. *J Exp Med* 178: 1531–1539

35   Tokman MG, Carey KD, Quimby FW (1995) The pathogenesis of experimental toxic shock syndrome: the role of IL-2 in the induction of hypotension and release of cytokines. *Shock* 3: 145–151

36   Tilg H, Trehu E, Atkins MB, Dinarello CA, Mier JW (1994) Interleukin-6 (IL-6) as an anti-inflammatory cytokine: induction of circulating IL-1 receptor antagonist and soluble tumor necrosis factor receptor p55. *Blood* 83: 113–118

37   Hack C, de Groot E, Felt-Bersma R, Nuijens J, Strack Van Schijndel R, Eerenberg-Belmer A, Thijs L, Aarden L (1989) Increased plasma levels of interleukin-6 in sepsis. *Blood* 74: 1704–1710

38   Helfgott DC, Tatter SB, Santhanam U, Clarick RH, Bhardwaj N, May LT, Sehgal PB (1989) Multiple forms of IFN-beta 2/IL-6 in serum and body fluids during acute bacterial infection. *J Immunol* 142: 948–953

39   Fong Y, Moldawer LL, Marano M, Wei H, Tatter SB, Clarick RH, Santhanam U, Sherris D, May LT, Sehgal PB, et al. (1989) Endotoxemia elicits increased circulating beta 2-IFN/IL-6 in man. *J Immunol* 142: 2321–2324

40   Yoshizawa KI, Naruto M, Ida N (1996) Injection time of interleukin-6 determines fatal outcome in experimental endotoxin shock. *J Interferon Cytokine Res* 16: 995–1000

41   Chang M, Williams A, Ishizawa L, Knoppel A, van de Ven C, Cairo MS (1996) Endogenous interleukin-11 expression is increased and prophylactic use of exogenous IL-11 enhances platelet recovery and improves survival during thrombocytopenia associated with experimental group B streptococcal sepsis in neonatal rats. *Blood Cells Mol & Dis* 22: 57–67

42   Villiger PM, Geng Y, Lotz M (1993) Induction of cytokine expression by leukemia inhibitory factor. *J Clin Invest* 91: 1575–1581

43   Modur V, Feldhaus MJ, Weyrich AS, Jicha DL, Prescotte SM, Zimmerman GA, McIntyre TM (1997) Oncostanin M is a proinflammatory mediator. *In vivo* effects correlate with endothelial cell expression of inflammatory cytokines and adhesion molecules. *J Clin Invest* 100: 158–168

44   Waring P, Wycherley K, Cary D, Nicola N, Metcalf D (1992) Leukemia inhibitory factor levels are elevated in septic shock and various inflammatory body fluids. *J Clin Invest* 90: 2031–2037

45   Villers D, Dao T, Nguyen JM, Bironneau E, Godard A, Moreau M, De Groote D, Nicolas F, Soulillou JP, Anegon I (1995) Increased plasma levels of human interleukin for DA1a cells / leukemia inhibitory factor in sepsis correlate with shock and poor prognosis. *J Infect Dis* 171: 232–236

46   Guillet C, Fourcin M, Chevalier S, Pouplard A, Gascan H (1995) ELISA detection of circulating levels of LIF, OSM and CNTF in septic shock. *Ann NY Acad Sci* 762: 407–412

47   Jansen PM, de Jong IW, Hart M, Kim KJ, Aarden LA, Hinshaw LB, Taylor FB, Hack CE (1996) Release of leukemia inhibitory factor in primate sepsis. Analysis of the role of TNFα. *J Immunol* 156: 4401–4407

48   Endo S, Inada K, Arakawa N, Yamada Y, Takakuwa T, Nakae H, Takakuwa T, Namiki M, Inoue Y, Shimamura T et al (1996) Interleukin-11 in patients with disseminated intravascular coagulation. *Res Com Mol Pathol Pharmac* 91: 253–256

49   Broaddus VC, Boylan AM, Hoeffel JM, Kim KJ, Sadick M, Chuntharapai A (1994) Neutralization of IL-8 inhibits neutrophils influx in a rabbit model of endotoxin-induced pleurisy. *J Immunol* 152: 2960–2967

50   Gimbrone MA, Obin MS, Brock AF, Luis EA, Hass PE, Hébert CA, Yip YK, Leung DW, Lowe DG, Kohr WJ, et al. (1989) Endothelial interleukin-8: a novel inhibitor of leukocyte-endothelial interactions. *Science* 246: 1601–1603

51   Cunha FQ, Cunha Tamashiro WMS (1992) Tumour necrosis factor-alpha and interleukin-8 inhibit neutrophil migration *in vitro* and *in vivo*. *Mediators Inflam* 1: 397–401

52   Zisman DA, Kunkel SL, Strieter RM, Tsai WC, Bucknell K, Wilkowski J, Standiford TJ (1997) MCP-1 protects mice in lethal endotoxemia. *J Clin Invest* 99: 2832–2836

53   Friedland J, Suputtamongkol Y, Remick D, Chaowagul W, Strieter R, Kunkel S, White N, Griffin G (1992) Prolonged elevation of interleukin-8 and interleukin-6 concentrations in plasma and of leukocyte interleukin-8 m-RNA levels during septicemic and localized Pseudomonas pseudomallei infection. *Infect Immun* 60: 2402–2408

54   Hack C, Hart M, Strack van Schijndel R, Eerenberg A, Nuijens J, Thijs L, Aarden L (1992) IL-8 in sepsis: relation to shock and inflammatory mediators. *Infect Immun* 60: 2835–2842

55   Miller E, Cohen, AB, Nagao S, Griffith D, Maunder R, Martin T, Weiner-Kronish J, Sticherling M, Christophers E, Matthay A (1992) Elevated levels of NAP-1/Interleukin-8 are present in the airspaces of patients with the adult respiratory distress syndrome and are associated with increased mortality. *Am J Respir Dis* 148: 427–432

56   Marty C, Misset B, Tamion F, Fitting C, Carlet J, Cavaillon J-M (1994) Circulating IL-

8 concentrations in patients with multiple organ failure of septic and nonseptic origin. *Crit Care Med* 22: 673–679

57 Endo S, Inada K, Ceska M, Takakuwa T, Yamada Y, Nakae H, Kasai T, Yamashita H, Taki K, Yoshida M (1995) Plasma interleukin 8 and polymorphonuclear leukocyte elastase concentrations in patients with septic shock. *J Inflamm* 45: 136–142

58 Redl H, Schlag G, Bahrami S, Schade U, Ceska M, Stütz P (1991) Plasma interleukin-8 and neutrophil elastase in a primate bacteremia model. *J Infect Dis* 164: 383–388

59 Bossink AW, Paemen L, Jansen PM, Hack CE, Thijs LG, Van Damme J (1995) Plasma levels of the chemokines MCP-1 and -2 are elevated in human sepsis. *Blood* 86: 3841–3847

60 Heinzel FP (1990) The role of interferon-gamma in the pathology of experimental endotoxemia. *J Immunol* 145: 2920–2924

61 Doherty GM, Lange JR, Langstein HN, Alexander HR, Buresh CM, Norton JA (1992) Evidence for IFN-γ as a mediator of the lethality of endotoxin and TNF-α. *J Immunol* 149: 1666–1670

62 Silva AT, Cohen J (1992) Role of interferon-gamma in experimental Gram-negative sepsis. *J Infect Dis* 166: 331–335

63 Nansen A, Pravsgaard Christensen J, Marker O, Randrup Thomsen A (1997) Sensitization to lipopolysaccharide in mice with asymptomatic viral infection: role of T cell-dependent production of interferon-γ. *J Infect Dis* 176: 151–157

64 Döcke WD, Randow F, Syrbe U, Krausch D, Asadullah K, Reinke P, Volk HD, Kox W (1997) Monocyte deactivation in septic patients: restoration by IFNγ treatment. *Nature Med* 3: 678–681

65 Zimmer S, Pollard V, Marshall GD, Garofalo RP, Traber D, Prough D, Herndon DN (1996) The 1996 Moyer Award. Effects of endotoxin on the Th1/Th2 response in humans. *J Burn Care Rehabil* 17: 491–496

66 Jansen PM, van der Pouw Kraan TCTM, de Jong IW, van Mierlo G, Wijdenes J, Chang AA, Aarden LA, Taylor FB, Hack CE (1996) Release of IL-12 in experimental *Escherichia coli* septic shock in baboons: relation to plasma levels to IL-10 and IFN-gamma. *Blood* 87: 5144–5151

67 Wysocka M, Kubin M, Vieira LQ, Ozmen L, Garotta G, Scott P, Trinchieri G (1995) Interleukin-12 is required for interferon-gamma production and lethality in lipopolysaccharide-induced shock in mice. *Eur J Immunol* 25: 672–676

68 Basu S, Dunn AR, Marino MW, Savoia H, Hodgson G, Lieschke GJ, Cebon J (1997) Increased tolerance to endotoxin by granulocyte-macrophage colony stimulating factor deficient mice. *J Immunol* 159: 1412–1417

69 François B, Trimoreau F, Vignon P, Fixe P, Praloran V, Gastinne H (1997) Thrombocytopenia in the sepsis syndrome: role of hemophagocytosis and macrophage colony-stimulating factor. *Am J Med* 103: 114–120

70 Waring PM, Presneill J, Maher DW, Layton JE, Cebon J, Waring LJ, Metcalf D (1995) Differential alterations in plasma colony-stimulating factor concentrations in meningococcaemia. *Clin Exper Immunol* 102: 501–506

71 Gessler P, Kirchmann N, Kientsch-Engel R, Haas N, Lasch P, Kachel W (1993) Serum concentrations of granulocyte colony-stimulating factor in healthy term and preterm neonates and in those with various diseases including bacterial infections. *Blood* 82: 3177–3182

72 Cairo MS, Suen Y, Knoppel E, Dana R, Park L, Clark S, van de Ven C, Sender L (1992) Decreased G-CSF and IL-3 production and gene expression from mononuclear cells of newborn infants. *Pediat Res* 31: 574–578

73 Bernhagen J, Calandra T, Mitchell RA, Martin SB, Tracey KJ, Voelter W, Manogue KR, Cerami A, Bucala R (1993) MIF is a pituitary-derived cytokine that potentiates lethal endotoxaemia. *Nature* 365: 756–759

74 Calandra T, Bernhagen J, Metz CN, Spiegel LA, Bacher M, Donnelly T, Cerami A, Bucala R (1995) MIF as a glucocorticoid-induced modulator of cytokine production. *Nature* 376: 68–71

75 Bacher M, Meinhardt A, Lan HY, Mu W, Metz CN, Chesney JA, Calandra T, Gemsa D, Donnelly T, Atkins RC, et al. (1997) Migration inhibitory factor expression in experimentally induced endotoxemia. *Am J Pathol* 150: 235–246

76 Girardin E, Roux-Lombard P, Grau GE, Suter P, Gallati H, Dayer JM (1992) Imbalance between tumour necrosis factor-alpha and soluble TNF receptor concentrations in severe meningococcaemia. *Immunology* 76: 20–23

77 Van Zee KJ, Kohno T, Fischer E, Rock CS, Moldawer LL, Lowry SF (1992) Tumor necrosis factor soluble receptors circulate during experimental and clinical inflammation and can protect against excessive TNFα *in vitro* and *in vivo*. *Proc Natl Acad Sci USA* 89: 4845–4849

78 Pruitt JH, B WM, Edwards PD, Harward RRS, Seeger JW, Martin TD, Smith C, Kenney JA, Wesdorp RIC, Meijer S, et al. (1996) Increased soluble IL-1 type II receptor concentrations in postoperative patients and in patients with sepsis syndrome. *Blood* 87: 3282–3288

79 Marchant A, Devière J, Byl B, De Groote D, Vincent J, Goldman M (1994) Interleukin-10 production during septicaemia. *Lancet* 343: 707–708

80 Derkx B, Marchant A, Goldman M, Bijlmer R, van Deventer S (1995) High levels of IL-10 during the initial phase of fulminant meningococcal septic shock. *J Infect Dis* 171: 229–232

81 Bone RC, Grodzin CJ, Balk RA (1997) Sepsis: A new hypothesis for pathogenesis of the disease process. *Chest* 121: 235–243

82 Donnelly SC, Strieter RM, Reid PT, Kunkel SL, Burdick MD, Armstrong I, Mackenzie A, Haslett C (1996) The association between mortality rates and decreased concentrations of interleukin-10 and interleukin-1 receptor antagonist in the lung fluids of patients with the adult respiratory distress syndrome. *Ann Intern Med* 125: 191–196

83 Zeni F, Vindimian M, Pain P, Gery P, Tardy B, Bertrand JC (1995) Antiinflammatory and proinflammatory cytokines in patients with severe sepsis. *J Infect Dis* 172: 1171–1172

84 Karres I, Kremer JP, Sterckholzer U, Kenney JS, Ertel W (1996) TGF-β1 inhibits syn-

thesis of cytokines in endotoxin-stimulated human whole blood. *Arch Surg* 131: 1310–1317

85 Astiz M, Saha D, Lustbader D, Lin R, Rackow E (1996) Monocyte response to bacterial toxins, expression of cell surface receptors, and release of anti-inflammatory cytokines during sepsis. *J Lab Clin Med* 128: 597–600

86 Marie C, Cavaillon J-M, Losser M-R (1996) Elevated levels of circulating transforming growth factor-β1 in patients with the sepsis syndrome. *Ann Intern Med* 125: 520–521

87 Junger WG, Hoyt DB, Redl H, Liu FC, Loomis WH, Davies J, Schlag G (1995) Tumor necrosis factor antibody treatment of septic baboons reduces the production of sustained T-cell suppressive factors. *Shock* 3: 173–178

88 Fischer E, Van Zee KJ, Marano MA, Rock CS, Kenney JS, Poutsiaka DD, Dinarello CA, Lowry SF, Moldawer LL (1992) Interleukin-1 receptor antagonist circulates in experimental inflammation and in human disease. *Blood* 79: 2196–2200

89 Cavaillon JM, Müller-Alouf H, Alouf JE (1997) Cytokines in streptococcal infections. An opening lecture. *Adv Exper Med Biol* 418: 869–879

90 Marie C, Cavaillon JM (1997) Negative feedback in inflammation: the role of antiinflammatory cytokines. *Bull Inst Pasteur* 95: 41–54

91 Halstensen A, Ceska M, Brandtzaeg P, Redl H, Naess A, Waage A (1993) IL-8 in serum and cerebrospinal fluid from patients with meningococcal disease. *J Infect Dis* 167: 471–475

92 Holzheimer RG, Schein M, Wittmann DH (1995) Inflammatory response in peritoneal exudate and plasma of patients undergoing planned relaparotomy for severe secondary peritonitis. *Arch Surg* 130: 1314–1319

93 Marie C, Losser MR, Fitting C, Kermarrec N, Payen D, Cavaillon J-M (1997) Cytokines and soluble cytokines receptors in pleural effusions from septic and nonseptic patients. *Am J Respir Crit Care Med* 156: 1515–1522

94 Williams PA, Bohnsack JF, Augustine NH, Drummond WK, Rubens CE, Hill HR (1993) Production of tumor necrosis factor by human cells *in vitro* and *in vivo*, induced by group B streptococci. *J Pediatr* 123: 292–300

95 Parsons PE, Moore EE, Moore FA, Iklé DN, Henson PM, Worthen GS (1992) Studies on the role of TNF in adult respiratory distress syndrome. *Am Rev Respir Dis* 146: 694–700

96 Suter PM, Suter S, Girardin E, Roux-Lombard P, Grau GE, Dayer JM (1992) High bronchoalveolar levels of tumor necrosis factor and its inhibitors, interleukin-1, interferon, and elastase, in patients with adult respiratory distress syndrome after trauma, shock, or sepsis. *Am Rev Respir Dis* 145: 1016–1022

97 Cavaillon JM, Muñoz C, Fitting C, Misset B, Carlet J (1992) Circulating cytokines: the tip of the iceberg? *Circ Shock* 38: 145–152

98 Darbonne WC, Rice GC, Mohler MA, Apple T, Hébert CA, Valente AJ, Baker JB (1991) Red blood cells are a sink for interleukin-8, a leukocyte chemotaxin. *J Clin Invest* 88: 1362–1369

99 Marie C, Fitting C, Cheval C, Losser MR, Carlet J, Payen D, Foster K, Cavaillon J-M

(1997) Presence of high levels of leukocyte-associated interleukin-8 upon cell activation and in patients with sepsis syndrome. *Infect Immun* 65: 865–871

100 Marie C, Muret J, Fitting C, Losser M-R, Payen D, Cavaillon J-M (1998) Reduced ex vivo interleukin-8 production by neutrophils in septic and non-septic systemic inflammatory response syndrome. *Blood* 91: 3439–3446

101 Nakamura H, Fujishima S, Soejima K, Waki Y, Nakamura M, Ishizaka A, Kanazawa M (1996) Flow cytometric detection of cell-associated cytokines in alveolar macrophages. *Eur Respir J* 9: 1181–1187

102 Yentis SM, Rowbottom AW, Riches PG (1995) Detection of cytoplasmic IL-1β in peripheral blood mononuclear cells from intensive care unit patients. *Clin Exp Immunol* 100: 330–335

103 Jason J, Larned J (1997) Single cell cytokine profiles in normal humans: comparison of flow cytometric reagents and stimulations protocols. *J Immunol* Methods 207: 13–22

104 Andersson J, Abrams J, Björk L, Funa K, Litton M, Agren K, Andersson U (1994) Concomitant *in vivo* production of 19 different cytokines in human tonsils. *Immunology* 83: 16–24

105 Björk L, Fehniger TE, Andersson U, Andersson J (1996) Computerized assessment of production of multiple cytokines at the single-cell level using image analysis. *J Leuk Biol* 59: 287–295

106 Donnelly S, Strieter R, Kunkel S, Walz A, Robertson C, Carter D, Grant I, Pollock A, Haslett C (1993) Interleukin-8 and development of adult respiratory distress syndrome in at-risk patients groups. *Lancet* 341: 643–647

107 Laszik Z, Nadasdy T, Johnson LD, Lerner MR, Brackett D, Silva FG (1994) Renal interleukin-1 expression during endotoxemia and Gram-negative septicemia in conscious rats. *Circ Shock* 43: 115–121

108 Koenig JI, Snow K, Clark BD, Toni R, Cannon JG, Shaw AR, Dinarello CA, Reichlin S, Lee SL, Lechan RM (1990) Intrinsic pituitary interleukin-1β is induced by bacterial lipopolysaccharide. *Endocrinol* 126: 3053–3058

109 Tanaka N, Kita T, Kasai K, Nagano T (1992) The immunocytochemical localization of tumour necrosis factor and leukotriene in the rat liver after treatment with lipopolysaccharide. *Int J Exp Path* 73: 675–683

110 Schmauder-Chock EA, Chock SP, Patchen ML (1994) Ultrastructural localization of tumour necrosis factor-alpha. *Histochem J* 26: 142–151

111 Shindoh C, Hida W, Ohkawara Y, Yamauchi K, Ohno I, Takishima T, Shirato K (1995) TNFα mRNA expression in diaphragm muscle after endotoxin administration. *Am J Resp Crit Care Med* 152: 1696–1696

112 Redl H, Bahrami S, Leichtfried G, Schlag G (1992) Special collection and storage tubes for blood endotoxin and cytokine measurements. *Clin Chem* 38: 764–765

113 Riches P, Gooding R, Millar BC, Rowbottom AW (1992) Influence of collection and separation of blood samples on plasma IL-1, IL-6 and TNF concentration. *J Immunol Methods* 153: 125–131

114 Hoffmann JN, Hartl WH, Faist E, Jochum M, Inthorn D (1997) Tumor necrosis factor

measurement and use of different anticoagulants: possible interference in plasma samples and supernatants from endotoxin-stimulated monocytes. *Inflamm Res* 46: 342–347

115 Cannon JG, van der Meer JW, Kwiatkowski D, Endres S, Lonnemann G, Burke JF, Dinarello CA (1988) Interleukin-1 beta in human plasma: optimization of blood collection, plasma extraction, and radioimmunoassay methods. *Lymphokine Res* 7: 457–467

116 Exley AR, Cohen J (1990) Optimal collection of blood samples for the measurements of tumor necrosis factor-α. *Cytokine* 2: 353–356

117 Schins RP, van Hartingsveldt B, Borm PJ (1996) *Ex vivo* cytokine release from whole blood. A routine method for health effect screening. *Exp Toxicol Pathol* 48: 494–496

118 Cannon JG, Nerad JL, Poutsiaka DD, Dinarello CA (1993) Measuring circulating cytokines. *J Appl Physiol* 75: 1897–1902

119 Engelberts I, Stephens S, Francot G, Van Der Linden C, Buurman W (1991) Evidence for different effects of soluble TNF-receptors on various TNF measurements in human biological fluids. *Lancet* 338: 515–516

120 Dinarello CA, Cannon JG (1993) Cytokine measurements in septic shock. *Ann Intern Med* 119: 853–854

121 Ledur A, Fitting C, David B, Hamberger C, Cavaillon JM (1995) Variable estimates of cytokine levels produced by commercial ELISA kits: results using international cytokine standards. *J Immunol Methods* 186: 171–179

122 Engervall P, Andersson B, Björkholm M (1995) Clinical significance of serum cytokine patterns during start of fever in patients with neutropenia. *Brit J Haematol* 91: 838–845

123 Chapiro J, Maillet F, Charpentier A, Lemonnier M, Misset J, Cavaillon JM (1996) Stimulation of cytokine production by Gram-positive bacteria in a neutropenic patient: difficulty of establishing a cytokine profile-bacterial family relationship. *Brit J Haematol* 95: 435–436

124 Ossege LM, Sindern E, Voss B, Malin JP (1996) Expression of TNF-alpha and TGF-1 in cerebrospinal fluid cells in meningitis. *J Neurol Sci* 144: 1–13

125 Tran Van Nhieu J, Misset B, Lebargy F, Carlet J, Bernaudin JF (1993) Expression of tumor necrosis factor-α gene in alveolar macrophages from patients with the adult respiratory distress syndrome. *Am Rev Respir Dis* 147: 1585–1589

126 Rieckmann P, Albrecht M, Ehrenreich H, Weber T, Michel U (1995) Semi-quantitative analysis of cytokine gene expression in blood and cerebrospinal fluid cells by reverse transcriptase polymerase chain reaction. *Res Exp Med* 195: 17–29

127 Navikas V, Haglund M, Link J, He B, Lindqvist L, Fredrikson S, Link H (1995) Cytokine mRNA profiles in mononuclear cells in acute aseptic meningoencephalitis. *Infect Immun* 63: 1581–1586

128 Giroir BP, Johnson JH, Brown T, Allen GL, Beutler B (1992) The tissue distribution of tumor necrosis factor biosynthesis during endotoxemia. *J Clin Invest* 90: 693–698

129 Ulich TR, Guo K, Yin S, del Castillo J, Yi ES, Thompson RC, Eisenberg SP (1992) Endotoxin-induced cytokine gene expression *in vivo*. IV. Expression of interleukin-1 alpha/beta and interleukin-1 receptor antagonist mRNA during endotoxemia and during endotoxin-initiated local acute inflammation. *Am J Pathol* 141: 61–68

130 Meyer TA, Wang J, Tiao GM, Ogle CK, Fischer JE, Hasselgren PO (1995) Sepsis and endotoxemia stimulate intestinal interleukin-6 production. *Surgery* 118: 336–342

131 Byerley L, Alcock N, Fletcher Starnes H (1992) Sepsis-induced cascade of cytokines mRNA expression: correlation with metabolic changes. *Am J Physiol* 261: E728–E735

132 Messer J, Eyer D, Donato L, Gallati H, Matis J, Simeoni U (1996) Evaluation of interleukin-6 and soluble receptors of tumor necrosis factor for early diagnosis of neonatal infection. *J Pediatr* 129: 574–580

133 Schonbohn H, Schuler M, Kolbe K, Peschel C, Huber C, Bemb W, Aulitzky WE (1995) Plasma levels of IL-1, TNF alpha, IL-6, IL-8, G-CSF, and IL1-RA during febrile neutropenia: results of a prospective study in patients undergoing chemotherapy for acute myelogenous leukemia. *Ann Hematol* 71: 161–168

Soluble TNF receptors

Maarten G. Bouma and Wim A. Buurman

Department of Surgery, Maastricht University, P.O. Box 616, NL-6200 MD Maastricht, The Netherlands

TNF as a principal mediator of sepsis

Over the last decade, numerous basic biological as well as experimental and clinical studies have firmly established the significance of tumor necrosis factor (TNF) as a principal proximal mediator of sepsis. Originally identified as a tumoricidal agent, TNF is now recognized as a major inflammatory cytokine with pleiotropic activities on many cell types and organs, which is involved in the local physiological host immune response to invading micro-organisms as well as in the pathophysiology of systemic inflammatory conditions, such as sepsis [1–4]. Highly elevated systemic levels of TNF, as observed during sepsis and septic shock, induce a wide range of immunological and metabolic sequelae, that result in tissue injury, eventually culminating in multiple organ dysfunction with high mortality. The accumulated evidence for the central involvement of TNF in the pathogenesis of septic shock has led many researchers, molecular biologists and clinicians alike, to investigate the complex mechanisms that regulate the production and release of TNF, and that determine its biological effects. The goals of such research efforts are to gain more insight into the pathophysiology of critical illnesses, to develop sensitive and rapid diagnostic tests, and ultimately to provide new therapeutic strategies from which the critically-ill may benefit.

One of the major insights that has emerged during recent years has been that under physiological circumstances, TNF activity is tightly controlled and locally restricted. In this respect, the soluble TNF receptors (sTNFR) have been recognized as exerting an important regulatory control on the biological actions of TNF, not only in the normal host defense against infection, but also in systemic inflammatory disorders that are related to infectious as well as non-infectious etiologies.

In this chapter we will review the mediators that are involved in the systemic release of sTNFR during sepsis, as well as the potential roles of sTNFR in the regulation of the biological activity of TNF during systemic inflammatory responses. Moreover, we will discuss the diagnostic and prognostic significance of enhanced sTNFR levels during critical illnesses, including severe sepsis and septic shock.

Cytokines in Severe Sepsis and Septic Shock, edited by H. Redl and G. Schlag[†]
© 1999 Birkhäuser Verlag Basel/Switzerland

TNF receptors

TNF interacts with at least two distinct transmembrane cellular receptors, with molecular masses of 55 kDa (TNFR-P55) and 75 kDa (TNFR-P75), which display similar binding affinities for TNF (reviewed in [5]). Both receptors are present on virtually every cell type, excluding erythrocytes and unstimulated T-lymphocytes. Whereas the TNFR-P55 is constitutively expressed at low levels, predominantly in the vascular system and in almost all organs, the TNFR-P75 is strongly induced during the course of an inflammatory response and mainly expressed by activated lymphocytes and monocytes. Both receptors display a four-fold cysteine-rich repeat in their extracellular domain which defines them as members of a larger family of receptor proteins, the so-called TNF receptor family, which also comprises CD27, OX 40 and the Fas antigen. In contrast, their transmembrane and intracytoplasmatic domains do not share sequence homology [6] and are therefore presumed to mediate cellular signalling via different signal transduction pathways. Although the inflammatory, cytotoxic activity of TNF seems to be transduced primarily by the P55 receptor, and the immunostimulatory, proliferative responses to TNF are supposed to be mediated by the TNFR-P75, the single involvement of either receptor in these TNF-induced responses remains controversial. The concept proposed by Tartaglia and Goeddel [7] that both receptors signal distinct TNF activities and that, at low TNF concentrations, TNFR-P75 functions as a catcher of TNF and delivers it to the TNFR-P55, may largely reconcile the controversies. In favor of this "passing-on" model, Leeuwenberg et al. [8] recently provided further experimental evidence by demonstrating the exclusive role of the TNFR-P55 in signaling TNF-induced endothelial cell activation, and a facilitating effect thereon of the TNFR-P75. Similarly, Barbara et al. [9] have supported the capacity of TNFR-P75 to potentiate the effect of TNFR-P55 in experiments using TNF mutants, selectively reactive with either TNFR-P55 or TNFR-P75. The non-signaling functions of TNFR-P75 have recently been reviewed by Van Tits et al. [10].

Soluble TNF receptors

Shedding of TNFR

Both membrane TNF receptors also exist in corresponding soluble forms, which are produced by proteolytic cleavage of the extracellular domains of the membrane receptors, and are shed into the circulation. Whereas sTNFR are detectable at the low ng/ml range in serum and urine of normal healthy individuals, with sTNFR-P75 being more abundant than sTNFR-P55, their concentrations increase significantly in acute or chronic infectious and inflammatory conditions [11], as well as in non-inflammatory diseases such as cancer [12]. Although the exact mechanisms that control the systemic release of sTNFR under these conditions are largely unclear, a variety of stimuli that induce shedding of TNFR from the cell surface have been identified, several of which are involved in the pathogenesis of the sepsis syndrome.

First, TNF itself is a principal modulator of systemic sTNFR release. *In vitro* stimulation of neutrophils and monocytes with TNF causes shedding of sTNFR from these cells [13–15], while infusion of TNF in humans results in highly increased sTNFR serum levels [16, 17]. Moreover, enhanced TNF levels during experimental endotoxemia and clinical sepsis correlate well with elevated sTNFR concentrations [11, 18–20]. However, although TNF is considered to be a principal trigger for sTNFR release, it is not essential for sTNFR shedding. Vossen et al. [21] have recently provided evidence that murine T cell activation by an anti-CD3 monoclonal antibody (mAb) induces shedding of both sTNFR relatively independent of the presence of TNF. In a similar murine study, Bemelmans et al. [22] found that anti-CD3 mAb-induced sTNFR release could only be partly reduced by neutralizing TNF using an anti-TNF mAb. Also, shedding of sTNFR by anti-CD3 mAb-activated human peripheral blood mononuclear cells *in vitro* is not affected by TNF [23].

Lipopolysaccharide (LPS), is a second important inducer of sTNFR shedding. *In vitro* stimulation of human monocytes with LPS from *Escherichia Coli* or *Neisseria Meningitidis* selectively induces the release of the TNFR-P75, but not of the TNFR-P55, together with an upregulation of membrane expression of both receptors after 24–48 h [24, 25]. In contrast, exposure of human endothelial cells to *Neisseria Meningitidis* LPS results in a dose-dependent shedding of TNFR-P55, but not TNFR-P75, from these cells [24]. The importance of LPS in the induction of sTNFR release *in vivo* has been clearly demonstrated in a large number of animal as well as human experimental endotoxemia and sepsis models, where administration of endotoxin or *E. Coli* resulted in significantly enhanced circulating sTNFR levels [11, 18, 20, 26–29]. While in most of these endotoxemia models endogenous TNF would be a likely mediator of LPS-induced release of sTNFR, Bemelmans et al. [27] demonstrated that LPS-induced sTNFR release in mice could not be inhibited by neutralizing TNF, suggesting a direct action of LPS on shedding of sTNFR without TNF as intermediate. Consistent with the latter is the observation that administration of LPS to C3H/HeJ mice, which do not produce TNF in response to LPS [30], directly induces shedding of sTNFR in these animals [31].

Interleukin-1 (IL-1) is another important endogenous pro-inflammatory mediator involved in the pathogenesis of septic shock that has been shown to induce release of sTNFR. As reported by Van der Poll et al. [32], infusion of IL-1α into baboons induces rapid increases in levels of both sTNFR. In the same study inhibition of endogenous IL-1 attenuated sTNFR-P55 release in baboons during experimental *E. Coli* sepsis and in patients with clinically defined sepsis, suggesting the intermediate involvement of endogenous IL-1 in sTNFR release in response to endotoxin. In addition, IL-1 also partly mediates anti-CD3 mAb-induced shedding of sTNFR from monocytes *in vitro* [23].

In addition to endotoxin, TNF, and IL-1, which are all considered to be proximal mediators of the sepsis syndrome, a variety of other inflammatory stimuli have also been recognized as inducers of sTNFR shedding. Stimulation of human neutrophils *in vitro* with various physiological polypeptides such as fMLP, C5a, GM-CSF, and elastase was found to result in a rapid decrease of cell surface expressed TNFR with an accompanying release of sTNFR [33-35]. Moreover, several cytokines, including IL-2, IL-6, IL-10 and Leukemia Inhibiting Factor, have been found to be involved in enhanced release of sTNFR *in vitro* or *in vivo* [13, 23, 27, 36, 37]. Adhesion of neutrophils, a crucial event during inflammatory responses, induces shedding of sTNFR [38]. Recently, Scannell et al. [39] demonstrated that hypoxia, a condition that is intimately associated with shock states, triggers the release of sTNFR by a human macrophage cell line *in vitro*, a finding which may have its clinical correlate in severely traumatized patients, in whom highly elevated levels of both sTNFR have been detected [40, 41].

In conclusion, it is apparent that the regulation of sTNFR release is the result of a complex interplay between the various inflammatory mediators and a variety of immunocompetent cell types that are involved in the pathogenesis of the sepsis syndrome. The complexity of this regulatory system is underscored by the observations that a given mediator may have opposing effects on shedding of TNFR by different cell types [24], and that blocking of individual mediators does not seem to be sufficient to completely inhibit the release of sTNFR [27].

Kinetics of sTNFR release during sepsis

From a large number of animal and human studies it has become evident that endotoxemia or clinical sepsis gives rise to an early systemic increase in TNF which subsequently subsides within hours. In most of the experimental studies, a stereotypical monophasic transient appearance of TNF is observed, with peak levels occurring within 90 to 120 minutes after endotoxin administration. This is followed by a rapid systemic clearance resulting in undetectable levels after four to six hours [3, 18, 20, 27, 42, 43]. Moreover, a contemporaneous release of both sTNFR is observed in these studies which displays, however, a different pattern of kinetics for both receptors. In the mouse, the TNFR-P55 peaks early after 30 minutes and gradually declines to normal levels therafter, whereas the TNFR-P75 reaches maximal levels after four to eight hours and subsequently diminishes over a relatively long period of approximately 24 hours [27]. A largely similar pattern is observed in human conditions of endotoxemia and sepsis, where both sTNFR persist in the circulation for an extended period of time, particularly in relationship to the more abbreviated systemic presence of TNF [43]. As postulated by Carpenter et al. [31], endotoxin may cause shedding of sTNFR *in vivo* in two separate ways. A first, immediate response involves shedding of sTNFR by neutrophils, whereas in a second, late response mononuclear cells are the main source of sTNFR. Consistent with the latter is the observation of Leeuwenberg et al. [23], who found the release of sTNFR by monocytes to be a relatively late and ongoing event. Moreover, they reported that after initial shedding of sTNFR, LPS-activated mononuclear cells strongly re-expressed both receptors on their cell surface, which was accompanied by the release of sTNFR-P75, but not sTNFR-P55 [25]. As stipulated by Carpenter and coworkers [31], the pattern of sTNFR release in response to endotoxin may be composed of two overlapping processes, i.e. an early peak derived from rapid shedding by neutrophils which is replaced by more protracted release of sTNFR by mononuclear cells. Together, these findings may begin to explain the kinetics of sTNFR release as observed during septic conditions *in vivo*.

Biological functions of sTNFR

With regard to the possible role of sTNFR as modulators of TNF function *in vivo*, several concepts have emerged. First, sTNFR compete with cell-associated receptors for TNF binding, thus reducing TNF bioactivity [5]. Alternatively, binding of sTNFR with free circulating TNF results in direct inhibition of TNF bioactivity [20, 44, 45]. Consequently, the highly increased levels of circulating sTNFR, as observed during septic conditions, are thought to protect the host from the unwanted toxicity of excessive TNF present under these circumstances [11, 20]. By binding and inactivating TNF in the systemic circulation, sTNFR might confine TNF to its local source of production and restrict TNF activity locally. Moreover, it has been suggested that by releasing the extracellular part of the TNFR, cells may be temporarily less sensitive or unresponsive to the deleterious effects of TNF [25]. In addition, internalization of membrane-bound TNFR in response to LPS, as described by Ding et al. [46], may also lead to a TNF-refractory state. Therefore, down-modulation of cellular TNFR expression, either by shedding or by internalization, could represent another physiological mechanism to limit the bio-effects of TNF. Furthermore, sTNFR play an important role in the clearance of TNF from the systemic circulation. The kidney has been identified as the major clearance organ for TNF/sTNFR complexes [47], although the liver, at least in mice, also seems to play a role in clearance of TNF complexed to sTNFR [48]. Consistent with the central role of the kidney in sTNFR clearance are the observations of enhanced sTNFR levels positively correlating with plasma creatinine levels in patients with acute or chronic renal failure [44, 49], as well as in patients with the sepsis syndrome [50].

Whereas it has been teleologically reasoned that the highly increased induction of sTNFR release by a variety of inflammatory mediators, e.g. in the setting of sepsis, may function to protect the host from the deleterious actions of excessive TNF and to prevent a vicious cycle of TNF self-propagation, the presence of lesser quantities of sTNFR may, in contrast, act to prolong the biological effects of TNF. Aderka et

125

al. [45] have postulated that low amounts of sTNFR stabilize the trimeric structure of TNF by slowing down its decomposition to biologically inactive monomeric structures, thus serving as a slow release reservoir of bio-active TNF, which prolongs TNF activity. It seems therefore, that the biological role of sTNFR in inflammation is dose-dependent [51, 52].

In conclusion, circulating sTNFR are considered to have a buffering function, acting either as inhibitors or as carrier proteins for TNF, depending on their concentration. During sepsis, the increased presence of sTNFR in a large molar excess over TNF may function mainly as an endogenous inhibitory and clearance mechanism of TNF bioactivity, which in severe cases may still be insufficient to prevent the lethal consequences of high systemic TNF concentrations [11].

Diagnostic and prognostic significance of sTNFR

As it has become evident that the sTNFR play an important role as modulators of TNF bioactivity in an agonist/antagonist pattern, determination of sTNFR in plasma or serum has become a new tool to gain information about various pathological conditions that are characterized by TNF-mediated immune activation [53]. However, the *diagnostic* significance of elevated sTNFR, in as much as they reflect the activation state of the TNF/TNFR system, may be of limited value due to its non-specific character, and has led critics to place it in one class with measurements of blood sedimentation rate [54]. Nevertheless, sTNFR levels may provide valuable information about disease severity and inflammatory activity in a variety of clinical entities. For example, Rogy et al. [42] have demonstrated a good correlation between circulating sTNFR-P55 and initial APACHE II scores in septic, critically-ill patients in the intensive care unit. After trauma, sustained systemic elevation of sTNFR mirrors the clinical patient status, with higher levels in the most critically ill patients gradually declining as the clinical condition improves [41]. Recently, De Beaux et al. [55] and Kaufmann et al. [56] have reported that elevated sTNFR-P55 levels, particularly in combination with C-reactive protein levels, accurately reflect the clinical severity of acute pancreatitis. Thus, determination of sTNFR may be useful for monitoring inflammatory responses and the severity of tissue injury.

There is a growing number of well-documented experimental and clinical studies to demonstrate that systemic sTNFR levels have accurate *prognostic* significance in critical illnesses. Markedly increased concentrations of sTNFR have been determined in patients with severe meningococcaemia, and were demonstrated to correlate with TNF levels and the outcome of disease in terms of mortality [19, 57]. Likewise, sTNFR-P55 levels were found to be signifcantly higher in non-survivors compared with survivors in critically-ill patients with sepsis [42]. Froon et al. [50] also detected higher plasma sTNFR-P55 peak concentrations in non-survivors of the sepsis syndrome, but emphasized the influence of impaired renal function on sTNFR levels in these patients. In severely injured patients serum concentrations of sTNFR early after trauma correlate with patient outcome, with higher receptor levels in non-survivors than in survivors [41]. Elevated sTNFR-P55 levels have been shown to correlate positively with the development of multiple organ failure and with mortality in patients with clinically severe acute pancreatitis [55, 56]. Similarly, Bemelmans et al. [58] identified both sTNFR, rather than TNF, as good prognostic factors for mortality after surgery in mice with biliary obstruction. Recently, it has been suggested that early postoperative serum concentrations of sTNFR-P55 are good predictors for mortality in postcardiac surgical patients at high risk for sepsis and may prove useful, in combination with APACHE II scores, for early sepsis severity and mortality risk stratification, thereby allowing for a more specific initiation of supplemental sepsis therapy [59]. In addition, it was established very recently that *pre*operative sTNFR levels in patients undergoing coronary artery bypass grafting represent a strong independent risk factor for postoperative complications (E.J. Fransen et al., unpublished observations).

Although in the aforementioned studies elevated systemic sTNFR levels were found to correlate well with initial serum TNF concentrations, the determination of sTNFR may have certain advantages over TNF measurement in monitoring inflammatory states and predicting clinical outcome. Compared to circulating TNF, which is only shortly present and can therefore be easily missed, sTNFR are detectable for a more prolonged period of time. In addition, sTNFR are very stable, and their determination seems to be less prone to artefacts than that of TNF [60]. Also, the presence of sTNFR may have a masking effect on measurement of TNF, depending on the specific TNF-assay used [61], which can easily lead to misinterpretation of results and may severely hamper cross-laboratory comparison of data concerning TNF levels. However, with regard to the interpretation of enhanced sTNFR levels there is also one important caveat to be remembered. As sTNFR are mainly cleared by the kidney, renal impairment may considerably influence systemic sTNFR concentrations [47, 50]. The presence of renal failure may result in an unproportional elevation of circulating sTNFR, that does not directly reflect the inflammatory state, but rather the degree of renal failure.

References

1   Bemelmans MHA, Van Tits LJH, Buurman WA (1996) Tumor necrosis factor: function, release and clearance. *Crit Rev Immunol* 16: 1–11

2   Strieter RM, Kunkel SL, Bone RC (1993) Role of tumor necrosis factor-α in disease states and inflammation. *Crit Care Med* 21: S447–S463

3   Tracey KJ, Cerami A (1993) Tumor necrosis factor: An updated review of its biology. *Crit Care Med* 21: S415–S422

4   Beutler B, Grau GE (1993) Tumor necrosis factor in the pathogenesis of infectious diseases. *Crit Care Med* 21: S423–S435

5   Bazzoni F, Beutler B (1996) The tumor necrosis factor ligand and receptor families. *N Eng J Med* 334: 1717–1725

6   Dembic Z, Loetscher H, Gubler U, Pan YCE, Lahm HW, Gentz R, Brockhaus M, Lesslauer W (1990) Two human TNF receptors have similar extracellular, but distinct intracellular, domain sequences. *Cytokine* 2: 231–237

7   Tartaglia LA, Goeddel DV (1992) Two TNF receptors. *Immunol Today* 13: 151–153

8   Leeuwenberg JFM, Van Tits LJH, Jeunhomme TMMA, Buurman WA (1995) Evidence for exclusive role in signalling of tumour necrosis factor p55 receptor and a potentiating function of p75 receptor on human endothelial cells. *Cytokine* 7: 457–462

9   Barbara JAJ, Smith WB, Gamble JR, Van Ostade X, Vandenabeele P, Tavernier J, Fiers W, Vadas MA, Lopez AF (1994) Dissociation of TNF-α cytotoxic and proinflammatory activities by p55 receptor- and p75 receptor-selective TNF-α mutants. *EMBO J* 13: 843–850

10   Van Tits LJ, Bemelmans MH, Steinshamn S, Waage A, Leeuwenberg JF, Buurman WA (1994) Non-signaling functions of TNF-R75: findings in man and mouse. *Circ Shock* 44: 40–44

11   Van der Poll T, Jansen J, Van Leenen D, Von der Möhlen M, Levi M, Ten Cate H, Gallati H, Ten Cate JW, Van Deventer SJ (1993) Release of soluble receptors for tumor necrosis factor in clinical sepsis and experimental endotoxemia. *J Infect Dis* 168: 955–960

12   Aderka D, Engelmann H, Hornik V, Skornick Y, Levo Y, Wallach D, Kushtai G (1991) Increased serum levels of soluble receptors for tumor necrosis factor in cancer patients. *Cancer Res* 51: 5602–5607

13   Joyce DA, Gibbons DP, Green P, Steer JH, Feldmann M, Brennan FM (1994) Two inhibitors of pro-inflammatory cytokine release, interleukin-10 and interleukin-4, have contrasting effects on release of soluble p75 tumor necrosis factor receptor by cultured monocytes. *Eur J Immunol* 24: 2699–2705

14   Porteu F, Hieblot C (1994) Tumor necrosis factor induces a selective shedding of its p75 receptor from human neutrophils. *J Biol Chem* 269: 2834–2840

15   Higuchi M, Aggarwal BB (1994) TNF induces internalization of the p60 receptor and shedding of the p80 receptor. *J Immunol* 152: 3550–3558

16   Lantz M, Malik S, Slevin ML, Olsson I (1990) Infusion of tumor necrosis factor (TNF) causes an increase in circulating TNF-binding protein in humans. *Cytokine* 2: 402–406

17   Lantz M, Gullberg U, Nilsson E, Olsson L (1990) Characterization *in vitro* of a human tumor necrosis factor-binding protein. *J Clin Invest* 86: 1396–1442

18   Spinas GA, Keller U, Brockhaus M (1992) Release of soluble receptors for tumor necrosis factor (TNF) in relation to circulating TNF during experimental endotoxinemia. *J Clin Invest* 90: 533–536

19   Girardin E, Roux-Lombard P, Grau GE, Suter P, Galati H, Dayer JM (1992) Imbalance

between tumour necrosis factor-α and soluble TNF receptor concentrations in severe meningococcocaemia. *Immunology* 76: 20–23

20 Van Zee KJ, Kohno T, Fischer E, Rock CS, Moldawer L, Lowry SF (1992) Tumor necrosis factor soluble receptors circulate during experimental and clinical inflammation and can protect against excessive tumor necrosis factor-alpha in vitro and *in vivo*. *Proc Natl Acad Sci USA* 89: 4845–4849

21 Vossen ACTM, Tibbe GJM, Buurman WA, Benner R, Savelkoul HFJ (1996) Soluble tumor necrosis factor receptor release after anti-CD3 monoclonal antibody treatment in mice is independent of tumour necrosis factor-α release. *Eur Cytokine Netw* 7: 751–755

22 Bemelmans MHA, Abramowicz D, Gouma DJ, Goldman M, Buurman WA (1994) *In vivo* T cell activation by anti-CD3 mAb induces soluble TNF receptor release in mice: effects of pentoxifylline, methylprednisolone, anti-TNF and anti-INF-γ antibodies. *J Immunol* 153: 499–506

23 Leeuwenberg JFM, Jeunhomme TMMA, Buurman WA (1994) Slow release of soluble TNF receptors by monocytes *in vitro*. *J Immunol* 152: 4036–4043

24 Lien E, Liabakk NB, Johnsen AC, Nonstad U, Sundan A, Espevik T (1995) Polymorphonuclear granulocytes enhance lipopolysaccharide-induced soluble p75 tumor necrosis factor receptor release from mononuclear cells. *Eur J Immunol* 25: 2714–2717

25 Leeuwenberg JFM, Dentener MA, Buurman WA (1994) Lipopolysaccharide-mediated soluble TNF receptor release and TNF receptor expression by monocytes. Role of CD14, LPS Binding Protein, and Bactericidal/Permeability-increasing Protein. *J Immunol* 152: 5070–5076

26 Redl H, Schlag G, Paul E, Bahrami S, Buurman WA, Strieter RM, Kunkel SL, Davies J, Foulkes R (1996) Endogenous modulators of TNF and IL-1 response are under partial control of TNF in baboon bacteremia. *Am J Physiol* 271: R1193–R1198

27 Bemelmans MHA, Gouma DJ, Buurman WA (1993) LPS-induced sTNF-receptor release *in vivo* in a murine model: investigation of the role of TNF, IL-1, LIF, and IFN-γ. *J Immunol* 151: 5554–5562

28 Steinshamn S, Bemelmans MHA, Buurman WA, Waage A (1995) Granulocytopenia reduces release of soluble TNF receptor p75 in endotoxin-stimulated mice: a possible mechanism of enhanced TNF activity. *Cytokine* 7: 50–56

29 Redl H, Schlag G, Schiesser A, Davies J (1995) Thrombomodulin release in baboon sepsis: its dependence on the dose of Escherichia coli and the presence of tumor necrosis factor. *J Infect Dis* 171: 1522–1527

30 Beutler B, Krochin N, Milsark IW, Luedke C, Cerami A (1986) Control of cachectin (tumor necrosis factor) synthesis: mechanisms of endotoxin resistance. *Science* 232: 977–980.

31 Carpenter A, Evans TJ, Buurman WA, Bemelmans MH, Moyes D, Cohen J (1995) Differences in the shedding of soluble TNF receptors between endotoxin-sensitive and endotoxin-resistant mice in response to lipopolysaccharide or live bacterial challenge. *J Immunol* 155: 2005–2012

32 Van der Poll T, Fischer E, Coyle SM, Van Zee KJ, Pribble JP, Stiles DM, Barie PS, Buur-

man WA, Moldawer LL, Lowry SF (1995) Interleukin-1 contributes to increased concentrations of soluble tumor necrosis factor receptor type I in sepsis. *J Infect Dis* 172: 577–580

33 Porteu F, Nathan C (1990) Shedding of tumor necrosis factor receptors by activated human neutrophils. *J Exp Med* 172: 599–607

34 Ding AH, Porteu F (1992) Regulation of tumor necrosis factor receptors on phagocytes. *P Soc Exp Biol Med* 200: 458–465

35 Porteu F, Brockhaus M, Wallach D, Engelmann H, Nathan C (1991) Human neutrophil elastase releases a ligand-binding fragment from the 75-kDa tumor necrosis factor (TNF) receptor. *J Biol Chem* 266: 18846–18853

36 Landmann R, Keilholz U, Scheibenbogen C, Brockhaus M, Gallati H, Denz H, Bargetzi M, Ludwig C. (1994) Relationship between soluble tumor necrosis factor (TNF) receptors and TNF alpha during immunotherapy with interleukin-2 and/or interferon alpha. *Cancer Immunol Immunother* 38: 113–118

37 Tilg H, Trehu E, Atkins MB, Dinarello CA, Mier JW (1994) Interleukin-6 (IL-6) as an anti-inflammatory cytokine: induction of circulating IL-1 receptor antagonist and soluble tumor necrosis factor receptor p55. *Blood* 83: 113–118

38 Lantz M, Björnberg F, Olsson I, Richter J (1994) Adherence of neutrophils induces release of soluble tumor necrosis factor receptor forms. *J Immunol* 152: 1362–1369

39 Scannell G, Waxman K, Kaml GJ, Ioli G, Gatanaga T, Yamamoto R, Granger GA (1993) Hypoxia induces a human macrophage cell line to release tumor necrosis factor-α and its soluble receptors *in vitro*. *J Surg Res* 54: 281–285

40 Tan LR, Waxman K, Scanell G, Loli G, Granger GA (1993) Trauma causes early release of soluble receptors for tumor necrosis factor. *J Trauma* 34: 634–638

41 Cinat ME, Waxman K, Granger GA, Pearce W, Annas C, Daughters K (1994) Trauma causes sustained elevation of soluble tumor necrosis factor receptors. *J Am Coll Surg* 179: 529–537

42 Rogy MA, Coyle SM, Oldenburg HS, Rock CS, Barie PS, Van Zee KJ, Smith CG, Moldawer LL, Lowry SF (1994) Persistently elevated soluble tumor necrosis factor receptor and interleukin-1 receptor antagonist levels in critically ill patients. *J Am Coll Surg* 178: 132–138

43 Lowry SF, Van Zee KJ, Rock CS, Thompson WA, Oldenburg HSA, Rogy MA, Moldawer LL (1993) Tumor necrosis factor as a mediator of sepsis. In: G Schlag, H Redl, DL Traber (eds): *Shock, sepsis and organ failure*. Springer-Verlag, Berlin, Heidelberg, 3–17

44 Peetre C, Thysell H, Grubb A, Olsson I (1988) A tumor necrosis factor binding protein is present in human biological fluids. *Eur J Haematol* 41: 414–419

45 Aderka D, Engelmann H, Maor Y, Brakebusch C, Wallach D (1992) Stabilization of the bioactivity of tumor necrosis factor by its soluble receptors. *J Exp Med* 175: 323–329

46 Ding AH, Sanchez E, Srimal S, Nathan CF (1989) Macrophages rapidly internalize their tumor necrosis factor receptors in response to lipopolysaccharide. *J Biol Chem* 264: 3924–3929

47 Bemelmans MHA, Gouma DJ, Buurman WA (1993) Influence of nephrectomy on tumor necrosis factor clearance in a murine model. *J Immunol* 150: 2007–2017

48 Bemelmans MHA, Gouma DJ, Buurman WA (1994) Tissue distribution and clearance of soluble murine TNF receptors in mice. *Cytokine* 6: 608–615

49 Brockhaus M, Bar-Khayim Y, Gurwicz S, Frensdorff A, Haran N (1992) Plasma tumor necrosis factor soluble receptors in chronic renal failure. *Kidney Int* 42: 663–667.

50 Froon AHM, Bemelmans MHA, Greve JW, Van der Linden CJ, Buurman WA (1994) Increased plasma concentrations of soluble tumor necrosis factor receptors in sepsis syndrome: correlation with plasma creatinine values. *Crit Care Med* 22: 803–809

51 Mohler KM, Torrance DS, Smith CA, Goodwin RG, Stremler KE, Fung VP, Madani H, Widmer MB (1993) Soluble tumor necrosis factor receptors are effective therapeutic agents in lethal endotoxemia and function simultaneously as both TNF carriers and TNF antagonists. *J Immunol* 151: 1548–1561

52 Olsson I, Gatanaga T, Gullberg U (1993) Tumor necrosis factor binding proteins (soluble TNF receptor forms) with possible roles in inflammation and malignancy. *Eur Cytokine Network* 4: 169–180

53 Diez-Ruiz A, Tilz GP, Zangerle R, Baier-Bitterlich G, Wachter H, Fuchs D (1995) Soluble receptors for tumour necrosis factor in clinical laboratory diagnosis. *Eur J Haematol* 54: 1–8

54 Brockhaus M (1997) Soluble TNF receptor: what is the significance? *Intensive Care Med* 23: 808–809

55 De Beaux AC, Goldie AS, Ross JA, Carter DC, Fearon KC (1996) Serum concentrations of inflammatory mediators related to organ failure in patients with acute pancreatitis. *Br J Surg* 83: 349–353

56 Kaufmann P, Tilz GP, Lueger A, Demel U (1997) Elevated plasma levels of soluble tumor necrosis factor receptor (sTNFRp60) reflect severity of acute pancreatitis. *Intensive Care Med* 23: 841–848

57 Van Deuren M, Van der Ven-Jongekrijg J, Demacker PMN, Bartelink AK, Van Dalen R, Sauerwein RW, Gallati H, Vannice JL, Van der Meer JW (1994) Differential expression of proinflammatory cytokines and their inhibitors during the course of meningococcal infections. *J Infect Dis* 169: 157–161

58 Bemelmans MHA, Greve JW, Gouma DJ, Buurman WA (1996) Increased concentrations of tumour necrosis factor (TNF) and soluble TNF receptors in biliary obstruction in mice; soluble TNF receptors as prognostic factors for mortality. *Gut* 38: 447–453

59 Pilz G, Fraunberger P, Appel R, Kreuzer E, Werdan K, Walli A, Seidel D (1996) Early prediction of outcome in score-identified, postcardiac surgical patients at high risk for sepsis, using soluble tumor necrosis factor receptor-p55 concentrations. *Crit Care Med* 24: 596–600

60 Engelberts I, Möller A, Schoen GJM, Van der Linden CJ, Buurman WA (1991) Evaluation of measurement of human TNF in plasma by ELISA. *Lymphokine Cytokine Res* 10: 69–76

61 Engelberts I, Stephens S, Francot GJM, Van der Linden CJ, Buurman WA (1991) Evidence for different effects of soluble TNF-receptors on various TNF measurements in human biological fluids. *Lancet* 338: 515–516

Relevance of surrogate tests in intensive care patients or "Heisenberg at the ICU"

Wolfgang Strohmaier[1] and Franz Tatzber[2]

[1]Ludwig Boltzmann Institute for Experimental and Clinical Traumatology, Donaueschingen-strasse 13, A-1200 Vienna, Austria
[2]Institute for Biochemistry, Schubertstrasse 1, A-8010 Graz, Austria

It was in 1927 that W.K. Heisenberg made the discovery for which he is best known – that of the Uncertainty Principle [1]. This states that it is impossible to specify precisely both the position and the simultaneous momentum (= mass multiplied by velocity) of a particle. There is always a degree of uncertainty in either, and as one is determined with greater precision, the other can only be found less exactly. Heisenberg's Uncertainty Principle negates cause and effect; it maintains that the result of an action can be expressed only in terms of the probability that a certain effect will occur.

Seventy years later this principle is still valid, and can easily be transferred to a focus of interest which has emerged in the recent years. Critical care medicine has developed into a highly specialized and sophisticated field of research and thereby attracted scientists far beyond physicians. Biochemistry, biology and molecular biology have produced an avalanche of sometimes controversial new insights into physiological and pathophysiological mechanisms together with the tools to measure and quantify almost every item of interest. The increasing amount of data available, in combination with subtle statistical evaluation, has enabled the creation of scoring systems [2] which were needed for several purposes, e.g. comparison of patients. The description of the status of a patient beyond his hemodynamic or respiratory situation was thought essential for successful intensive care medicine. Strong motivation for these extensive efforts may have come from the insight that the diseases of the decade, systemic inflammatory response syndrome (SIRS), multiple organ dysfunction syndrome (MODS) and multiple organ failure (MOF) are actually a consequence of successful resuscitation of critically ill and severely traumatized patients with state-of-the-art intensive care. We face the situation that every effort and immediate accomplishment may only postpone the problem and possibly shift it to a higher level of complexity. The situation is aggravated by the fact that critical care medicine at the Intensive Care Unit (ICU) has remained almost entirely supportive, although substantial progress has been made, e.g. in ventilation techniques or "kinetic therapy". However, mortality associated with MOF, especially septic MOF, is unchanged. This has led to further attempts to better understand what is really going on in the early phase after a traumatic event. Extensive measurement of more parameters at shorter intervals together with careful retrospective evaluation was expected to lead from diagnosis via monitoring to prognosis. This probably is the point when Heisenberg appears on the scene: If "position" means present condition and "momentum" translates to progredience (e.g. age connected to condition at admission), then the principle reads as follows: It is probably impossible to diagnose the stage of disease at a given point in time with ultimate precision (unless resources are unlimited) simultaneously with short-term changes. In other words, the more parameters are more frequently measured, and the more compartments are included in diagnosis, the more uncertainties arise. This is accompanied by increasing problems with overall validity, since the meaningfulness of a single parameter or a even a sophisticated score is always inversely proportional to the heterogeneity of the patient cohort. Due to the variety of events which may lead to SIRS, sepsis and MOF via the activation of a large number of cellular and humoral cascades and mediator networks, a multitude of parameters comprising key players of the aforementioned systems as well as several metabolites have recently been discussed in terms of their diagnostic and prognostic power [3]. In a review by Cavaillon et al. [4] circulating cytokines were called the "tip of the iceberg". The authors wanted to express their opinion that the presence or the absence of circulating cytokines cannot be considered to resemble a bioactive or a resting organism, respectively.

This paper discusses three parameters that have been shown to contribute to the clinical picture of a patient, especially with regard to the diagnosis of infection and/or the onset of a septic event. Interestingly, only one of them can be assigned to a defined source; however, there is increasing evidence for the usefulness of these surrogate markers (SM): 2-amino-4-hydroxy-6-(D-erythro-1',2',3'-trihydroxy-propyl)-pteridine, vulgo neopterin (Neo); Procalcitonin (PCT); and auto-antibodies against oxidized low- density lipoprotein (oxLDLAb). It is beyond the scope of this paper to deal in depth with the principal difficulties of biochemical/immunological monitoring in the posttraumatic and/or septic course, despite the reasonable assumption that these problems in turn have played a part in the introduction and evaluation of surrogate markers. At least in our opinion it remains speculative to what extent the above parameters can serve as surrogate endpoints according to the definition given by Fleming et al. [5].

Neopterin

Neopterin is a member of the ubiquitous family of unconjugated pteridines and was originally discovered in the larvae of bees, in worker bees, and in royal jelly [6, 7]. All members of this family are derived from guanosinetriphosphate (GTP) [8]. The first step is catalyzed by the enzyme GTP-cyclohydrolase I, which cleaves the imidazole ring of the purine. After molecular conversion by Amadori rearrangement,

134

the key precursor 7,8-dihydroneopterin triphosphate in the biosynthesis of folate, riboflavin, methanopterin, tetrahydropterin and Neo is produced. The molecular next of kin to Neo, the biopterins, have gained widespread interest since tetrahy-drobiopterin is the essential co-factor for aromatic amino acid monoxygenases and thus for neurotransmitter synthesis, as well as for nitric oxide synthases (NOS) [9]. A possible biological function was recently suggested [10] by those who demon-strated *in vitro* induction of inducible (i) NOS expression by Neo in rat vascular smooth muscle cells. The same group [11] had previously proposed a redox state-dependent NF-κB translocation to the nucleus as an explanation for this impact of Neo on iNOS expression.

Increased concentrations of urinary Neo were first reported in patients with an extremely rare variant of atypical phenylketonuria [12, 13]; in the same year raised Neo levels were found in the urine of patients with malignancy and viral infection [14]. Subsequently it was shown that antigenic stimulation of human peripheral blood mononuclear cells (PBMC) leads to Neo release into cell culture medium [15, 16] and finally, that human macrophages produce Neo *in vitro* upon stimulation by IFNγ [17]. It is of major importance to mention that IFNγ is the most potent stim-ulus when highly purified macrophage preparations or cell lines (e.g. THP-1) [18] are used. *In vivo*, or in PBMCs in the presence of T-lymphocytes, lipopolysaccha-ride (LPS) also is a very potent trigger of Neo production via the release of IFNγ and cytokines by activated T-lymphocytes. However, the ultimate proof for this hypoth-esis *in vivo* did not come until Woloszcuk [19] improved the methods for measur-ing IFNγ. He drastically reduced the detection limit and demonstrated that an increase in IFNγ is invariably followed by an increase in Neo. The same holds true for TNF which, though being a potent costimulator, is almost inactive in inducing pteridine synthesis in purified macrophages as a single agent. Since that time, urine and blood Neo levels have been shown to be elevated in several different categories of diseases (for details see [20]). That macrophages might not be the single source of Neo was suggested by Andert et al. [21], who showed release of Neo in cultured endothelial cells upon stimulation with IFNγ. This may result in a remarkable con-tribution to the total amount of Neo as there are at least ten times more endothelial cells than macrophages. Since Neo is cleared via the kidneys in a creatinine-like fashion [22], Neo values are influenced by kidney function, so optional correction for creatinine should be kept in mind.

In 1987 we reported on a strong correlation between Neo levels and the occur-rence of septic events in intensive care patients [23]. We could clearly discriminate between survivors and non-survivors in these 21 patients as early as day one. An investigation on 56 patients by Pacher et al. [24] was in agreement; in that study Neo testing (96% sensitivity and 73% specificity for Neo; ≤ 40 nmol/L) yielded an overall accuracy of 83%. Neo also precisely predicted the MOF score (if ≥ 5) according to Goris when measured one day before the evaluation ($r = 0.75$, $p \leq 0.0001$). In this study Neo always differentiated between septic and non-septic survivors and non-survivors as well. Similar findings regarding early increased Neo concentrations were reported by Faist et al. [25] who additionally demonstrated that freshly isolated monocytes stimulated *ex vivo* with LPS are exhausted in surgical patients. Faist concluded that resident, tissue-bound macrophages are responsible for the high serum levels. Further validation of Neo as a prognostic parameter came from Nast-Kolb et al. [26]. He reported clear discrimination between survivors and non-survivors starting as early as day two post trauma in a 14 day observation period. One hundred patients with severe polytrauma (mean injury severity score (ISS) = 37) were studied. Both Neo and soluble interleukin (IL)-2 receptor were identified as significant predictors of shock states in Gram-negative sepsis by Delogu et al. [27]. Slightly divergent data were presented in a prospective study, in 56 patients, evaluating various inflammatory mediators as predictors of MOF after blunt trauma (ISS ≥ 33) [28]. Since the authors used the Neo/creatinine ratio in their calculations the significant changes indicating MOF were found much later in the course. One might speculate that in these patients a rise in Neo due to the kidney failure is mathematically eliminated by the use of the Neo/creatinine ratio. This approach relates the late increase exclusively to overwhelming macrophage activation, an assumption in line with Nast-Kolb et al. [26]. However, one important pathophysiological conclusion can be drawn from the work so far: the central involvement of monocytes and macrophages in inflammatory processes. This seems even more important, if one considers "the macrophages" as an active compartment.

Evidence for the clinical association of endotoxin, septicemia, and Neo in humans came from an experiment performed by Bloom et al. [29]: a bolus of 4 ng/kg BW endotoxin was administered intravenously into healthy subjects. All individuals responded with a two- to three-fold increase in Neo within 24 h. In comparison to TNFα, this increase had a delay of at least 6 h, but remained for some 72 h. This experiment also provided insight into the kinetic characteristics of Neo and the mediators presently discussed as diagnostic or prognostic parameters, mainly TNFα and IL-6. After a single stimulus the cytokines rapidly increase to their respective maxima at 2 to 4 h and decline just as quickly, revealing virtually baseline (= zero) levels after 6 to 8 h. This has been shown in rats [30] and baboons [31]. In further baboon experiments [32] this time course was confirmed. It was also shown that significant rises in Neo are restricted to septic animals, while trauma settings induce only minor changes. Unfortunately, Neo data from animal experiments are only available for primates and subprimates, since other animal species produce only negligible amounts of Neo.

For well over ten years now, Neo has been assessed routinely in the trauma ICU at the Lorenz Böhler Trauma Hospital and it is an accepted part of the monitoring. Moreover, it has turned out that additional applications are possible. First, selective puncture of corresponding veins and arteries allows for comparison of their respective concentration and this arterio-venous difference contributes information on the existence or, sometimes even more important, the absence of septic foci [33]. Second, in 1996 Strohmaier et al. [34] showed that Neo blood levels can provide a reliable basis for the decision on whether to use or not to use antibiotics in our ICU. After a two-year evaluation period with 536 patients enrolled and the definition of a few exceptions (e.g. open head fracture), we ended up with the present procedure: In cases of suspected infection, antibiotics are given only if serum Neo levels exceed 40 nmol/L. This approach is supported by bedside infection screening using Gram-stained smears [35]. The cut-off value of 40 nmol/L serves as a discriminator between colonization, which remains untreated, and systemic infection. The main results of this strategy are a profound reduction in infectious episodes and isolated micro-organisms, especially pseudomonads and staphylococci, and in treatment costs.

Despite the significant progress achieved in transplantation medicine in recent years, rejection of transplants remains a major problem. Besides the immunological problems of graft rejection due to the recognition of non-self MHC structures, infection as a consequence of prolonged immunosuppression of the recipient is a critical problem. A large body of data has been collected by different research groups during recent years showing the behavior and the possible applications of Neo in various situations involving allograft transplantation. Independent groups have confirmed that measurement of Neo in body fluids of recipients of solid organ as well as bone marrow grafts is of clinical relevance and value for the prognosis of immunological rejection and infection [20]. A large amount of knowledge was accrued from renal transplantation. The first reports on the use of Neo as a marker for the immunological state of recipients came from Fuchs et al. [15] and Margreiter et al. [36]. Almost ten years later Reibnegger et al. [37] evaluated 294 kidney graft recipients. By means of advanced statistical techniques and the introduction of a logarithmic likelihood ratio function, a flow diagram for the interpretation of individual Neo values was developed. With regard to Neo in liver transplantation the above findings generally apply [38] for the prediction of impending risk of immunological complications such as rejection and/or infection. Moreover, by means of multivariate Cox regression, a peak Neo concentration around day seven was identified as being a significant predictor for graft survival.

The determination of Neo and creatinine in combination with β-2 microglobulin in heart-transplanted patients [39] offers a simple tool to aid differentiation between rejection and infection. Neo values alone have been successfully used to guide the decision as to whether to perform endomyocardial biopsy [40].

Procalcitonin

Procalcitonin (PCT) is a 116 amino acid polypeptide and represents the pro-hormone of the 32 amino-acid-long calcitonin (CT). PCT itself is synthesized as a 16 kDa, 141 amino acid pre-PCT [41, 42]. Cleavage of the active hormone calcitonin takes place in the C-cells of the thyroid gland by specific proteolysis [41, 43].

The calcitonin gene family comprises four members, of which CALC-I is the gene of interest [44]. According to the suggestions of Nylen et al. [43], and Becker et al. [44], cytokines and endotoxin suppress proteolytic cleavage of PCT to CT in the Golgi vesicles, which leads to the secretion of unprocessed PCT. The origin of most of the circulating PCT has not been identified yet since an infection-associated rise in PCT has been shown in a thyroidectomized patient with septicemia [45].

An increase in serum PCT was experimentally induced by intravenous injection of 4 ng/kg endotoxin [46]. The volunteers responded with consecutive peaks of TNF and IL-6 after 1.5 and 3 h respectively. PCT was undetectable until 2 h post injection, measurable at 4 h, and then rose sharply to a plateau at 6 to 8 h, where it remained until at least 24 h. At this time TNF and IL-6 were no longer detectable. No elevation of CT levels was measured during the experiment. The same group [47] expanded their investigations by giving repeated doses of 4 ng/kg BW endotoxin (*Salmonella abortus equi*) at 0 h, 24 h and 48 h. Interestingly, the initially reached plateau was only slightly exceeded and the decrease toward baseline at 72 h was not affected. This time course was confirmed by Redl et al. (manuscript in preparation) in septic baboons. In another set of experiments, severe head trauma also produced a massive, albeit transient, increase in PCT. The rapid appearance of such high concentrations suggested a specific role for PCT in host defense. There are two short reports [48, 49] showing that both PCT and CT are able to decrease prostaglandin and thromboxane B2 substantially in lymphocytes *ex vivo*. The authors speculate that this is achieved by blocking cyclooxygenase. The hypothesis of a protective role is fostered by the finding that patients who survive classical heatstroke reveal higher PCT levels than non-survivors [50].

The first report on high serum PCT levels in patients with sepsis or infection came from Assicot et al. [45]. They prospectively investigated 79 children (age range: newborn to 12 years) with suspected infections. While PCT was undetectable (≤ 0.1 ng/mL) in children without infection, severe bacterial infection was always accompanied by massively increased PCT levels (6 to 60 ng/mL). The study also suggested that PCT levels may respond to successful antibiotic treatment with a substantial decrease. In this study population, PCT also clearly discriminated between systemic and local infection. Again, serum concentrations of the mature hormone CT were normal in all subjects, whatever PCT concentrations were found. The use of serum PCT as a marker of neonatal sepsis was also previously suggested by Gendrel et al. [51]. Moreover, new applications of PCT have been suggested. Reith et al. [52] reported on significantly declining plasma PCT concentrations in patients with peritonitis after successful focal assanation. When the surgical removal of the septic foci failed and the patients died, mean PCT levels remained high. Brunkhorst et al. [53] clearly discriminated between an infectious and a non-infectious etiology of ARDS. In a series of 17 consecutive patients with very similar Murray scores, PCT distinguished between the septic and the non-septic origin of ARDS. TNF and Neo yielded equivalent results, while IL-6 and C-reactive protein (CRP) proved insufficient. Scoring the patients by means of the APACHE II also clearly discriminated septic from non-septic etiology. Another group of patients very vulnerable to infection are burns victims. Nylen et al. [54] investigated 41 patients and demonstrated a preferential release of PCT from the lung; he concluded that serum PCT levels might have prognostic power regarding severity of inhalational injury. Circulating PCT was measured in 40 burns patients with total body surface area (TBSA) $\geq 30\%$ by Carsin et al. [55] up to one week after admission and compared to IL-6, TNFα and endotoxin. All patients without any proven infection had increased IL-6 and PCT levels in combination with undetectable TNF and endotoxin. PCT levels proved to possess prognostic value for mortality and to correlate with IL-6 and the severity of skin burn injury, but were not associated with inhalation injury.

After a case report on highly elevated PCT concentrations in a liver transplant recipient with disseminated candidiasis [56], Hammer et al. [57] claimed PCT to be a new marker for the differential diagnosis of acute rejection and bacterial infection in heart-transplanted patients. The main conclusion that rejection alone does not lead to increased PCT levels deserves further confirmation.

Antibodies against oxidized low-density lipoprotein (LDL)

Lipid peroxidation (LPO) is currently regarded as the initial step to chemical modification of low density lipoprotein (LDL) and represents the key event in atherosclerosis. LPO is not restricted to atherosclerotic processes but occurs in a large variety of inflammatory disorders, especially cardiovascular ones [58]. The mechanisms of LDL oxidation have been extensively reviewed by Jialal and Devaraj [59] and Esterbauer and Juergens [60]. LPO products of LDL are detectable in humans and animals and give clear evidence that lipoproteins undergo LPO *in vivo* and yield a wide range of oxidation products [61]. Briefly, free radical action depletes lipids of their protective antioxidants like tocopherol. This loss of chain-breaking agents gives way to lipid hydroperoxides in the LDL particle and probably in other cell membranes. The end products of this chain reaction are oxLDL plus highly reactive aldehydes, predominantly hexanal, malondialdehyde (MDA) and 4-hydroxynonenal (4-HNE).

Autologous oxLDL is more immunogenic in guinea pigs than the native form [62], and even minor modifications render the native LDL more immunogenic [63]. In healthy subjects the IgG antibodies against oxLDL are clearly detectable, Poisson distributed, and inversely correlated to age. Normal titers measured in plasma are assumed to range between 100 and 500 U/mL and include about two thirds of the above study population (for review see [64]).

The physiological significance of antibodies against oxLDL is not fully established. LPO occurs in healthy conditions as well as in pathological states, although to a much lesser extent. OxLDL has several direct effects on the endothelial cells and causes dysfunction and increased permeability of the vessel wall [65–67]. Moreover, oxidized lipoproteins are potent inhibitors of endothelium-dependent vascular relaxation [68]. Therefore a scavenger-like role for oxidatively damaged cell membranes and lipoproteins may be postulated. This assumption is supported by the experimental *in vitro* depletion of oxLDLAb from sera by incubation with aged erythrocytes [64]. Whole blood incubation with endotoxin or direct oxidation of erythrocyte membranes with superoxide also led to the quantitative consumption of oxLDLAb. Further evidence for a protective function can be deduced from a comparative study performed by Tatzber et al. [69]. With a special modification of the genuine test system with protein A it was possible to measure oxLDLAb titers in various animal species and to display a close attachment to nutrition: in the sera from herbivores like rats and rabbits, animals which are usually well supplied with antioxidants and do not develop atherosclerosis, no antibodies were found. Omnivores like pigs and baboons showed clearly detectable levels, but healthy carnivorous animals like cats and dogs exhibited the highest titers. Another finding possibly related to the clinical situation was the discovery that accidentally severely cachectic dogs were depleted of oxLDLAb but refeeding restored normal values within six weeks.

In how far these effects and actions together with the pathogenic interaction of oxLDL- antibody complexes with monocytes/macrophages and the endothelium play a role in acute inflammation remains unclear, although the involvement of oxygen and its reactive species in these conditions is generally accepted. Several human studies have documented either a dramatic loss of antioxidant capacity [70], the occurrence of conjugated dienes [71], and/or highly increased levels of LPO products such as thiobarbituric-acid reactive species (TBARS) [72] and MDA [73]. This latter article by Khoschsorur et al. [73] was the first to describe a correlation between oxLDLAb and MDA in transplantation patients ($r = 0.61$; $p \leq 0.001$) together with the finding that septic episodes and/or courses were accompanied by persisting low oxLDLAb levels. A significant consumption of Ab was also shown [58, 64], together with increasing concentrations with the onset of recovery. In a total of 23 patients (16 with sepsis, seven with SIRS), Ziervogel et al. [74] investigated the prognostic power of oxLDLAb serum titers. Septic survivors produced significantly increasing antibody levels together with decreasing PCT concentrations. Non-survivors exhibited precisely inverse courses. The findings were identical in the SIRS patients, although PCT turned out to be a weaker prognostic marker. Comparison to Neo showed results similar to oxLDLAb in both groups.

Head to head

A critical valuation of these surrogate markers is not an easy task. At present a valid comparison is only possible for PCT and Neo. Both molecules show fast enough stimulation to serve as early onset markers together with a sufficient half-life time for stable monitoring. Neo measurement in acute inflammation was introduced over ten years earlier than PCT and oxLDLAb, and therefore more data have been collected and validated. Further studies with precisely defined entry criteria are necessary not only to compare all three parameters but particularly to elaborate statistical dependencies among them because there is an evident connection at least between Neo, oxLDLAb and macrophages. Additionally, there may exist subpopulations of patients where the different markers may reveal different prognostic power. For example, there seems to be a slight superiority for PCT in terms of bacterial infection in severely ill patients prone to develop septicemia, but this could be outweighed by oxLDLAb in conditions more involving oxidative stress and LPO.

The radioimmunoassay for Neo is by far the quickest method (1 h), followed by PCT (2.5 h) and oxLDLAb (3.5 h). The use of Neo in routine laboratories is certainly limited due to radioactivity; a switch to the existing ELISA technique would probably prolong the procedure. The PCT luminescence immunoassay requires specialized equipment.

Conclusion and prospects

In one of his last printed statements Roger C. Bone [75] expressed this view: "Our concept of the pathogenesis of sepsis is undergoing revision because of the disappointing results of several pharmacologic randomized, placebo-controlled clinical trials. These trials were based on the assumption that a single proinflammatory mediator can modulate the events that define sepsis in a heterogenous group of patients. Drugs, as administered, did not improve outcome in sepsis and SIRS. Although the evidence available at that time suggested that such a strategy should be successful, hindsight indicates that this was a simplistic approach. Instead, it should be emphasized that for patients with sepsis the predominant state, over time, may be inflammatory, anti-inflammatory, or both." The close relation between this statement and the attempts to fully understand what is happening at any point of time in every patient is obvious. Advanced biochemistry, molecular biology and biophysics develop and provide tools to measure and quantify almost every item of interest. Monitoring of severely ill patients routinely comprises about 50 parameters, and this number is easily doubled in research units. Nonetheless, the situation also clearly shows the limits, because – in a very benevolent view – with a few exceptions the step from diagnosing an already present clinical condition to its prognosis remains unaccomplished. One pathway to the solution of this problem is certainly the search for new parameters; another, the ongoing evaluation and perhaps the combination of established measurements. These efforts need the support of extensive pathophysiological research, because improved knowledge about the patients' underlying disease may facilitate the finding and/or choice of the appropriate marker or set of markers.

It remains an unresolved question as to what extent the theoretical approach influences the search for markers. Perhaps it was these considerations that helped come up with the so-called surrogate markers. In some cases they may prove to be of overall importance and display all effects of either progression of the disease or action of the therapeutic drug [76]. In other circumstances they reveal independence from most common clinical parameters and therefore from underlying individual irregularities, thus possibly describing a "meta condition" as yet not precisely defined: Just as in the Uncertainty Principle, where often there is "no yet proven link between cause and effect and the results can be expressed only in terms of probability that a certain effect will occur".

Appendix

As it should be, research is overtaking authors of reviews. In a very recent report peripheral blood mononuclear cells were identified to express PCT mRNA and that this expression is modulated by bacterial LPS and sepsis related cytokines [77]. Additionally, an interesting experiment was performed by Nylen et al. [78]. When septic animals were treated with an antiserum reactive to PCT, mortality was decreased. These findings suggest that PCT is more than a marker of bacterial sepsis, it can be seen as an active player in inflammatory processes.

References

1   Heisenberg W (1927) Über den anschaulichen Inhalt der quantentheoretischen Kinematik und Mechanik. *Zeitschr Physik* 7: 235–246

2   Roumen RMH (1993) *Clinical studies in patients at risk for ARDS and MOF.* Thesis, Katholieke Univ. Nijmegen, Netherlands

3   Redl H, Schlag G (1996) Biochemical/immunological monitoring in the posttraumatic course. In: Risberg B (ed): *Trauma care – an update.* Pharmacia and Upjohn Sverige AB, Göteborg, 80–87

4   Cavaillon JM, Munoz C, Fitting C, Misset B, Carlet J (1992) Circulating cytokines: the tip of the iceberg? *Circ Shock* 38: 145–152

5   Fleming TR, DeMets DL (1996) Surrogate end points in clinical trials: are we being misled? *Ann Intern Med* 125: 605–613

6   Rembold H, Buschmann L (1963) Struktur und Synthese des Neopterins. *Chem Ber* 96: 1406–1410

7   Rembold H, Buschmann L (1963) Untersuchungen über die Pteridine der Bienenpuppe (apis mellifica). *Justus Liebig Ann Chem* 662: 72–82

8   Brown GM (1971) The biosynthesis of pteridines. *Adv Enzymol* 35: 5–77

9   Kaufman S (1963) The structure of phenylalanine hydroxylation cofactor. *Proc Natl Acad Sci USA* 50: 1085–1093

10   Schobersberger W, Hoffmann G, Grote J, Wachter H, Fuchs D (1995) Induction of inducible nitric oxide synthase expression by neopterin in vascular smooth muscle cells. *FEBS Lett* 377: 461–464

11   Hoffmann G, Schobersberger W, Frede S, Pelzer L, Fandrey J, Wachter H, Fuchs D, Grote J (1996) Neopterin activates transcription factor nuclear factor-kappa B in vascular smooth muscle cells. *J Neurol Neurosurg Psychiatry* 61: 211–212

12   Kaufman S, Holtzman NA, Milstien S, Butler IJ, Krumholz A (1975) Phenylketonuria due to a deficiency of dihydropteridine reductase. *N Engl J Med* 293: 785–790

13   Niederwieser A, Curtius H-C, Bettoni O, Bieri J, Schircks M, Viscontini M, Schaub J (1979) Atypical phenylketonuria caused by 7,8-dihydrobiopterin synthetase deficiency. *Lancet* I: 131–133

14   Wachter H, Hausen A, Grassmayr K (1979) Erhöhte Ausscheidung von Neopterin im Harn von Patienten mit malignen Tumoren und mit Viruserkrankungen. *Hoppe Seyler's Z Physiol Chem* 360: 1957–1960

15   Fuchs D, Hausen A, Huber C, Margreiter R, Reibnegger G, Spielberger M, Wachter H (1982) Pteridinausscheidung als Marker für alloantigen-induzierte Lymphozytenproliferation. *Hoppe Seyler's Z Physiol Chem* 363: 661–664

16   Huber C, Fuchs D, Hausen A, Margreiter R, Reibnegger G, Spielberger M, Wachter H (1983) Pteridines as a new marker to detect human T cells activated by allogeneic or modified self major histocompatibility complex (MHC) determinants. *J Immunol* 130: 1047–1050

17   Huber C, Batchelor JR, Fuchs D, Hausen A, Lang A, Niederwieser D, Reibnegger G, Swetly P, Troppmair J, Wachter H (1984) Immune response associated production of neopterin. Release from macrophages primarily under control of interferon gamma. *J Exp Med* 160: 310–316

18   Werner-Felmayer G, Werner ER, Fuchs D, Hausen A, Reibnegger G, Wachter H (1990) Tetrahydrobiopterin-dependent formation of nitrite and nitrate in murine fibroblasts. *J Exp Med* 172: 1599–1607

19   Woloszczuk W (1985) A sensitive immunoradiometric assay for gamma interferon, suitable for its measurements in serum. *Clin Chem* 31: 1090–1093

20   Wachter H, Fuchs D, Hausen A, Reibnegger G, Weiss G, Werner ER, Werner-Felmayer G (eds) (1992) *Neopterin – Biochemistry, methods, clinical application.* Walter de Gruyter, Berlin, New York

21   Andert SE, Griesmacher A, Zuckermann A, Mueller MM (1992) Neopterin release from human endothelial cells is triggered by interferon gamma. *Clin Exp Immunol* 88: 555–558

22   Estelberger W, Weiss G, Petek W, Paletta B, Wachter H, Reibnegger G (1993) Determination of renal clearance of neopterin by a pharmacokinetic approach. *FEBS Lett* 329: 13–16

23 Strohmaier W, Redl H, Schlag G, Inthorn D (1987) D-erythro-neopterin plasma levels in intensive care patients with and without septic complications. *Crit Care Med* 15: 757–760

24 Pacher R, Redl H, Frass M, Petzl DH, Schuster E,Woloszczuk W (1989) Relationship between neopterin and granulocyte elastase plasma levels and the severity of multiple organ failure. *Crit Care Med* 17: 221–226

25 Faist E, Storck M, Hültner L, Redl H, Ertel W, Walz A, Schildberg FW (1992) Functional analysis of monocyte activity through synthesis patterns of proinflammatory cytokines and neopterin in patients in surgical intensive care. *Surgery* 112: 562–572

26 Nast-Kolb D, Waydhas C, Jochum M, Duswald KH, Machleidt W, Spannagl M, Schramm W, Fritz H, Schweiberer L (1992) Biochemical factors as objective parameters for assessing the prognosis in polytrauma. *Unfallchirurg* 95: 59–66

27 Delogu G, Casula MA, Mancini P, Tellan G, Signore L (1995) Serum neopterin and soluble interleukin-2 receptor for prediction of a shock state in gram-negative sepsis. *J Crit Care* 10: 64–71

28 Roumen RMH, Redl H, Schlag G, Sandtner W, Koller W, Goris RJA (1993) Scoring systems and blood lactate concentrations in relation to the development of adult respiratory distress syndrome and multiple organ failure in severely traumatized patients. *J Trauma* 35: 349–355

29 Bloom JN, Suffredini AF, Parrillo JE, Palestine A (1990) Serum neopterin levels following intravenous endotoxin administration to normal humans. *Immunobiology* 181: 317–323

30 Bahrami S, Redl H, Leichtfried G, Yu Y, Schlag G (1994) Similar cytokine but different coagulation responses to lipopolysaccharide in D-galactosamine-sensitized versus nonsensitized rats. *Infect Immun* 62: 99–105

31 Schlag G, Redl H, Hallström S, Radmore K, Davies J (1991) Hyperdynamic sepsis in baboons. I. Aspects of hemodynamics. *Circ Shock* 34: 311–318

32 Strohmaier W, Werner ER, Wachter H, Redl H, Schlag G (1996) Pteridine and nitrite/nitrate formation in experimental septic and traumatic shock. *Shock* 6: 254–258

33 Strohmaier W, Mauritz W, Gaudernak T, Grünwald C, Schüller W, Schlag G (1992) Septic focus localized by determination of arterio-venous difference in neopterin blood levels. *Circ Shock* 38: 219–221

34 Strohmaier W, Poigenfürst J, Mauritz W (1996) Neopterin blood levels: a basis for deciding to use antibiotics in intensive care unit (ICU) patients. *Pteridines* 7: 1–4

35 Huemer G, Graninger W, Mauritz W (1992) Bed-side infection screening of ICU patients using Gram stained smears. *Eur J Anaesthesiol* 9: 229–233

36 Margreiter R, Fuchs D, Hausen A, Huber C, Reibnegger G, Spielberger M, Wachter H (1983) Neopterin as a new biochemical marker for diagnosis of allograft rejection. *Transplantation* 36: 650–653

37 Reibnegger G, Aichberger C, Fuchs D, Hausen A, Spielberger M, Werner ER, Margreiter R, Wachter H (1991) Posttranslant neopterin excretion in renal allograft recipients:

reliable diagnostic aid of acute rejection and predictive marker of long-term graft survival. *Transplantation* 52: 58–63

38 Tilg H, Vogel W, Aulitzky WE, Schönitzer D, Margreiter R, Dietze O, Judmaier G, Wachter H, Huber C (1989) Neopterin excretion after liver transplantation and its value in differential diagnosis of complications. *Transplantation* 48: 594–599

39 Schmitt F, Myara I, Benoit MO, Guillemain T, Amrein C, Dreyfus G, Paris M, Moatti N (1989) Monitoring of heart allograft rejection by simultaneous measurement of serum beta-2 microglobulin and urinary neopterin. *Ann Biol Clin* 47: 237–241

40 Hölzel WGE, Havel M, Laczkovics A, Müller MM (1988) Diagnostic validity of multivariate combinations of biochemical analytes as markers for rejection and infection in the follow-up of patients with heart transplants. *J Clin Chem Clin Biochem* 26: 667–671

41 Petitjean S, Assicot M (1993) Étude de l'immunoreactivité calcitonine-like au cours des processus infectieux. Diplome d'études approfondies de biotechnologie.

42 LeMoullec JM, Julienne A, Chenais J, Lasmoles F, Guliana JM, Milhaud G, Moukhtar MS (1984) The complete sequence of human preprocalcitonin. *FEBS Lett* 167: 93–97

43 Nylen E, Snider R, Thompson K, Rohatgi P, Becker K (1996) Pneumonitis-associated hyperprocalcitoninemia. *Am J Med Sci* 312: 12–18

44 Becker KL, Gazdar AF, Carney BN, Snider RH, Moore CF, Silva OL (1994) Small cell lung carcinoma cell line express mRNA for calcitonin and alpha- and beta-calcitonin gene related peptide. *Cancer Lett* 81: 19–25

45 Assicot M, Gendrel D, Carsin H, Raymond J, Guilbaud J, Bohuon C (1993) High serum procalcitonin concentration in patients with sepsis and infection. *Lancet* 341: 515–518

46 Dandona P, Nix D, Wilson MF, Aljada A, Love J, Assicot M, Bohuon C (1994) Procalcitonin increase after endotoxin injection in normal subjects. *J Clin Endocrinol Metab* 79: 1605–1608

47 Assicot M, Mackensen A, Petitjean S, Engelhardt R, Bohuon C (1998) Kinetics of the appearance of procalcitonin following endotoxin adminstration; *submitted*

48 Meisner M, Tschaikowsky K, Spiessl C, Schüttler J (1996) Procalcitonin – a marker or modulator of the acute immune response? *Intens Care Med* 22 (Suppl 1): 14

49 Meisner M, Tschaikowsky K, Spiessl C, Schüttler J (1998) Hemmung der Arachidonsäure-induzierten Prostaglandin-Produktion in humanen Lymphozyten durch Procalcitonin. *Der Anästhesist; in press*

50 Nylen ES, Al Arifi A, Becker KL, Snider RHj, Alzeer A (1997) Effect of classic heatstroke on serum procalcitonin. *Crit Care Med* 25: 1362–1365

51 Gendrel D, Assicot M, Raymond J, Moulin F, Francoual C, Badoual J, Bohuon C (1996) Procalcitonin as a marker for the early diagnosis of neonatal infection. *J Pediatr* 128: 570–573

52 Reith HB, Lehmkuhl R, Beier W, Högy B, und die Studiengruppe Peritonitis (1995) Procalcitonin – ein prognostischer Infektionsparameter bei der Peritonitis. *Chir Gastroenterol* 11 (Suppl 2): 47–50

53 Brunkhorst FM, Forycki ZF, Wagner J (1995) Frühe Identifizierung der biliären akuten

Pankreatitis durch Procalcitonin-Immunreaktivität – vorläufige Ergebnisse. *Chir Gastroenterol* 11 (Suppl 2): 42–46

54 Nylen ES, O'Nell WO, Jordan MH, Snider RH, Moore CF, Lewis M, Silva OL, Becker KL (1992) Serum procalcitonin as an index of inhalation injury in burns. *Horm Metab Res* 24: 439–442

55 Carsin H, Assicot M, Feger F, Roy O, Pennacino I, LeBever H, Ainaud P, Bohuon C (1997) Evolution and significance of circulating procalcitonin levels compared with IL-6, TNF alpha and endotoxin levels early after thermal injury. *Burns* 23: 218–224

56 Gerad Y, Hober D, Petitjean S, Assicot M, Bohuon C, Mouton Y, Wattre P (1995) High serum procalcitonin level in a 4-year old liver transplant recipient with disseminated candidiasis. *Infection* 23, Vol 5: 310–311

57 Hammer C, Staehler M (1996) Procalcitonin (PCT) – a new marker for differntial diagnosis of acute rejection and bacterial infection of heart transplanted patients. *Clin Intens Care* 7 (Suppl 1): 39

58 Tatzber F, Esterbauer H (1995) Autoantibodies to oxidized low density lipoprotein. In: Bellomo G, Finardi G, Maggi E, Rice-Evans C (eds): *Free radicals, lipoprotein oxidation and atherosclerosis*. The Richelieu Press, London, 245–262

59 Jialal I, Devaraj S (1996) Low density lipoprotein oxidation antioxidants and atherosclerosis: a clinical biochemistry perspective. *Clin Chem* 42: 498–506

60 Esterbauer H, Juergens G (1993) Mechanistic and genetic aspects of susceptibility of LDL to oxidation. *Current Opinion Lipidol* 4: 114–124

61 Esterbauer H, Zollner H, Schaur RJ (1989) Aldehydes formed by lipid peroxidation: mechanism of formation, occurrence and determination. In: Vigo-Pelfrey C (ed): Membrane lipid peroxidation. CRC Press, Boca Raton, 239–268

62 Witztum JL, Steinbrecher UP, Fisher M, Kesaniemi A (1983) Nonenzymatic glucosylation of homologous low density lipoprotein and albumin render them immunogenic in the guinea pig. *Proc Natl Acad Sci USA* 80: 2757–2761

63 Berliner JA, Territo MC, Sevanian A et al (1990) Minimally modified low density lipoprotein stimulates monocyte endothelial interactions. *J Clin Invest* 85: 1260–1266

64 Tatzber F, Esterbauer H, Temml C, Reiger J, Khoschsorur G, Wonisch W, Schmidl E, Lapin A (1996) Antibodies to oxidised LDL in health and disease. Biochemical and clinical implications. In: Finardi G, Bellomo G, Maggi E (eds): *Lipoprotein oxidation and atherosclerosis. Biological and clinical aspects*. Pavia (Italy): 32–38

65 Hessler JR, Robertson ALj, Chisolm GM (1979) LDL-induced cytotoxicity and its inhibition by HLD in human vascular smooth muscle and endothelial cells in culture. *Atherosclerosis* 32: 213–229

66 Hessler JR, Morel DW, Lewis LJ, Chisolm GM (1983) Lipoprotein oxidation and lipoprotein-induced cytotoxicity. *Arteriosclerosis* 3: 215–222

67 Morel DW, Hessler JR, Chisolm GM (1983) Low density lipoprotein cytotoxicity induced by free radical peroxidation of lipid. *J Lipid Res* 24: 1070–1073

68 Chin JH, Azhar S, Hoffman BB (1989) Inactivation of endothelial derived relaxing factor by oxidized lipoproteins. *J Clin Invest* 89: 10–18

69 Tatzber F, Wonisch W, Schmidl E, Esterbauer H (1997) Quantitative determintion of oLAb titers in various animal species. *BioFactors* 6: 125–130

70 Redl H, Gasser H, Schlag G, Marzi I (1993) Involvement of oxygen radicals in shock related cell injury. *Br Med Bull* 49: 556–565

71 Gasser H, Paul E, Redl H, Schlag G, Traber DL, Herndon D (1991) Loss of plasma antioxidants after burn injury. *Circ Shock* 34: 13A

72 Richard C, Lemonnier F, Thibault M, Couturier M, Auzcpy P (1990) Vitamin E deficiency and lipoperoxidation during adult respiratory distress syndrome. *Crit Care Med* 18: 4–9

73 Khoschsorur G, Tatzber F, Freigassner M, Tscheliessnigg KH, Iberer F, Lamprecht M, Uranüs S, Petek W (1996) Inverse correlation of malondialdehyde (MDA) and anti-Cu^{2+} oxidised low-density lipoprotein (LDL) immunoglobulin G (IgG) antibodies in transplantation patients. *Mol Sci Res* 24: 851–854

74 Ziervogel G, Sterz B, Reiger J, Stettner H, Köller U (1997) Autoantibodies against oxydated LDL and procalcitonin as prognostic markers for patients suffering from sepsis and SIRS. Berichte ÖGKC 20: 59A

75 Bone RC (1997) Current topics in critical care medicine. *Crit Care Int* 7: 4

76 Lagakos SW (1993) Surrogate markers in AIDS clinical trials: conceptual basis, validation, and uncertainties. *Clin Infect Dis* 16 (Suppl 1): 22–25

77 Oberhoffer M, Russwurm S, Stonans I, Stonane E, Vogelsang H, Junker U, Jäger L, Reinhart K (1998) Human peripheral blood mononuclear cells express mRNA for procalcitonin; modulation by lipopolysaccharides and sepsis related cytokines. *Crit Care* 2 (suppl 1): P35

78 Nylen ES, Whang KT, Snider RH Jr, Steinwald PM, White JC, Becker KL (1998) Mortality is increased by procalcitonin and decreased by an antiserum reactive to procalcitonin in experimental sepsis. *Crit Care Med* 26 (2): 1001–1006

Actions
(selected events)

Nitric oxide and endothelin-1 in circulatory shock involving cytokines

Christoph Thiemermann and Timothy D. Warner

The William Harvey Research Institute, St. Bartholomew's and the Royal London School of Medicine and Dentistry, Charterhouse Square, London EC1M 6BQ, UK

Introduction

The vascular endothelium regulates the tone of the underlying smooth muscle and the reactivity of blood platelets and neutrophils by the release of mediators, in particular nitric oxide (NO), prostacyclin and endothelin-1 (ET-1). The first two of these are potent vasodilators which also inhibit platelet and neutrophil aggregation and adhesion, while ET-1 is the most potent mammalian vasoconstrictor peptide yet found. Unlike NO (which keeps the vasculature in a constant state of active vasodilation) and ET-1, prostacyclin is less important for the regulation of vascular tone under physiological and even pathophysiological conditions. Thus, the discovery of two potent vasoactive mediators NO and ET-1 has stimulated an enormous amount of research into the regulation of vascular tone in health and disease.

NO is generated from L-arginine by a family of enzymes collectively called NO synthases (NOS), which contain an oxygenase domain (containing the catalytic center) and a reductase domain. The synthesis of NO from L-arginine and molecular oxygen involves the generation of N^G-hydroxy-L-arginine and water (first step) and subsequently the oxidation of N^G-hydroxy-L-arginine in the presence of molecular oxygen to form NO, L-citrulline and water. When generated, NO diffuses to adjacent cells where it activates soluble guanylate cyclase, resulting in the formation of cGMP, which in turn mediates many (but not all) of the effects of NO. NO is generated by many mammalian cells by at least three different isoforms of NOS. The NOS in endothelial cells (eNOS or NOS III) and neuronal cells (nNOS or NOS I) are expressed constitutively, and both enzymes require an increase in intracellular calcium for activation. Activation of macrophages and many other cells with pro-inflammatory cytokines or endotoxin results in the expression of a distinct isoform of NOS (inducible NOS; iNOS or NOS II), the activity of which is functionally independent of changes in intracellular calcium [1–5]. Thus, it is not surprising that NO has many biological functions in the cardiovascular, nervous and immune systems. For instance, activation of eNOS by shear stress results in a continuous release of picomolar amounts of NO which helps to regulate blood pressure and organ blood

Cytokines in Severe Sepsis and Septic Shock, edited by H. Redl and G. Schlag[†]
© 1999 Birkhäuser Verlag Basel/Switzerland

flow by causing vasodilatation and opposing the effects of circulating cate-cholamines. NO also reduces the adhesion of platelets and polymorphonuclear leukocytes (PMNs) to the endothelium [3]. The latter effect of NO is, at least in part, due to the prevention by NO of the expression of the adhesion molecules P-selectin and intercellular adhesion molecule (ICAM-1) on the surface of endothelial cells. In addition to preventing the adhesion of platelets to endothelial cells, NO also directly attenuates the activation of platelets. These effects of NO are associated with and/or due to prevention of the expression of P-selectin (on platelets), secretion of platelet granules, intracellular calcium flux, as well as binding of glycoprotein IIb/IIIa to fibrinogen [6].

Although much research has focused on the release of vasodilator autacoids including NO, the endothelium also produces vasoconstrictor substances. One of these has been postulated to be angiotensin II, another superoxide anion, and a third, a prostaglandin endoperoxide. Despite these suggestions it would, however, be fair to say that only one vasoconstrictor factor, ET-1, has been properly identi-fied. ET-1, a member of the 21-amino acid endothelin family of peptides (ET-1, ET-2, ET-3 and sarafotoxins), is a potent vasoconstrictor produced by the endothelium from its precursor big-endothelin-1 by endothelin-converting enzyme-1 [8, 9]. Two distinct endothelin receptors have been cloned and expressed, namely ET_A and ET_B. The vasoconstrictor effects of ET-1 are primarily mediated by activation of the ET_A receptor, which is present on vascular smooth muscle cells. Activation by ET-1 of the ET_B receptor located on endothelial cells results in a release of nitric oxide (NO) and prostacyclin to cause vasodilatation [9, 10]. ET_B receptors also exist on vascu-lar smooth muscle cells of certain blood vessels of a variety of species including rats, pigs, dogs and man, where they mediate vasoconstriction. In healthy humans or ani-mals ET-1 is generally reported to circulate at particularly low concentrations. This suggests that ET-1 may only have minor roles within the healthy circulation, even bearing in mind its particularly short circulating half-life (3 to 7 min). In marked comparison to the healthy animal, substantial elevations in the circulating and/or tissue levels of ET-1 have been noted in a variety of cardiovascular disorders includ-ing septic shock. Taken together these observations suggest that the endothelin sys-tem is largely dormant in the healthy adult body, and particularly within the healthy adult circulation, but that it becomes activated in circulatory shock [11]. This chap-ter reviews the roles of NO and ET-1 in the pathophysiology of circulatory shock in animals and man.

Role of NO in the pathophysiology of septic shock

Since the discovery in 1990 that an enhanced formation of endogenous NO con-tributes to (i) the hypotension caused by endotoxin and TNFα [12–14], (ii) the vas-cular hyporesponsiveness to vasoconstrictor agents (also termed 'vasoplegia') [15,

16], and (iii) the protection of liver integrity in rodents with sepsis [17], there has been an ever increasing interest in the role of NO in the pathophysiology of animals and man with septic shock. The overproduction of NO in animal models of circulatory shock is due to an early activation of eNOS (which is transient) and the delayed induction of iNOS activity (resulting in the formation of nanomolar amounts of NO) in macrophages (host defence), vascular smooth muscle (hypotension, vascular hyporeactivity, maldistribution of blood flow) and parenchymal cells [18]. The finding that inhibitors of NOS activity attenuate the hypotension and vasoplegia caused by endotoxin in animals (see above), together with the discovery that mice in which the iNOS gene has been inactivated by gene-targeting (iNOS knockout mice) exhibit only a minor fall in blood pressure when challenged with endotoxin [19, 20], support the hypothesis that an overproduction of NO by iNOS contributes to the circulatory failure in septic shock. It is less clear whether increased formation of NO also contributes to the organ injury and dysfunction caused by endotoxin. The formation of NO by eNOS (and potentially also by iNOS) also exerts beneficial effects in shock including vasodilatation, prevention of platelet and leukocyte adhesion, maintenance of microcirculatory blood flow and augmentation of host defence (Tab. 1). Thus, it is not surprising that basic and clinical scientists have advocated the use of contrasting therapeutic approaches including inhibition of NOS activity, enhancement of the availability of NO (NO-donors, NO-inhalation) or a combination of both approaches. The following paragraphs highlight some of the effects and side effects of inhibitors of NOS activity (Tab. 1) in animal models of septic shock. For a more detailed review of (i) the many roles of NO in the pathophysiology of septic or other forms of shock, (ii) the mechanisms leading to the induction of iNOS (Fig. 1) and (iii) a more detailed account of the chemistry and pharmacology (iso-enzyme selectivity) of NOS inhibitors, the interested reader is referred to recent reviews of these topics [4, 5, 21, 22].

Table 1 - The possible effects of administration of NOS inhibitors in septic shock, both beneficial and adverse effects are shown.

Beneficial	Adverse
Increased blood pressure	Excessive vasoconstriction
Restores responsiveness to pressor agents	Pulmonary hypertension
Cardiac output return to baseline values	Fall in cardiac output
Decreased production of peroxynitrite	Increased platelet adhesiveness
Attenuation of inhibition of mitochondrial respiration	Increased neutrophil adhesion
Improved organ function	Worsened organ function
Improved survival	

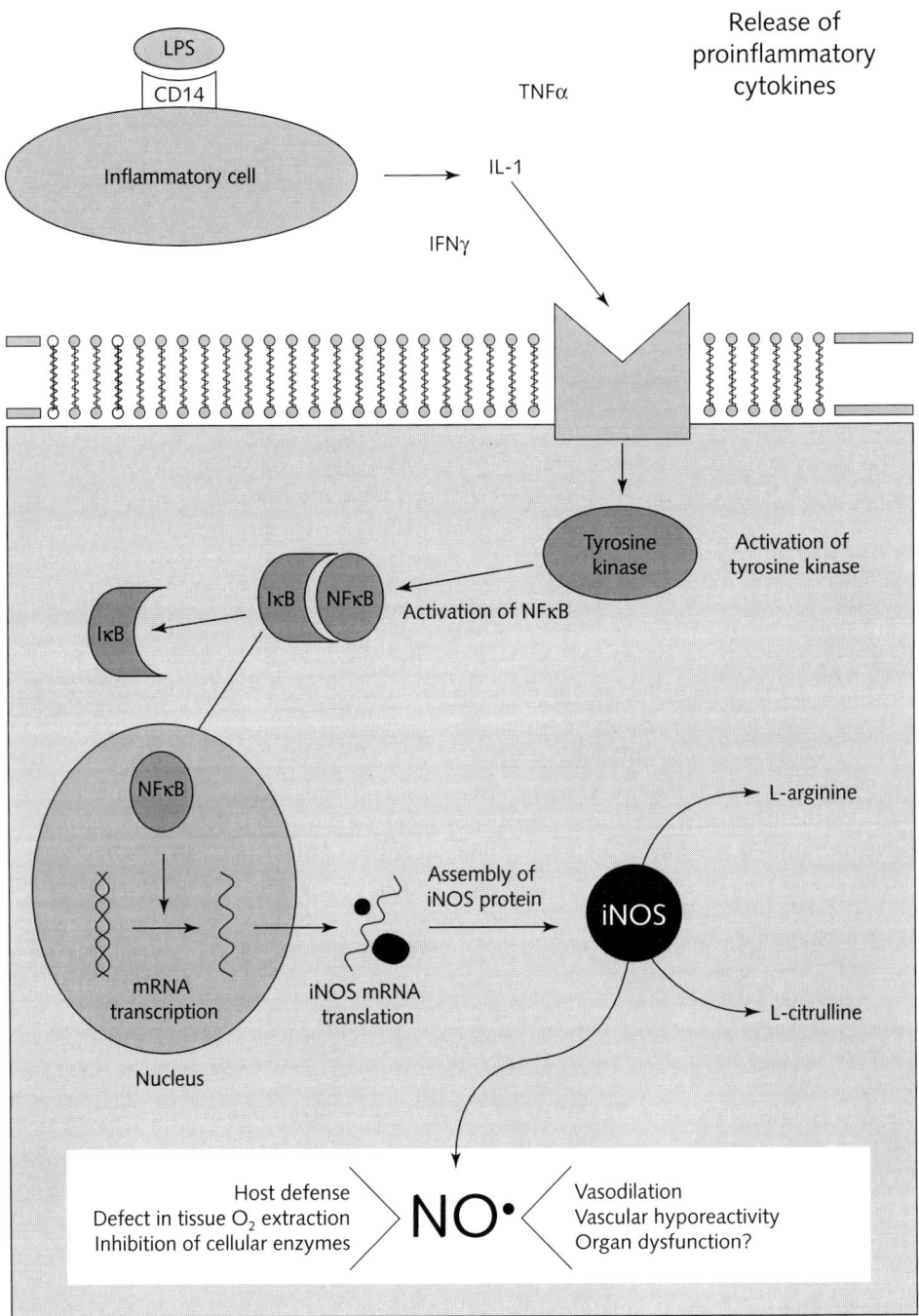

Inhibition of NOS activity in animal models of shock: Effects and side effects

Although there is good evidence that endotoxemia or sepsis in rodents results in the induction of iNOS (in various tissues) leading to an increase in the plasma levels of nitrite/nitrate (from 20 to up to 600 µM), there is limited information regarding the time course of iNOS induction, the degree of iNOS activity (in tissues) or even the plasma levels of nitrite/nitrate in large animal models (pig, dog, sheep, baboon) of shock or in humans with sepsis and septic shock. Clearly, sepsis (or endotoxemia) results in an increase in the plasma levels of nitrite/nitrate in these species. However, it appears that the rise in the plasma levels of nitrite/nitrate in e.g. humans with septic shock is much smaller than in rodents [23]. When evaluating the role of NO or elucidating the effects of NOS inhibitors in animal models of shock, one needs to remember that (i) many of the models used are non-resuscitated, hypodynamic models of shock, (ii) the effects (and side effects) of non-selective inhibitors of NOS activity (see below) will greatly vary depending upon the degree of iNOS induction in the species, and (iii) any observed effects of the respective NOS inhibitor used will obviously depend on the chosen dose regimen and timing of the intervention.

The N-substituted L-arginine analogue, N^G-methyl-L-arginine (L-NMMA), was the first agent reported to inhibit NOS activity. Following the discovery in 1990 that L-NMMA exerted beneficial hemodynamic effects in animal models of endotoxemia (Fig. 2) [12–14], many subsequent studies aimed at elucidating the role of NO in septic shock have used the NOS inhibitor N^G-nitro-L-arginine methyl ester (L-NAME), rather than L-NMMA, as L-NAME is cheap and readily available. In contrast to L-NMMA, L-NAME is a relatively selective inhibitor of eNOS rather than iNOS activity [22] and, hence, higher doses of this agent may cause excessive vasoconstriction (particularly in the pulmonary, renal and myocardial vascular bed) and enhance the incidence of both microvascular thrombosis and neutrophil adhesion to the endothelium. Thus, L-NAME reduces oxygen delivery and exacerbates organ injury in many, but not all, animal models of endotoxic or septic shock (see [21]). These results are not necessarily solely due to the use of very large amounts of L-NAME, but rather a reflection of the fact that L-NAME is a more selective inhibitor

Figure 1

Mechanism(s) leading to the overproduction of nitric oxide (NO) in septic shock. The release of pro-inflammatory cytokines including tumour necrosis factor α (TNFα), IL-1 and interferon-γ (IFNγ) leads to the activation of (receptor-linked) protein tyrosine kinases and of the transcription factor NF-κB, which in turn causes the expression of iNOS protein. An enhanced formation of iNOS contributes to the circulatory failure (vasodilatation, vascular hyporeactivity), inhibition of certain enzymes, and possibly host defence and organ injury/dysfunction. LPS, lipopolysaccharide

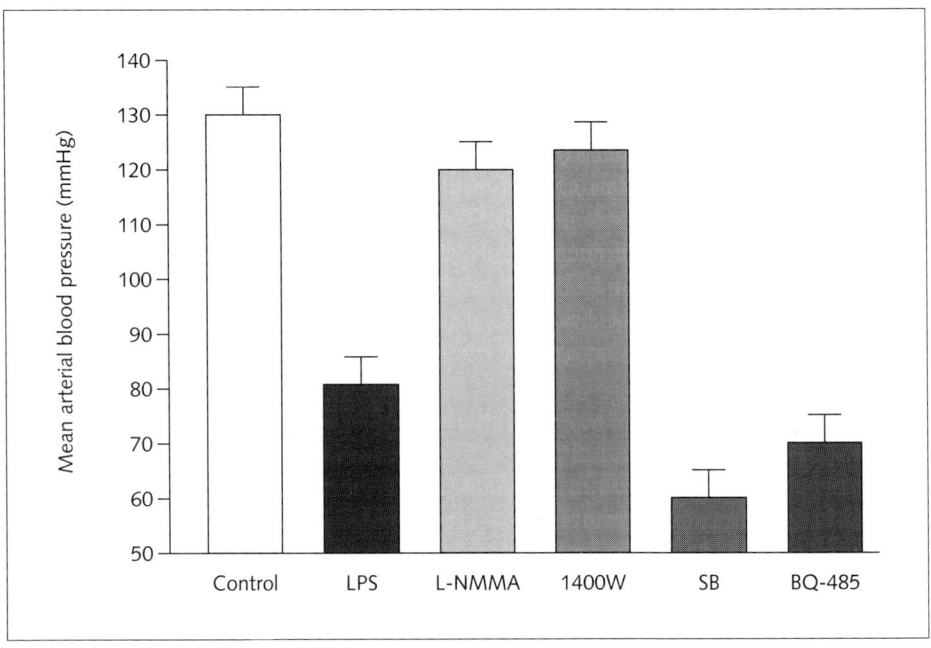

Figure 2
Comparison of the effects of the non-selective NOS inhibitor N^G-methyl-L-arginine (L-NMMA), the iNOS selective NOS inhibitor 1400W, the non-selective ET receptor antagonist SB209670 and the ET_A receptor antagonist BQ-485 on the fall in mean arterial blood pressure (MAP) caused by endotoxin in the anesthetised rat. Please note that the inhibition of NOS activity with either L-NMMA or 1400W restores blood pressure. In contrast, the non-selective blockade of ET receptors augments the hypotension caused by endotoxin in this rodent model of severe endotoxemia.

of eNOS than iNOS activity. Although L-NAME may be suitable for inhibiting the generation of NO by all three isoforms of NOS, this agent should not be used as a therapeutic intervention in diseases such as septic shock, where an overproduction of NO by iNOS has been implicated to be the underlying cause of the pathology.

In contrast to L-NAME, L-NMMA is an endogenous substance present in the urine of both animals and man. Although L-NMMA inhibits all isoforms of NOS to a variable degree, it is a more potent inhibitor of iNOS than eNOS activity. L-NMMA is a competitive inhibitor of the binding of L-arginine to NOS and, hence, excess of L-arginine reverses the inhibition of NOS activity by L-NMMA. The effects of L-NMMA in models of shock vary from "very beneficial" to "moderately beneficial with some adverse effects" to "detrimental" (often due to marked inhibition of eNOS activity) [21, 22]. Clearly, the observed result depends on the dose of L-NMMA as well as the model of shock used. When given after the onset of hypotension, infusions of relatively low doses of L-NMMA (3 to 10 mg/kg/h) have been convincingly demonstrated to exert beneficial hemodynamic effects in rodents, sheep, dogs and baboon models of endotoxemia and sepsis. For instance, in conscious baboons, administration of live *E. coli* bacteria resulted in a significant increase in the serum levels of biopterin, neopterin and nitrate, suggesting induction of GTP cyclohydrolase I and iNOS. In this model, infusion of L-NMMA (5 mg/kg/h) attenuated the rise in the serum levels of nitrate and creatinine, the hypotension and fall in peripheral vascular resistance and the substantial six day mortality caused by severe sepsis in this species (D. Rees and H. Redl, personal communication). These findings clearly document that the circulatory failure caused by septic shock in baboons is largely mediated by an enhanced formation of NO by iNOS and that inhibition of iNOS with L-NMMA improves outcome in this model.

Selective inhibition of iNOS activity in experimental endotoxemia

The observed beneficial effects of L-NMMA in animal models of septic shock stimulated the search for selective inhibitors of iNOS activity. In the last years several compounds have been tested including aminoguanidine, certain isothiourea-derivatives (e.g. aminoethyl-isothiourea), amidines (e.g. 1400W) and amino acid analogues (L-NIL). As an extensive review of the chemistry and pharmacology of selective inhibitors of iNOS activity is not possible within this monograph, the interested reader is referred to a recent review of this topic [22]. Aminoguanidine was the first relatively selective inhibitor of iNOS activity discovered [24]. Although aminoguanidine is a more potent inhibitor of iNOS than eNOS activity *in vitro* and *in vivo*, aminoguanidine is not a very potent inhibitor of iNOS activity. Although a variety of studies document beneficial effects of aminoguanidine on the circulatory failure and the multiple organ dysfunction caused by endotoxin in animals, the interpretation of the mechanism(s) by which aminoguanidine exerts these beneficial effects is difficult, as aminoguanidine is not a specific inhibitor of iNOS activity. Indeed, aminoguanidine has many other pharmacological properties including inhibition of (i) histamine metabolism, (ii) polyamine catabolism, (iii) the formation of advanced glycosylation end products, and of (iv) catalase activity (as well as other copper- or iron-containing enzymes). Interestingly, aminoguanidine also prevents the expression of iNOS protein by a hitherto unknown mechanism (see [21]). Thus, aminoguanidine has to be regarded as an agent which (i) is a relatively selective, but not very potent inhibitor of iNOS activity, (ii) reduces the formation of NO by two distinct mechanisms, namely prevention of the expression of iNOS protein and inhibition of iNOS activity, and (iii) exerts many other effects, which appear to be unrelated to the inhibition of iNOS activity (non-specific effects).

S-substituted isothioureas (ITUs) are non-amino acid analogues of L-arginine and also potent inhibitors of iNOS activity with variable isoform selectivity [25–27]. The most potent isothioureas are those with only short alkyl chains on the sulphur atom and no substituents on the nitrogen atoms. In 1994, we demonstrated that S-methyl-ITU reverses the circulatory failure caused by endotoxin in the rat. This beneficial hemodynamic effect of S-methyl-ITU was associated with an attenuation of the liver injury and hepatocellular dysfunction caused by endotoxin in rats as well as an increase in the survival rate of mice challenged with a high dose of endotoxin [26]. Similarly, aminoethyl-ITU exerts beneficial hemodynamic effects and attenuates the degree of liver injury/dysfunction caused by endotoxin in the rat [28]. In pigs with endotoxemia, injection of aminoethyl-ITU restores hepatic arterial blood flow (from reduced to normal levels) and increases hepatic oxygen consumption, without affecting cardiac output [29]. Having stressed that some of the beneficial effects of aminoguanidine in shock may not be due to its ability to inhibit iNOS activity (e.g. non-specific effects), it should be noted that S-substituted isothioureas are also likely to elicit effects which are unrelated to inhibition of NOS activity. For instance, aminoethyl-ITU is a scavenger of peroxynitrite and exerts beneficial effects in models of disease/pathology known to be mediated by oxygen-derived free radicals (see [21]). Interestingly, dimethyl-ITU (which does not inhibit iNOS activity) is a weak radical scavenger which inhibits the activation of the transcription factor NF-κB. In rats challenged with either endotoxin or live *Salmonella typhimurium*, dimethyl-ITU attenuates the formation of TNFα and improves survival [30]. The ability of aminoethyl-ITU to scavenge peroxynitrite and to prevent the expression of certain proteins (possibly by attenuating the activation of NF-κB) may well contribute to or even account for the beneficial effects of this isothiourea-derivative in animal models of shock.

S-substituted ITUs and guanidines contain the amidine function (–CH(=NH)NH$_2$), a feature which they have in common with O-substituted isoureas and amidines themselves. In 1996, we reported that certain amidines inhibit NOS activity [31]. Recently, an analogue of acetamidine termed 1400W [N-(3-(aminomethyl)benzyl)acetamidine] has been reported to be a slow, tight-binding inhibitor of human iNOS. The inhibition by 1400W of the activity of human iNOS is potent, dependent on the co-factor NADPH, and either irreversible or extremely slowly reversible. Most notably, 1400W was approximately 5000-fold more potent as an inhibitor of iNOS activity than of eNOS activity (human). In a rat model of vascular injury caused by endotoxin, 1400W is 50-fold more potent as an inhibitor of iNOS than eNOS activity and attenuates the vascular leak syndrome [32]. Interestingly, selective inhibition of iNOS activity with 1400W attenuates the circulatory failure (Fig. 2), but not the liver injury/dysfunction (Fig. 3), caused by endotoxin in the rat [33]. In addition to 1400W, L-NIL is a highly selective and potent inhibitor of iNOS activity in the rat [34] and mouse [35]. Like 1400W, L-NIL attenuates the delayed hypotension, but does not reduce the degree

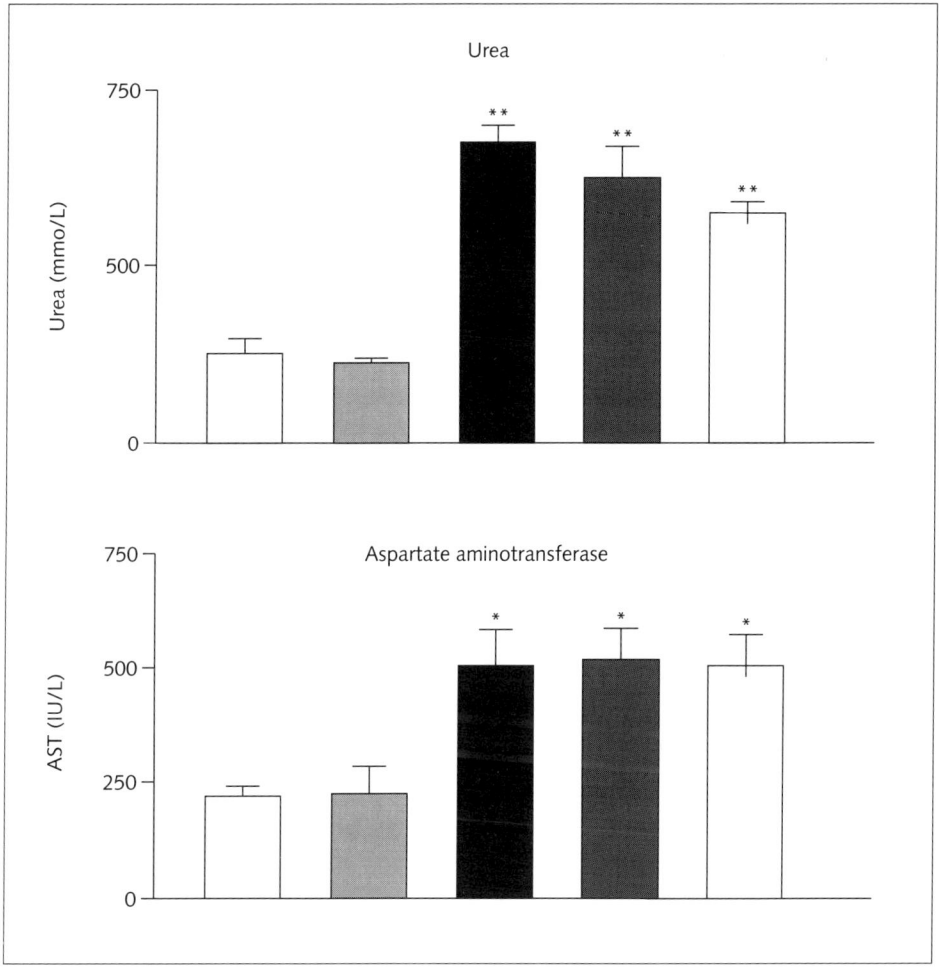

Figure 3
This figure shows the effects of the selective iNOS inhibitor 1400W on the rise in the serum
levels of urea (an indicator of the development of renal dysfunction) and aspartate amino-
transferase (AST, an indicator of hepatocellular injury) in anaesthetised rats challenged with
endotoxin (LPS, 6 mg kg⁻¹ i.v.). Animals received injections of saline rather than LPS and
were treated with infusions of either saline (vehicle for 1400W, open columns, n=10) or
1400W (10 mg kg⁻¹ bolus plus 10 mg kg⁻¹ h⁻¹ (horizontal stripes, n=3). Different groups of
LPS-rats were treated with (starting 2 h after LPS) (i) vehicle (saline control, black columns,
n=10) 1400W 3 mg kg⁻¹ bolus +3 mg kg⁻¹ h⁻¹ (diagonal stripes, n=8) (iii) 1400W 10 mg
*kg⁻¹ bolus + 10 mg kg⁻¹ h⁻¹ (checked column, n=5). *p < 0.01, **p < 0.001 when compared*
by ANOVA to rats which had received vehicle rather than LPS. There were no differences in
urea or AST between the LPS controls and 1400W treated rats.

of renal dysfunction, liver dysfunction or hepatocellular injury caused by endotoxin in the rat [33]. These findings support the view that selective inhibition of
iNOS activity might provide a useful approach in the restoration of blood pressure in patients with shock. Most notably, however, our data are also consistent
with the notion that – as in the case of iNOS knock out mice challenged with
endotoxin [19, 20] – enhanced formation of NO by iNOS primarily contributes
to the circulatory failure, but not to the liver injury or dysfunction caused by endotoxin.

Nitric oxide synthase inhibition in humans with septic shock

Although our understanding of the role of NO in animal models of circulatory
shock has improved substantially over the past years, our knowledge regarding the
biosynthesis and importance of NO in the pathophysiology of patients with septic
shock is still very limited. Although several studies support the view that septic
shock in man is associated with an enhanced formation of NO, it should be stressed
that the increase in the plasma levels of nitrite/nitrate elicited by endotoxin,
cytokines or bacteria in rodents (10-fold) is substantially higher than the observed
increases in the plasma levels of these metabolites of NO in other animal species
(pig, sheep etc) or humans. Early reports of beneficial hemodynamic effects of L-
NMMA in humans with septic shock ([36], see [23] for review) stimulated a phase
I, multi-center, open-label, dose-escalation (1, 2.5, 5, 10 or 20 mg/kg/h for up to
eight h) study using L-NMMA (546C88) in 32 patients with septic shock. In this
study, L-NMMA sustained blood pressure and enabled a reduction in vasopressor
(norepinephrine) support. The cardiac index fell to baseline values (possibly due to
an increase in peripheral vascular resistance) and left ventricular function was well
maintained. Moreover, L-NMMA increased oxygen extraction, while pulmonary
shunt was not worsened [37]. A recent, placebo-controlled multi-center study
involving 312 patients with septic shock, has evaluated the effects of L-NMMA on
the resolution of shock at 72 h (primary endpoint). The severity of illness according
to the SAPS II score was similar between placebo and the L-NMMA group. Infusion
of L-NMMA enhanced mean arterial blood pressure and systemic vascular resistance index and decreased cardiac output (from elevated towards normal levels). L-
NMMA had no effect on left ventricular systolic work index indicating that the fall
in cardiac output was not due to an impairment in cardiac contractility. In patients
treated with L-NMMA, there was a transient increase in mean pulmonary artery
pressure. Interestingly, L-NMMA did not affect the thrombocytopenia or the renal
dysfunction caused by sepsis. Most notably, 41% of patients treated with L-
NMMA, but only 21% of patients treated with placebo, recovered from shock within 72 h. There was also a strong trend for a reduction in mortality (at day 14) in
patients treated with L-NMMA.

Role of endothelin-1 in circulatory shock

There is good evidence that endotoxemia or sepsis leads to a substantial increase in the plasma levels of ET-1. Pronounced rises in the plasma levels of ET-1 occur in experimental endotoxemia or septicemia in rats, dogs, pigs, sheep and baboons [38]. More importantly, enhanced ET-1 serum levels have also been documented in humans with sepsis and septic shock [39, 40]. In man, the serum levels of ET-1 correlate positively with the severity of endotoxemia [39] and are lower in survivors than in non-survivors of septic shock [40]. In patients with sepsis, with or without adult respiratory distress syndrome (ARDS), plasma levels of ET-1 correlated positively with organ failure score and oxygen consumption, and negatively with the $PaO_2:FiO_2$ ratio [41]. There was, however, no correlation between plasma ET-1 and plasma creatinine levels suggesting that a reduction in the clearance of ET-1 does not account for the elevated plasma levels [41]. Although the elevation in the plasma levels of ET-1 are largely due to an enhanced formation of this peptide, there is some evidence that – at least in patients with a substantial impairment of renal function (anuria) – the plasma levels of ET-1 are significantly higher than in those patients without anuria. Thus, a reduction in ET-1 clearance may contribute to the high plasma levels of this peptide in patients with a severe impairment of renal function [38].

Regulation of endothelin formation by pro-inflammatory cytokines

It is often thought that the production of ET-1 is exclusively regulated at the level of gene transcription. In agreement with this view the production of ET-1 by cultured endothelial cells is increased by stimulants such as growth factors and vasoactive substances over the course of hours rather than minutes. ET-1 has, therefore, not been seen as a mediator of rapid responses within the vasculature. There are, however, certain stimuli that will quickly increase the circulating levels of ET-1. One of the first reports noting that ET-1 levels in the circulation could increase rapidly was from studies in humans in which it was shown that such changes followed rapid postural changes [42]. Surgery also appears to cause fairly rapid increases in the circulating levels of ET-1 both in humans [43] and in animals [44]. It appears, therefore, that *in vivo* the circulating levels of ET-1 can be regulated over short periods, i.e. minutes rather than hours [11].

Although the source of ET-1 in endotoxemia is not clear, there is evidence that the release of ET-1 may be triggered by pro-inflammatory cytokines. For instance, intravenous administration of TNFα to rats causes a rapid increase in the circulating levels of ET-1, that are unaffected by pre-treatment of the animals with phosphoramidon [45], suggestive of a release of ET-1 from pre-formed stores. When hearts are removed from rats treated 15 min previously with TNFα and perfused at constant flow *ex vivo* with Krebs' buffer, a profound coronary vasoconstriction is revealed [46]. This vasoconstriction is seen functionally as an increase in coronary perfusion pressure to more than double that seen in hearts removed from sham-treated animals. The coronary vasoconstriction can be positively correlated to the accompanying increase in the circulating level of ET-1, for it is greatly decreased when rats are pre-treated with an endothelin ET_A receptor antagonist or with antibodies directed against ET-1. Similarly, treatment of rats with IL-2 causes an increase in the plasma levels of TNFα which is associated with an increase in the coronary perfusion pressure [46]. More importantly, the coronary vasoconstriction seen in these IL-2-treated rats is reduced by antibodies directed against TNFα or by endothelin ET_A receptor antagonists. There is additional evidence supporting the notion that cytokines may increase the production of ET-1 over the short to medium term (minutes to hours). Intravenous infusion of live bacteria into young pigs causes, within 4 h, increases in the circulating levels of ET-1 which are markedly reduced if the animals are treated with an antibody directed against TNFα. In the baboon, the increase in the circulating concentration of big ET-1 caused by bacteremia/endotoxemia is also reduced by treatment with an anti-TNFα antibody [48]. Furthermore, in humans with sepsis there is a positive correlation between the circulating levels of TNFα and ET-1 [49]. Thus, cytokines, and in particular TNFα, can promote both an increase in the immediate release of ET-1 and also an up-regulation in the expression of ET-1 over periods of hours.

Pro-inflammatory cytokines including TNFα, IL-1 and interferon-γ can also stimulate the release/biosynthesis of ET-1 from a variety of cultured cells (e.g. endothelial cells, epithelial cells, mesangial cells, macrophages, astrocytes etc.) (Tab. 2). For instance, treatment of bovine, porcine or human endothelial cells with any of the above cytokines (or a combination thereof) leads – within hours – to a significant increase in ET-1 release by these cells [38]. However, it is not only the endothelium within the vascular wall that may respond to cytokines by up-regulating their production of ET-1. The vascular smooth muscle, which is not considered to be a source of ET-1 under normal conditions, can also be induced to release ET-1. Treatment of human vascular smooth muscle cells in culture, for instance, with the vasoconstrictor hormones angiotensin II or arginine-vasopressin, TGFβ, platelet-derived growth factor or epidermal-growth stimulates the expression of ET-1 [50]. Taken together, there is evidence that TNFα, IL-1 and interferon-γ stimulate the synthesis/release of ET-1 by a range of endothelial, epithelial and other cell types (Tab. 2).

Role of ET-1 in the hemodynamic alterations associated with sepsis

Vascular hyporeactivity to vasoconstrictors

Sepsis is associated with an impairment in the ability of the vascular smooth muscle to contract in response to a great variety of vasoconstrictors including noradrena-

Table 2 - Enhanced formation of ET-1 by various cells types (in culture) exposed tumour necrosis factor α (TNFα), interleukins (IL), interferon-γ (IFNγ) or to transforming growth factor β (TGFβ).

Cell type	Species	Cytokine
Endothelial	porcine	IL-1, TGFβ, TNFα
	bovine	TNFα, INFγ, IL-1β
	HUVEC	IL-1β
	rat	IL-1α, IL-1β, TNFα
Amnion	human	IL-1β, EGF, TNFα, IL-6
LLCPK1 (renal epithelium)	porcine	TGFβ, TNFα, IL-1β
Airway epithelium	human	IL-1, TNFα, IL-2
	guinea-pig	IL-8, TNFα, TGFβ
Mesenteric artery	rat	IL-2
Vascular smooth muscle	human	TGFβ
Mesangial	human	TGFβ
	rat	TNFα
Breast cancer	human	IL-6

line, adrenaline, serotonin and calcium. Interestingly, the contractile responses elicited by ET-1 in aortic rings of rats subjected to endotoxemia for several hours are not diminished [51]. Similarly, endotoxemia does not cause an impairment of the contractile responses caused by ET-1 in the rat mesentery [52]. In pithed rats, the pressor responses caused by injection of ET-1 are also not attenuated, while those of a variety of other vasoconstrictors are [53]. There is, however, some evidence that the contractile responses to ET-1 are impaired in the microcirculation of animals with sepsis. For instance, in rats made septic by coecal ligation and puncture, the vasoconstrictor responses elicited by ET-1 in the cremaster muscle are significantly reduced. Interestingly, inhibition of NO formation restores the contractile responses to ET-1 in this tissue [54]. Thus it is possible that an overproduction of NO by iNOS in vascular smooth muscle leads to a reduction in the constrictor/pressor responses elicited by ET-1 in some vascular beds (microcirculation?), but not in others (conductance vessels?). Nevertheless, it is possible that inhibitors of NOS activity may reduce vascular diameter by reducing the generation of NO and also by facilitating the vasoconstrictor responses to ET-1. It should be noted that endotoxemia (in the rat) also leads to an increase in the binding of ET-1 to membranes of the kidney. This has been attributed to an increase in receptor density, which in turn may amplify the effects of ET-1. Thus, elevated plasma levels of ET-1 together with

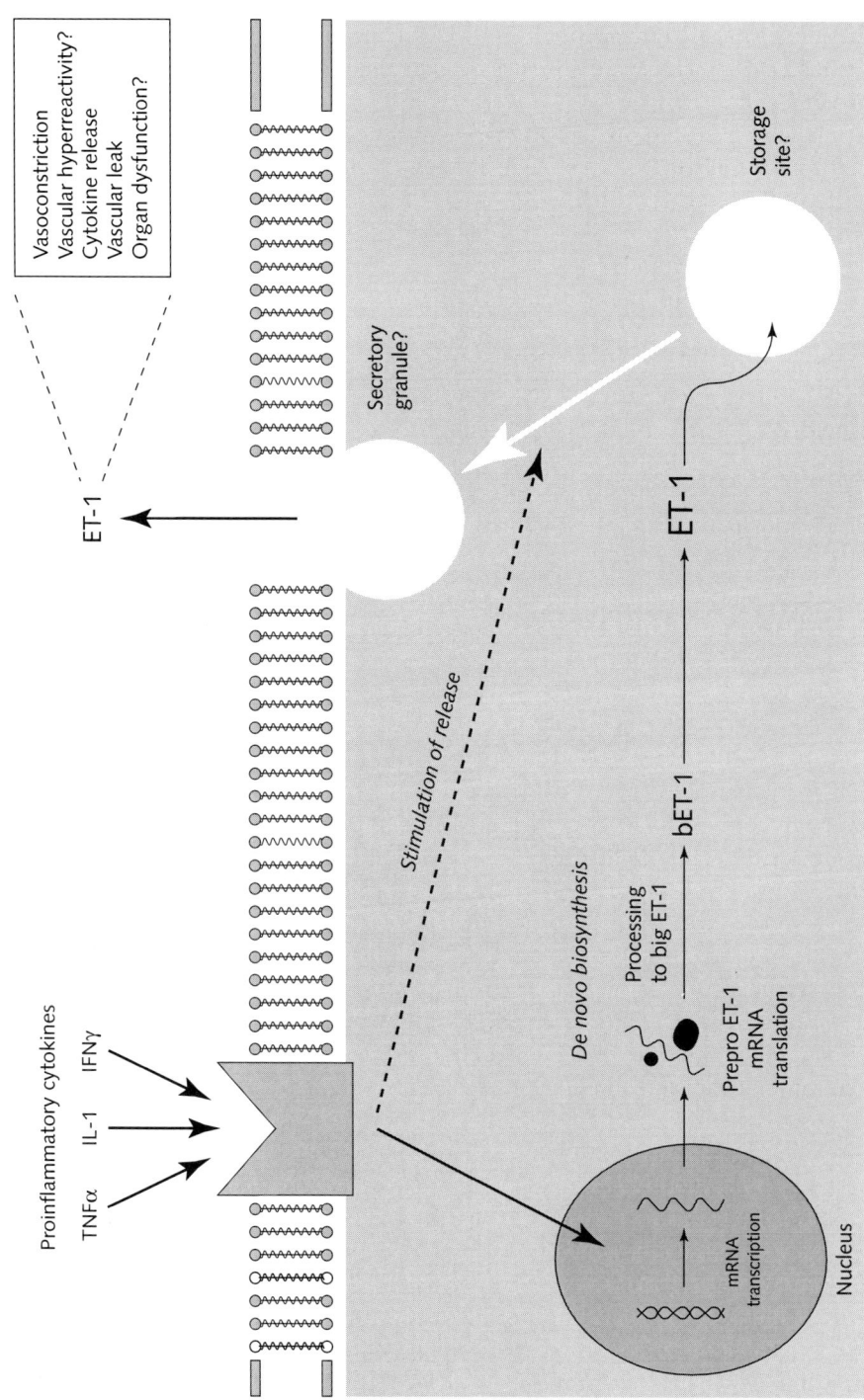

an increase in ET-receptor density may facilitate an ET-1 mediated excessive vaso-constriction (in some vascular beds) (Fig. 4).

ET-1 and alterations in systemic hemodynamics in shock

There is evidence that the enhanced formation of ET-1 in endotoxemia may serve to counteract the severe hypotension. For instance, infusion of ET-1 reduces the fall in both blood pressure and cardiac output caused by endotoxin in dogs (see [38]). Moreover, the non-selective ET_A/ET_B-receptor antagonist SB 209670 aggravates the fall in blood pressure caused by endotoxin in the conscious rat [55]. In the anaes-thetised rat, SB 209670 substantially aggravates the hypotension caused by endo-toxin (Fig. 2) resulting in a reduction in organ perfusion, an increase in organ injury/dysfunction and ultimately in an increase in mortality [56].

ET-1 and the alterations in regional hemodynamics associated with shock

Although the rapid release of ET-1 in endotoxemia helps to maintain blood pressure and organ perfusion (beneficial effects of ET-1), excessive rises in the plasma levels of ET-1 for longer periods are also associated with excessive vasoconstriction in some vascular beds (harmful effects of ET-1). For instance, there is evidence (in pigs and sheep) that the increase in pulmonary, splenic, portal and renal vascular resis-tance correlates positively with an increase in the plasma levels of ET-1 [38]. In con-scious rats, the release of ET-1 afforded by endotoxin contributes to the constriction of the mesenteric (and other) vascular bed(s) [55]. The delayed rise in pulmonary vascular resistance and the associated fall in cardiac output afforded by endotoxin in pigs is also due to an overproduction of ET-1, as it is reduced by the non-selec-tive ET-receptor antagonist bosentan [57, 58]. In pigs with endotoxemia, bosentan also restores cardiac index, increases the stroke volume index and improves systemic

Figure 4
This figure shows the mechanism(s) leading to the overproduction of endothelin-1 (ET-1) in septic shock. The release of pro-inflammatory cytokines including tumor necrosis factor α (TNFα), IL-1 and interferon-γ (IFNγ) leads to the enhanced formation of ET-1 by causing transcription/translation of the preproET-1 gene. Subsequently, preproET-1 is processed by endothelin-converting-enzyme (ECE) to form mature ET-1. ET-1 is secreted (in endothelial cells) via secretory granules which may serve as storage sites for ET-1. Please note that cytokines and other stimuli can auso cause a rapid (within minutes) release of ET-1, the mechanism(s) of which is unknown. Once released, ET-1 may contribute to vasoconstriction, vascular hyperreactivity, organ dysfunction, vascular leak syndrome, defect in tissue oxygen extraction and cytokine release

oxygen delivery and acid base balance. Interestingly, bosentan further augments the rise in the plasma levels of ET-1 caused by endotoxin [57]. The ET_A-receptor antagonist BMS 182874 also attenuates the rise in pulmonary vascular resistance in sheep with endotoxemia (see [38]).

Role of ET-1 in the organ dysfunction associated with endotoxemia or sepsis

Renal dysfunction

Within the kidney, ET-1 is generated by vascular endothelial cells (large vessels), glomerular endothelial cells, renal epithelial cells and proximal tubule cells [59]. The renal vasculature is particularly sensitive to the vasoconstrictor effects of ET-1, with a 10-fold greater response than that observed in bronchial, femoral and coronary arteries [60]. In the kidney, ET-1 causes a reduction in glomerular filtration rate (GFR) and an increase in renovascular resistance. The vasoconstriction is equipotent in the afferent and efferent arterioles, such that the glomerular hydrostatic pressure, the driving force for glomerular filtration, is unaltered [61]. Thus, it has been proposed that the reduction in GFR caused by ET-1 is due to mesangial cell contraction [61]. In a rodent model of endotoxemia, anti-ET antiserum was infused selectively into the left kidney via the renal artery, preventing the fall in GFR in the ipsilateral kidney, but not affecting the fall in GFR in the contralateral, control kidney [61]. Thus, it has been suggested that endogenous ET-1 may contribute to the development of the renal dysfunction associated with endotoxemia. There are, however, also other studies which suggest that the blockade of ET-receptors does not improve renal function in endotoxemia. For instance, the rise in blood urea nitrogen afforded by endotoxin in the rat is not attenuated by pretreatment of the animals with SB 209670 [62]. Similarly, SB 209670 does not affect the rise in the serum levels of creatinine and urea caused by endotoxin in the anaesthetised rat [56]. Selective blockade of ET_A receptors with BQ-485 or of ET_B receptors with BQ-788 did also not reduce the impairment in renal function caused by endotoxin in the rat [63].

Liver injury and dysfunction

In the anaesthetised rat, endotoxaemia for 6 h results in rises in the serum levels of glutamate-oxalate-transferase and glutamate-pyruvate-transferase (indicators of hepatocellular injury) and bilirubin and γ-glutamyl transferase (indicators of liver failure). Treatment of LPS-rats with the ET_B receptor antagonist BQ-788 attenuated the degree of liver injury and failure, while the ET_A receptor antagonist BQ-485 was without effect [63]. In this study, BQ-788 also attenuated the delayed hypotension and the vascular hyporeactivity to noradrenaline caused by endotoxin. The prevention of the hepatocellular dysfunction and injury caused BQ-788 in endotoxaemia may be due to an improvement in oxygen delivery to the liver secondary to

(i) inhibition of pre-sinusoidal constriction, (ii) inhibition of sinusoidal constriction, and (iii) improvement in perfusion pressure [63].

Concluding remarks

There is good evidence that sepsis and endotoxemia is associated with an enhanced formation of the vasoactive autacoids NO and ET-1. The generation of NO (presumably by iNOS) contributes to the fall in peripheral vascular resistance and the vascular hyporeactivity to vasoconstrictor agents. Inhibition of NOS activity restores blood pressure and pressor responses to noradrenaline in animals and man with sepsis. The question as to whether NO contributes to the multiple organ injury and the mortality associated with sepsis is less clear. Stimulation of the formation of ET-1 by pro-inflammatory cytokines accounts for the enhanced formation of these potent pressor peptides in animals and man with endotoxic/septic shock. The over-production of ET-1 may help to counteract the fall in peripheral vascular resistance associated with septic shock (beneficial effects), but exposure of certain vascular beds (mesenteric, liver, lung) to larger amounts of ET-1 (for longer time periods) may result in excessive vasoconstriction and reduction in oxygen supply. Inhibition of the effects of ET-1 may augment the hypotension associated with endotoxemia (in hypodynamic models of sepsis), while inhibition of NOS activity may predispose to vasoconstriction by ET-1. Whether blockade of the effects of ET-1 or inhibition of NOS activity will improve the therapy of patients with septic shock remains to be seen.

Acknowledgements
CT is a Senior Fellow of the British Heart Foundation (FS 918/96). This work was in part funded by a Biomed 2 grant awarded to CT by the European Commission.

References

1   Nathan C (1992) Nitric oxide as a secretory product of mammalian cells. *FASEB J* 6: 3051–3064
2   Dinerman JL, Lowenstein CJ, Snyder SH (1993) Molecular mechanism of nitric oxide regulation: potential relevance to cardiovascular disease. *Circ Res* 73: 217–222
3   Moncada S, Higgs A (1993) The L-arginine-nitric oxide pathway. *N Eng J Med* 329: 2202–2212
4   Morris SM, Billiar TR (1994) New insights into the regulation of inducible nitric oxide synthase. *Am J Physiol* 266: E829–839

5   Szabo C, Thiemermann C (1995) Regulation of the expression of the inducible isoform of nitric oxide synthase. *Adv Pharmacol* 34: 113–154

6   Loscalzo J, Welsch G (1995) Nitric oxide and its role in the cardiovascular system. *Prog Cardiovascular Dis* 38: 87–104

7   Rubanyi GM, Polokoff MA (1994) Endothelins: molecular biology, biochemistry, pharmacology, physiology and pathophysiology. *Pharmacol Rev* 46: 325–415

8   Yanagisawa M, Masaki T (1989) Molecular biology and biochemistry of endothelin. *Trends Pharmacol Sci* 10: 374–378

9   Warner TD (1994) Endothelin receptor antagonists. *Cardiovasc Drug Rev* 12: 105–122

10   Warner TD, Battistini B, Doherty AM, Corder R (1994) Endothelin receptor antagonists: actions and rationale for their development. *Biochem Pharmacol* 48: 625–635

11   Warner T, Klemm P (1996) What turns on the endothelins? Inflamm Res 45: 51–53

12   Thiemermann C, Vane JR (1990) Inhibition of nitric oxide synthesis reduces the hypotension induced by bacterial lipopolysaccharide in the rat. *Eur J Pharmacol* 182: 591–5

13   Kilbourn RG, Gross SS, Jubran A, Adams J, Griffith OW, Levi R, Lodato RF (1990) N^G-methyl-L-arginine inhibits tumour necrosis factor-induced hypotension: implications for the involvement of nitric oxide. *Proc Natl Acad Sci USA* 87: 3629–3632

14   Kilbourn RG, Juburan A, Gross SS, Griffith OW, Levi R, Adams J (1990) Reversal of endotoxin-mediated shock by N^G-monomethyl -L-arginine, an inhibitor of nitric oxide synthesis. *Biochem Biophys Res Commun* 172: 1132–1138

15   Julou-Schaeffer G, Gray GA, Fleming I, Schott C, Parratt JR, Stoclet JC (1990) Loss of vascular responsiveness induced by endotoxin involves the L-arginine pathway. *Am J Physiol* 259: H1038–1043

16   Rees DD, Cellek S, Palmer RMJ, Moncada S (1990) Dexamethasone prevents the induction of nitric oxide synthase and the associated effects on the vascular tone: an insight into endotoxic shock. *Biochem Biophys Res Commun* 173: 541–547

17   Billiar TR, Curran RD, Harbrecht BG, Stuehr DJ, Demetris AJ, Simmons RL (1990) Modulation of nitrogen oxide synthesis *in vivo*: N^G-monomethyl-L-arginine inhibits endotoxin-induced nitrite/nitrate biosynthesis while promoting hepatic damage. *J Leukoc Biol* 48: 565–569

18   Thiemermann C (1994) The role of L-arginine: nitric oxide pathway in circulatory shock. *Adv Pharmacol* 28: 45–79

19   MacMicking JD, Nathan C, Hom G, Chartrain N, Fletcher DS, Trumbauer M, Stevens K, Xie QW, Sokol K, Hutchinson M et al (1995) Altered responses to bacterial infection and endotoxic shock in mice lacking inducible nitric oxide synthase. *Cell* 82: 641–650

20   Wei X, Charles IG, Smith A, Ure J, Feng GJ, Huang FP, Xu D, Muller W, Moncada S, Liew FY (1995) Altered immune responses in mice lacking inducible nitric oxide synthase. *Nature* 375: 408–411

21   Thiemermann C (1998) The use of selective inhibitors of inducible nitric oxide synthase in septic shock. *Sepsis*; *in press*

22 Southan GJ, Szabo C (1996) Selective pharmacological inhibition of distinct nitric oxide synthase isoforms. *Biochem Pharmacol* 51: 383–394

23 Preiser JC, Vincent JL (1996) Nitric oxide involvement in septic shock: Do human beings behave like rodents? In: JL Vincent (ed): *1996 Yearbook of Intensive Care and Emergency Medicine*. Springer-Verlag, Berlin, 358–365

24 Corbett JA, Tilton RG, Chang K, Hasan KS, Ido Y, Wang JL, Sweetland MA, Lancaster JR, Williamson JR, McDaniel ML (1992) Aminoguanidine, a novel inhibitor of nitric oxide formation, prevents diabetic vascular dysfunction. Diabetes 41: 552–558

25 Garvey PE, Oplinger JA, Tanoury GJ, Sherman PA, Fowler M, Marshall S, Marmon MF, Paith JE, Furfine ES (1994) Potent and selective inhibition of human nitric oxide synthases. Inhibition by non-amino acid isothioureas. *J Biol Chem* 269: 26669–26676

26 Szabo C, Southan G, Thiemermann C (1994) Beneficial effects and improved survival in rodent models of septic shock with S-methyl-isothiourea sulfate, a novel, potent and selective inhibitor of inducible nitric oxide synthase. *Proc Natl Acad Sci USA* 91: 12472–12476

27 Southan G, Szabo C, Thiemermann C (1995) Isothioureas: potent inhibitors of nitric oxide synthases with variable isoform selectivity. *Br J Pharmacol* 114: 510–516

28 Thiemermann C, Ruetten H, Wu CC, Vane JR (1995) The multiple organ dysfunction syndrome caused by endotoxin in the rat: Attenuation of liver dysfunction by inhibitors of nitric oxide synthase. *Br J Pharmacol* 116: 2845–2851

29 Saetre T, Gundersen Y, Thiemermann C, Lilleansen P, Aasen AO (1997) Aminoethyl-isothiourea, a selective inhibitor of inducible nitric oxide synthase activity, improves liver circulation and oxygen metabolism in a porcine model of endotoxaemia. *Shock*; *in press*

30 Sprong RC, Aarsman CJM, Oirschot JFLM, Asbeck BS (1997) Dimethylthiourea protects rats against gram-negative sepsis and decreases tumour necrosis factor and nuclear factor κB activity. *J Lab Clin Med* 129: 470–481

31 Southan GJ, Szabo C, O'Conner MP, Salzman AC, Thiemermann C (1996) Amidines are potent inhibitors of constitutive and inducible nitric oxide synthases: Preferential inhibition of the inducible isoform. *Eur J Pharmacol* 291: 311–318

32 Garvey EP, Oplinger JA, Furfine ES, Kiff RJ, Laszlo F, Whittle BJR, Knowles RG (1997) 1400W is a slow, tight binding, and highly selective inhibitor of inducible nitric oxide synthase *in vitro* and *in vivo*. *J Biol Chem* 272: 4959–4963

33 Wray G, Miller CGM, Hinds C, Thiemermann C (1998) Selective inhibition of the activity of inducible nitric oxide synthase prevents the circulatory failure, but not the organ injury/dysfunction caused by endotoxin. *Shock*; *in press*

34 Faraci WS, Nagel AA, Verdries KA, Vincent LA, Xu H, Nichols LE, Labasi JM, Salter ED, Pettipher ER (1996) 2-Amino-4-methylpyridine as a potent inhibitor of inducible NO synthase activity *in vitro* and *in vivo*. *Br J Pharmacol* 119: 1101–1108

35 Moore WM, Webber RK, Jerome GM, Tjoeng FS, Misko TP, Currie MD (1994) L-N6-(1-iminoethyl)lysine: a selective inhibitor of inducible nitric oxide synthase. *J Med Chem* 37: 3886–3888

36   Petros A, Lamb G, Leone A, Moncada S, Bennett D, Vallance P (1994) Effects of a nitric oxide synthase inhibitor in humans with septic shock. *Cardiovasc Res* 28: 34–39

37   Watson D, Donaldson J, Grover R, Mottola D, Guntipalli K, Vincent JL (1995) The cardiopulmonary effects of 546C88 in human septic shock. *Int Care Med* 21: S117

38   Battistini B, Forget MA, Laight D (1996) Potential roles for endothelins in systemic inflammatory response syndrome with particular relationship to cytokines. *Shock* 5: 167–183

39   Pittet JF, Morel DR, Hemsen A, Gunning K, Lacroix JS, Suter PM, Lundberg JM (1991) Elevated plasma endothelin-1 concentrations are associated with the severity of illness in patients with sepsis. *Ann Surg* 213: 261–264

40   Takukawa T, Endo S, Nakae H, Kikichi M, Suzuki T, Inada K, Yoshida M (1994). Plasma levels of TNFα, endothelin-1 and thrombomodulin in patients with sepsis. *Res Commun Chem Pathol Pharmacol* 84: 261–269

41   Sanai L, Haynes WG, MacKenzie A, Grant IS, Webb DJ (1996) Endothelin production in sepsis and the adult respiratory distress syndrome. *Int Care Med* 22: 52–56

42   Kaufmann H, Oribe E, Oliver JA. (1991) Plasma endothelin during upright tilt: relevance for orthostatic hypotension. *Lancet* 338: 1542–1545

43   Haak T, Matheis G, Kohleisen M, Ngo H, Bayersdorf F, Usadel KH (1995) Endothelin during cardiovascular surgery: the effect of diltiazem and nitroglycerin. *J Cardiovasc Pharmacol* 26 (Suppl 3): S494–S496

44   Pollock DM, Divish BJ, Opgenorth TJ (1993) Stimulation of endogenous endothelin release in the anesthetized rat. *J Cardiovasc Pharmacol* 22 (Suppl 8): S295–S298

45   Vemulapalli S, Chiu PJS, Griscti K, Brown A, Kurowski S, Sybertz EJ (1994) Phosphoramidon does not inhibit endogenous endothelin-1 release stimulated by hemorrhage, cytokines and hypoxia in rats. *Eur J Pharmacol* 257: 95–102

46   Klemm P, Warner TD, Hohlfeld T, Corder R, Vane JR (1995) Endothelin 1 mediates ex vivo coronary vasoconstriction caused by exogenous and endogenous cytokines. *Proc Natl Acad Sci USA* 92: 2691–2695

47   Han JJ, Windsor A, Drenning DH, Leeper-Woodford S, Mullen PG, Bechard DE, Sugerman HJ, Fowler AA (1994) Release of endothelin in relation to tumor necrosis factor-α in porcine *Pseudomonas aeruginosa*-induced septic shock. *Shock* 1: 343–346

48   Redl H, Schlag G, Bahrami S, Burrman WA, Strieter RM, Kunkel SC, Daries J, Foulkes R (1994) Big-endothelin release in baboon bacteremia is partially TNF dependent. *J Lab Clin Med* 124: 796–801

49   Takakuwa T, Endo S, Nakae H (1994) Plasma levels of TNF-α, endothelin-1 and thrombomodulin in patients with sepsis. *Res Commun Chem Pathol Pharmacol* 84: 261–269

50   Resink TJ, Hahn AWA, Scott-Burden T, Powell J, Weber E, B̧hler F (1990) Inducible endothelin mRNA expression and peptide secretion in cultured human vascular smooth muscle cells. *Biochem Biophys Res Commun* 168: 1303–1310

51   Auget M, Delaflotte S, Chabrier PE, Braquet P (1990) Loss of contractile stability induced by phenylephrine and endothelin in the aorta of rats treated with endotoxin. *Arch Mal Coeur Vasc* 83: 1187–1190

52 Mitchell JA, Kohlhaas KL, Sorrentino R, Warner TD, Murad F, Vane JR (1993) Induction by endotoxin of nitric oxide synthase in the rat mesentery: Lack of effect on action of vasoconstrictors. *Br J Pharmacol* 109: 265–270

53 Guc MO, Furman BL, Parratt JR (1990) Endotoxin-induced impairment of vasopressor and vasodepressor responses in the pithed rat. *Br J Pharmacol* 101: 913–919

54 Hollenberg SM, Piotrowski MJ, Parillo JE (1997) Nitric oxide synthase inhibition reverses arteriolar hyporesponsiveness to endothelin-1 in septic rats. *Am J Physiol* 272: R969–974

55 Gardiner SM, Kemp PA, March JE, Bennett T (1995) Enhancement of the hypotensive and vasodilator effects of endotoxaemia in conscious rats by the endothelin antagonist, SB 209670. *Br J Pharmacol* 116: 1718–1719

56 Ruetten H, Thiemermann C, Vane JR (1996) Effects of endothelin receptor antagonist, SB 209670, on circulatory failure and organ injury in endotoxic shock in the anaesthetized rat. *Br J Pharmacol* 118: 198–204

57 Weitzberg E, Hemsen A, Rudehill A, Modin A, Wanacek M, Lundberg JM (1997) *Br J Pharmacol* 118: 617–626

58 Yamamoto S, Burman HP, O'Donnell CP, Cahill PA, Robotham JL (1997) Endothelin causes portal and pulmonary hypertension in porcine endotoxemic shock. *Am J Physiol* 272: H1239–1249

59 Miller CGM, Thiemermann C (1997) Nitric oxide in septic shock. In: MS Goligorsky, SS Gross (eds): *Nitric oxide and the kidney*. Chapman & Hall, New York, 271–306

60 Pernow J, Bouther J-F, Franco-Cereceda A, Lacroix JS, Matran R, Lundberg JM (1988) Potent selective vasoconstrictor effects of endothelin in the pig kidney *in vivo*. *Acta Physiol Scand* 134: 573–574

61 Kon V, Badr KF (1991) Biological actions and pathophysiologic significance of endothelin in the kidney. *Kidney Int* 40: 1–12

62 Wellings RP, Corder R, Vane JR (1995) Lack of effect of ET antibody or SB209670 on endotoxin-induced renal failure. *J Cardiovasc Pharmacol* 26 (Suppl 3): S476–478

63 Ruetten H, Thiemermann C (1996) Effect of selective blockade of endothelin ETB receptors on the liver dysfunction and injury caused by endotoxaemia in the rat. *Br J Pharmacol* 119: 479–486

Multistep processes in neutrophil homotypic aggregation and tissue injury

C. Wayne Smith[1], Scott I. Simon[1] and Hartmut Jaeschke[2]

[1]Baylor College of Medicine, Section of Leukocyte Biology, Children's Nutrition Research Center, 1100 Bates, Room 6014, Houston, TX 77030-2600, USA
[2]Pharmacia & Upjohn, Inc., Kalamazoo, MI, USA

This review will deal with two broad aspects of neutrophil function – the mechanisms of neutrophil aggregation, and the mechanisms of neutrophil mediated tissue injury using the liver as a specific example. Much of the work on neutrophil aggregation has been performed *in vitro*, which allows dissection of the molecular mechanisms involved, and much of the work regarding tissue injury reveals tissue specific features that could not have been predicted by studies of isolated neutrophils *in vitro*.

Neutrophil aggregation

Isolated blood neutrophils mixed in suspension will adhere to one another when stimulated with soluble chemotactic factors such as complement component C5a, formyl peptides, platelet activating factor (PAF), Interleukin-8 (IL-8), or leukotriene-B$_4$ (LTB$_4$). This process of homotypic aggregation has been used extensively as a model of neutrophil adhesion as well as a model of a potentially pathogenic process. Neutrophil aggregates have been observed in the blood and microvessels under conditions of complement activation and chemokine production *in vivo* such as that occurring during hemodialysis, systemic lupus erythematosus, and myocardial infarction [1–5]. Leukocyte-platelet aggregates have been observed by intravital microscopy following systemic inflammatory activation induced by cigarette smoke, a process linked to the induction of PAF-like oxidized phospholipids [6], and in ischemic episodes in cardiac tissue [7]. Accumulation of aggregates in microvessels may contribute to tissue-ischemia and injury. Neutrophil adhesion to other neutrophils may also provide a mechanism of recruitment at sites of inflammation. Recent studies have shown that neutrophils rolling on a substrate in a parallel plate flow chamber *in vitro* may recruit other neutrophils from the free stream, thereby providing an alternate means of marginating leukocytes at shear rates typical of venular blood flow [8–11]. Homotypic adhesion can thus occur under physiologically relevant shear conditions and, as will be discussed below, occurs efficiently only at venular shear rates ($\sim 100-1000$ s^{-1}). It has now become clear that the transition from tethering to cell arrest under hydrodynamic shear proceeds as a sequence of adhesive events involving several classes of adhesion molecules.

Homotypic adhesion and neutrophil emigration

In the systemic circulation as observed by intravital microscopy in the mesenteric or cremasteric vascular beds, leukocytes typically adhere to the endothelium in the post capillary venules, where shear rates have been estimated to be from less than 100 s^{-1} up to 1000 s^{-1}, depending on the blood flow rate and vessel diameter. The magnitude of the shear rate as well as interactions with red blood cells in the flow stream displace leukocytes from the central position where flow is greatest to the margin of the vessel where they can interact with the endothelium and adherent leukocytes. The shear rate determines key factors that influence the probability that leukocytes will adhere, including viscous forces that drive the cell motion, and the frequency and duration of collisions between cells and the vessel wall [12]. In this region of the microcirculation, the dominant cellular interaction observed is leukocyte rolling on the endothelial lining of the vessel wall [13, 14]. During acute inflammation, the number of rolling leukocytes markedly increases, but the number that adhere and emigrate into the extravascular tissue is low relative to the number of leukocytes passing through the vessel [15, 16]. The rolling behavior of leukocytes does not require activation of the leukocytes, but is largely mediated by members of the selectin family of adhesion molecules expressed on stimulated endothelial cells [17, 18]. The precise mechanisms that mediate the transition from cell rolling to stable adhesion are largely undefined but include stimulation of leukocytes by chemotactic factors presented on the endothelial surface (e.g. PAF and IL-8), and ligation of a leukocyte selectin (CD62L) and endothelial selectins (CD62P and CD62E). These events signal within seconds activation of a portion of the expressed CD18-integrins to adopt an active state characterized by high avidity binding to ligands (e.g. intercellular adhesion molecule-1 (ICAM-1)) on the endothelium [19–21]. The formation of these bonds in sufficient numbers enables the transition from rolling to shear-resistant adhesion [22].

The concept of a multistep cascade of molecular recognition, cell activation, and transition to firm adhesion that characterizes leukocyte adhesion to endothelium in systemic venules under conditions of shear also applies to adhesion between neutrophils [20]. The primary mechanism of capture is mediated by a selectin on one cell binding to sialylated and flucosylated ligands on another [23, 24]. The second step in homotypic neutrophil interactions is integrin-mediated shear resistant aggregation. Many of the same stimuli (e.g. PAF and IL-8) activate high avidity integrin binding and enable firm adhesion in both homotypic and heterotypic (i.e. to endothelium) adhesion [25–27].

Measurement of homotypic aggregation

Most of the early studies were conducted on an aggregometer with high concentrations of isolated neutrophils ($\sim 10^7$/ml) that were mixed with a magnetic stir bar in a cylindrical glass tube. Aggregation was revealed by the increase in light transmittance through the turbid cell suspension [2, 4, 28–31]. Protocols designed to obtain maximum aggregation used non-physiological stimulus conditions such as cytochalasin-B followed by chemotactic stimulation, or phorbol esters. While these studies demonstrated that homotypic neutrophil aggregation could occur, the stimuli provided poor sensitivity, and distorted normal cell physiology.

While mixing cell suspensions in conventional aggregometers provides a high intercellular encounter frequency, it does so by producing shear fields that are too complex to allow precise calculations of shear rate. Recent refinements in methodology have enabled studies of the interplay between shear rate and the underlying adhesive events. Rotational viscometry has been used to apply precise and uniform shear rates to cell suspensions, and the size distribution of aggregates has been detected by flow cytometry. This provides a marked increase in sensitivity for detecting aggregate formation, and the process can be mathematically modeled based on a theory that describes the interaction of spherical particles mixed in a linear shear field [32]. These approaches have enabled analysis of aggregation and disaggregation in terms of fluid shear rate (G) and shear stress (viscosity $\times$ G), and the kinetics of adhesion receptor activation and binding.

Stimulation of neutrophils ($\sim 10^6$ cells/ml) while being sheared in a cone and plate viscometer results in a reversible process over several minutes that is characterized by three distinct phases of aggregation (Fig. 1) [33, 34]. The first phase is detected within seconds of the addition of an agonist (e.g. formyl peptide). Under optimum conditions > 90% of the neutrophils can be recruited into aggregates within 30 seconds. While the rate and extent of aggregation is a function of the shear rate, the relationship is complex [34]. The uniform gradient in the velocity streamlines of a linear shear field cause the cells closer to the rotating cone surface to move faster than the cells near the stationary plate, resulting in cell-cell collisions and the formation of aggregates stable enough to be measured (Fig. 1). Aggregation rate coefficients can be mathematically derived from a system of differential equations that describe the recruitment of singlets into aggregates. The average adhesion efficiency can then be computed from the ratio of the aggregate rate coefficients to the total number of cell collisions estimated from the two body collision theory [35]. This aggregation efficiency is assumed to reflect the intrinsic biological properties of the cell that determine adhesivity and, as modeled, is independent of the experimental parameters such as the initial cell concentration and the shear rate. As shown in Figure 2, at shear rates of 400–800 s^{-1}, a peak efficiency of 80% (8 out of 10 collisions resulting in aggregation) occurs over the first phase of aggregation. However, at the highest (3000 s^{-1}) and lowest (100 s^{-1}) shear rates applied, the efficiency is

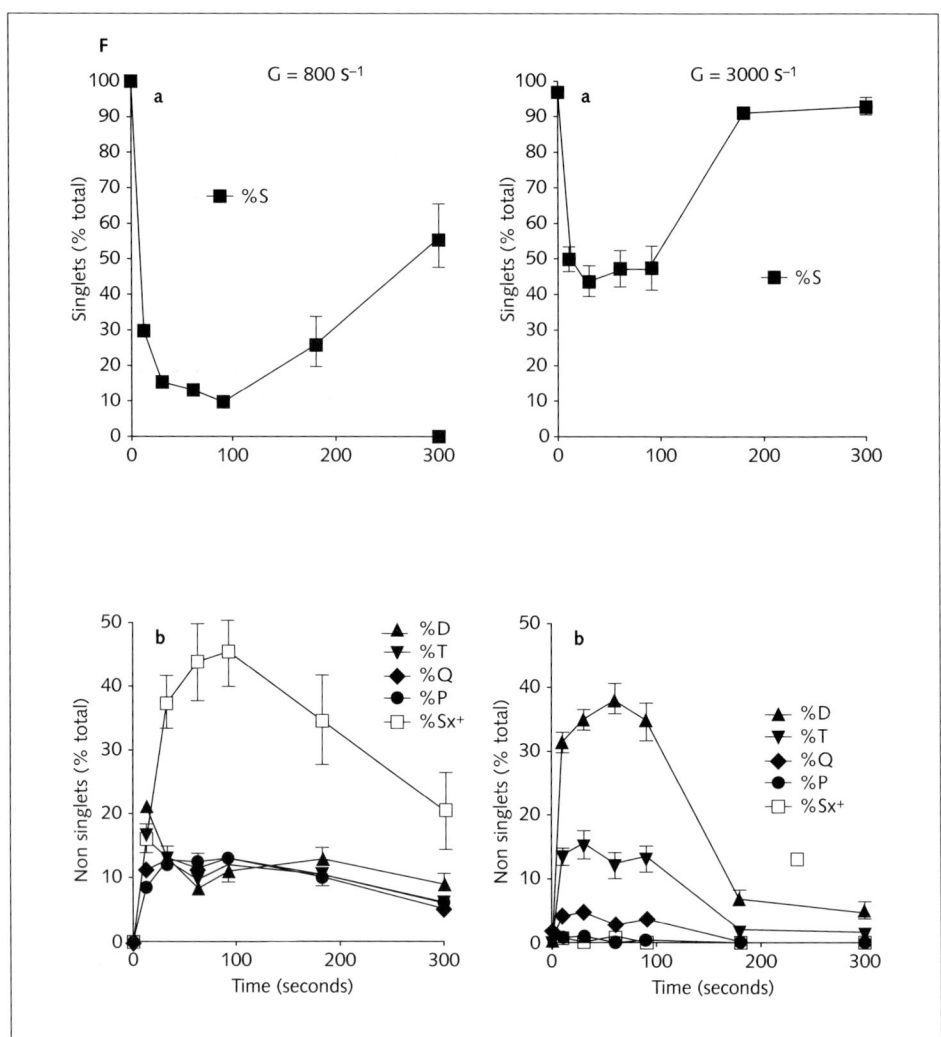

Figure 1
Kinetics of neutrophil aggregation at two shear rates.
Isolated neutrophils were incubated in 37°C buffer for 3 min, stimulated with 1 μM fMLP, and exposed to a constant shear in a cone plate viscometer. Samples were taken at various times and fixed with 2% glutaraldehyde and aggregate sizes were quantitated on a fluorescence flow cytometer. Singles and aggregates were calculated as percentage of total neutrophils. The distribution of (a) singlets and (b) doublets through sextuplets+, mean ± SEM are shown, for shear rates of 800 and 3000 s⁻¹, respectively.
%D, percent doublets; %T, percent triplets; %Q, percent quadruplets; %P, percent pentuplets; %Sx+, percent sextuplets or greater

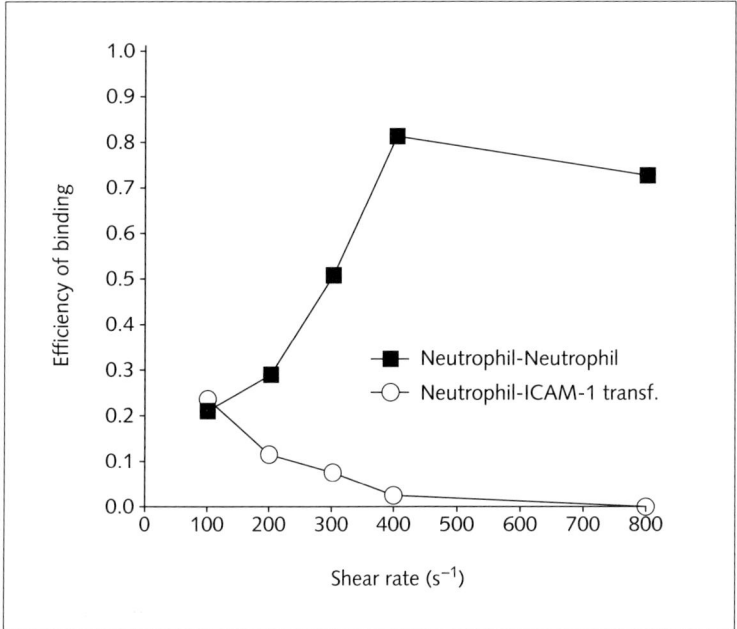

Figure 2
The efficiency of homotypic neutrophil binding to ICAM-1 transfectants over a range of shear.
Neutrophils in the presence or absence of ICAM-1 transfectants were stimulated with 1 μM FMLP and exposed to prescribed shear rates. The adhesion efficiency of neutrophil-neutrophil and neutrophil E3-ICAM-1 cells was determined from the kinetics of the mean particle distributions for n = 5 experiments. The decrease in efficiency with shear was also observed in neutrophil homotypic aggregation pretreated with anti-L-selectin [35].

only 20% [34]. The magnitude of neutrophil adhesion efficiency is remarkable when compared to other activation-dependent blood cell aggregation such as platelets that reach optimum efficiencies of ~25% with adenosine diphosphate (ADP) activation [36].

The boost in adhesion efficiency following chemotactic stimulation as shear increases up to 800 s⁻¹ was not observed in the absence of L-selectin or its counter structure P-selectin glycoprotein ligand-1 (PSGL-1). Blocking these receptors with Fab fragments to these receptors, or cleaving them with proteases [34], resulted in adhesion mediated solely by CD18 integrins. Integrin-mediated adhesion efficiency under these conditions was observed to decrease from a maximum level equal to control, untreated neutrophils at 100 s⁻¹, down to approximately zero by 400 s⁻¹.

This observation of integrin sufficient adhesion at low shears is also observed for neutrophils binding to ICAM-1 expressing cells (Fig. 2) and *in vivo* during tissue ischemia.

The second phase, characterized by aggregate stability, follows the time point of maximal aggregation. A steady state plateau phase is observed over a period of 1–2 minutes (Fig. 1). The stability of these aggregates has been demonstrated by stimulating cells for 30s and then diluting the suspension to reduce the encounter frequency by 2500 fold, thereby drastically limiting new aggregate formation. Following dilution, no significant change in aggregate distribution occurs over the period from 30 to 120s of stimulation. Formed aggregates are also observed to be resistant to shear stress as shown by an experiment in which the shear rate is boosted from the optimum level of 400 s^{-1} to 3000 s^{-1}. Stepping up the shear over the plateau phase does not cause premature disaggregation.

The third phase appears to reflect changes that are occuring during the period of aggregate stability. A rapid transition to disaggregation is consistently observed at 100–150 seconds (Fig. 1), and its rate is directly proportional to the magnitude of the shear stress applied [35]. The mechanism of disaggregation appears to involve both active cell shape change and a decrease in adhesion. The cells adopt a bipolar shape by the 2 min time point [35, 37]. This is accompanied by a three-fold reduction in the area of cell-cell contact, and coincides with the biphasic time course of F-actin formation [38]. Following these changes, the strength of intercellular adhesion is exceeded by the hydrodynamic forces, and disaggregation of virtually the entire population of aggregates proceeds within seconds.

Molecular interactions supporting homotypic neutrophil adhesion

Early studies on patients deficient in CD18-integrin (leukocyte adhesion deficiency I) [39], demonstrated the requirement for CD11b/CD18 (Mac-1, Complement receptor type 3) in homotypic aggregation [40, 41]. Simon et al. found that antibodies to L-selectin were as effective as those against CD18 in blocking aggregation. These studies were performed with isolated neutrophils and in diluted whole blood by fluorescence flow cytometry. A critical feature in achieving inhibition with anti-L-selectin was the use of Fab fragments rather than whole IgG. In fact, preincubation with whole IgG of anti-L-selectin monoclonal antibodies consistently resulted in aggregation in the absence of chemotactic stimulation. This response was mediated in part by Fc receptors since it was reduced by pretreating cells with Fab fragments of antibodies to the Fc receptors on neutrophils. Thus, it appeared that homotypic aggregation of neutrophils required both L-selectin and Mac-1.

Subsequent experiments have provided evidence that L-selectin is essential for transient adhesion, while CD18-integrin serves to stabilize adhesive interactions and enable aggregation. The dynamics of the molecular binding are illustrated in exper-

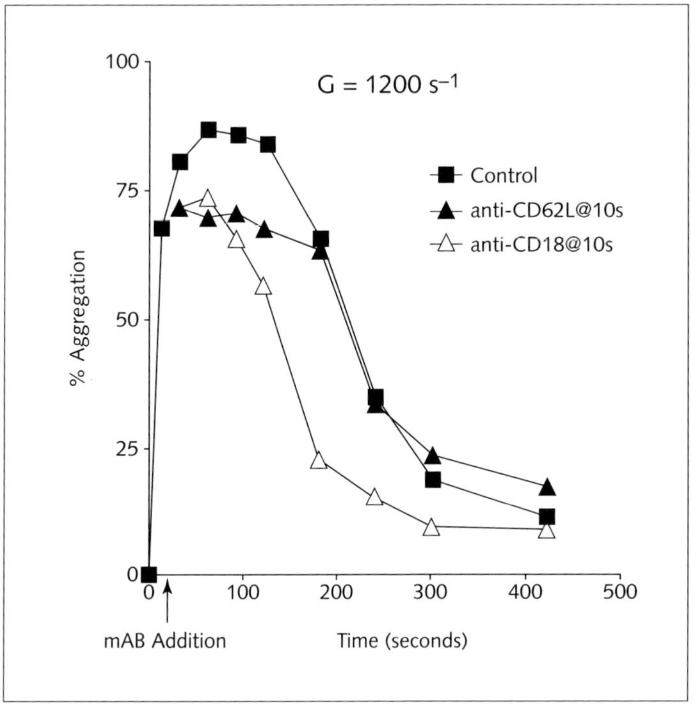

Figure 3
Inhibition of aggregate formation by addition of anti-CD62L or anti-CD18 mAbs after fMLP stimulation.
Neutrophils (10^6 cells/ml) were stimulated with 1 μM fMLP and exposed to $G = 1200\ s^{-1}$. After 10 s, suprasaturating concentrations of DREG-200 Fab (50 μg/ml) to CD62L or IB4 (50 μg/ml) to CD18 were added. The kinetics of aggreate formation are plotted for control, anti-CD62L, and anti-CD18. Samples were taken at indicated time points and fixed with 2% glutaraldehyde. Shown are the fraction of singlets forming aggregates. Kinetics are representative of four separate experiments.

iments where either L-selectin or Mac-1 is blocked by addition of monoclonal antibody (MAb) over the time course of chemotactic stimulation [34, 42]. There is a marked decrease in the extent of aggregation when either receptor is blocked at ten seconds following addition of stimulus, a time point when new aggregate formation is most rapid (Fig. 3). In contrast, addition of anti-L-selectin MAb at 30 seconds to existing aggregates at the beginning of the plateau phase does not alter the kinetics of adhesion. Addition of blocking antibody to CD18 at 10 or 30 seconds causes premature breakup of aggregates. These observations support the concept of a multistep process in which L-selectin is essential for the initial step in the formation of aggregates. Additional studies indicate that P-selectin glycoprotein ligand-1 (PSGL-1) serves as one counter-structure for L-selectin [9, 43]. Activated CD18-integrin then stabilizes the otherwise transient cell contacts, a process that is complete within 30 seconds. The high adhesion efficiency immediately after chemotactic stimulation is apparently a function of a fast and efficient rate of bond formation which vastly exceeds the rate of bond breakage. Adhesion efficiency decreases gradually over the initial 30 seconds after stimulation [35] such that neutrophils stimulated in the absence of shear do not aggregate if shear is introduced within 2–3 minutes. Although L-selectin contributes to the time-dependent change in efficiency, under conditions in which its shedding was blocked with an inhibitor of the metalloprotease, adhesivity still decreased to zero [35].

While the events just described seem to occur at shear rates where aggregation is most efficient (i.e. between 400 and 800 s^{-1}), the contributions of L-selectin appear to exhibit a shear threshold [44, 45]. Aggregation at low shears (e.g. 100 s^{-1}) is independent of L-selectin but requires expression and activation of the CD18-integrin. The role of Mac-1, LFA-1 and ICAM-3 have been studied using blocking MAbs [46]. ICAM-3 is expressed on neutrophils and has been shown to be a ligand for LFA-1 on resting and activated T cells [47]. When neutrophils are preincubated with either anti-LFA- 1 or anti-Mac-1 the efficiency of aggregation is inhibited by 30% over the initial 30 seconds following stimulation. Preincubation with a combination of MAbs to both LFA-1 and Mac-1 decreases adhesion efficiency to zero. Preincubation of PMN with anti-ICAM-3 also inhibits aggregation by 30%. In a series of blocking studies, the paradigm that has emerged is that homotypic aggregation at low shear is supported by LFA-1 interacting with ICAM-3, but the ligands recognized by Mac-1 remain to be discovered.

At shear rates optimal for homotypic aggregation (400 s^{-1}), the estimated duration of cell contact in the absence of firm adhesion is estimated to be 6 msec. This interval is insufficient for adhesion mediated through binding of Mac-1 and LFA-1 alone either between neutrophils or to ICAM-1-expressing target cells [47a]. However, given sufficient bonding time (e.g. at a shear rate 100 s^{-1} and corresponding encounter duration of ~25 msec) CD18-integrin dependent adhesion can form and moreover withstand high tensile stress (> 10 dynes/cm^2). At shear rates greater than 400 s^{-1} the encounter duration should still be well within the molecular association rate reported for selectins (~$10^7 s^{-1}$). Therefore, a critical function of the L-selectin bond, which has been reported to have a lifetime of 150 msec [44], is to enable sufficient Mac-1 and LFA-1 bonds to form stable adhesion. The importance of selectins in the transition to integrin-mediated arrest is apparent when one considers hydrodynamics alone. A leukocyte colliding with a vessel wall [12] at a venular shear rate of 100 s^{-1} would experience an encounter duration on the order of 1 ms, an interval insufficient for integrin dependent adhesion. A second potentially important mechanism for this transition is supported through ligation and clustering of L-selectin. This process results in intracellular signaling and rapid activation of CD18-integrins leading to neutrophil adhesion in shear flow [46, 48, 49].

These studies performed on neutrophils under defined shear rates support a model for integrin binding and anchoring that is dependent on contact duration. Neutrophil adhesion efficiency is limited at shear rates above 400 s^{-1} in sheared cell suspensions. The implications for neutrophil recruitment *in vivo* are that hydrodynamics and collisional geometries influence targeting of cells to sites of inflammation. This concept has been corroborated by observations *in vivo* under low flow conditions in which a shift towards integrin dependent adhesion is observed [50, 51]. At physological levels of shear the intrinsic binding kinetics and function of selectins and integrins may enable target adhesion as a function of the local shear rates and stress.

Neotrophil-induced hepatocyte necrosis

Neutrophils contribute to ischemia-reperfusion injury in most major organs, e.g., heart [52, 53], liver [54, 55], and intestine [56]. They cause liver injury during endotoxemia [57, 58], lung injury after complement activation [59], alcoholic hepatitis [60], and immune complex-mediated lung and kidney injury [61, 62]. In many cases there appears to be damage to vascular endothelial cells, with plasma protein leakage and edema formation. In addition, emigrating neutrophils can adhere to and injure parenchymal cells, often leading to parenchymal cell death. Neutrophil-induced parenchymal cell damage has been documented and extensively studied in the liver.

The mechanisms of liver injury by neutrophils can be divided into at least three steps – the initial sequestration of neutrophils in the hepatic vasculature; migration out of the sinusoids (if vascular lining cells are intact), and adherence-dependent cytotoxicity against hepatocytes. Each of these steps will be discussed separately. Other potential contributing factors to inflammatory liver injury, which will not be discussed in detail, include the activation of the resident Kupffer cells and newly-recruited macrophages, accumulation of cytotoxic lymphocytes, platelet aggregation, microcirculatory disturbances, or perfusion failure resulting in ischemic injury.

Sequestration of neutrophils in the liver vasculature

Neutrophils accumulate in sinusoids and in post-sinusoidal venules during ischemia-reperfusion [63, 64] and endotoxemia [57, 65] (Fig. 4). A variety of inflammatory mediators generated during reperfusion or endotoxemia have been shown to cause hepatic neutrophil sequestration. This includes activated complement factors [66], tumor necrosis factor α (TNFα) [67, 68], interleukin-1 (IL-1) [68], platelet-activat-

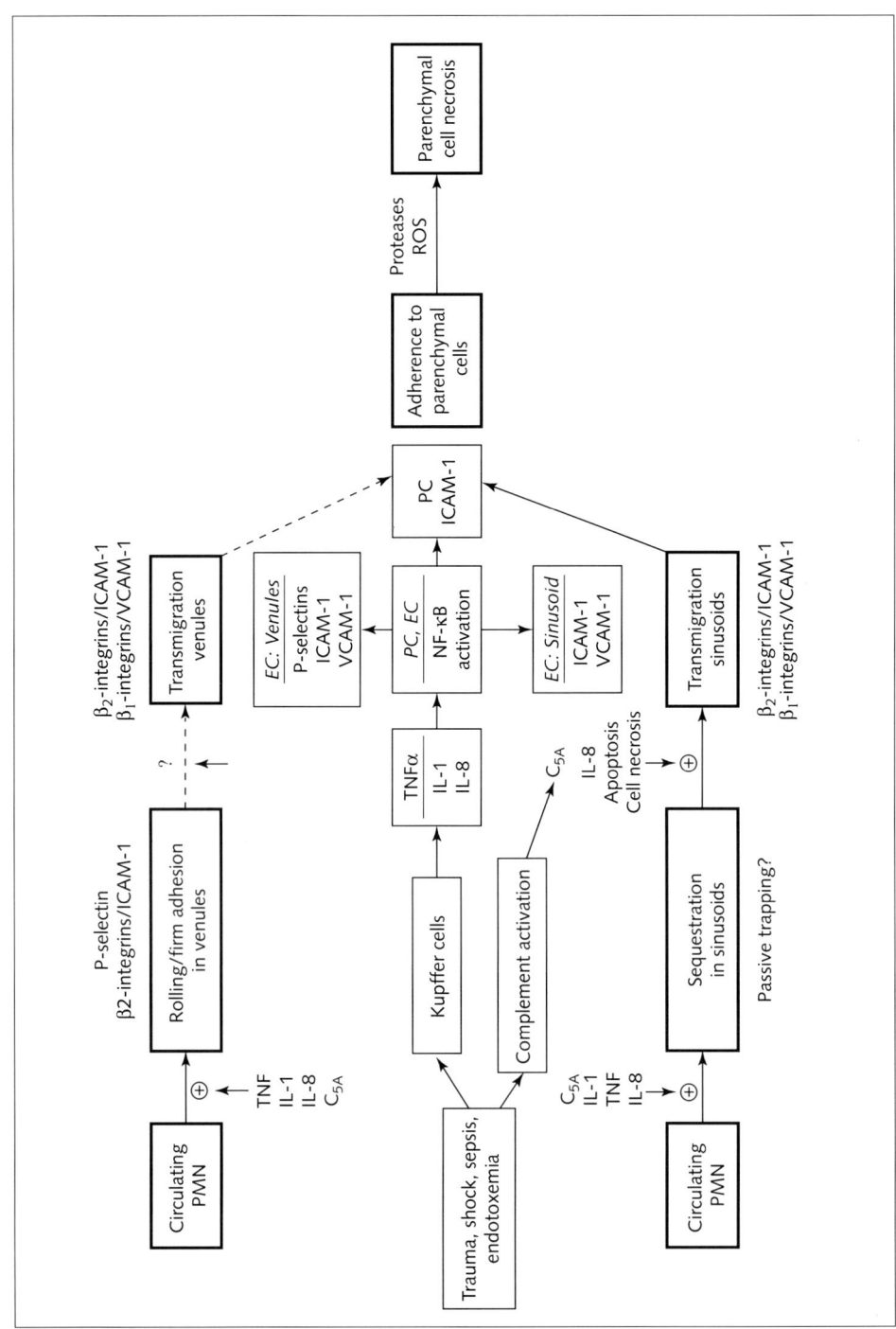

ing factor (PAF) [69], and chemokines such as cytokine-inducible neutrophil chemotactic factor (CINC) [70–72] and epithelial neutrophil activating protein-78 (ENA-78) [73, 74]. Because in most pathophysiological situations a combination of these mediators is formed, there may be additive effects [75]. The impact of any one individual mediator is often difficult to assess. For example, lack of TNFα in mice completely prevents hepatic neutrophil accumulation in response to a low dose of endotoxin [67, 68]. In contrast, TNFα antibodies do not prevent hepatic neutrophil accumulation after high doses of endotoxin in rats [76, 77]. Apparently, low dose endotoxin will generate only TNFα as the proximal mediator, whereas the high dose will also activate complement [75, 78], which is able to elicit neutrophil responses.

TNFα and complement factors increase surface expression and function of the CD18 integrin Mac-1 (CD11b/CD18) on neutrophils [78]. TNFα and IL-1β are responsible for transcriptional activation of intercellular adhesion molecule-1 (ICAM-1) [68, 79–81], vascular cell adhesion molecule-1 (VCAM-1) [82], E-selectin, and P-selectin [79, 83] in the liver. The increase of ICAM-1 mRNA levels and protein expression can be detected in all liver cell types including hepatocytes [79–81, 84–86], hepatic endothelial cells [79], Kupffer cells [79], stellate cells [87], and pit cells [88]. In contrast, VCAM-1 and selectins are only expressed on endothelial cells and Kupffer cells [79, 82, 83]. Detailed immunohistochemical analysis indicates that VCAM-1 can be induced on the entire hepatic endothelium [82]. P-Selectin is predominantly expressed on endothelial cells of larger vessels but is not found on sinusoidal cells [83]. The distribution of various adhesion molecules in experimental models agrees with those in human livers under pathophysiological conditions [89–91].

The functional importance of these adhesion molecules has been studied *in vitro* under flow conditions and *in vivo* in systemic vascular beds [92, 93]. In general, as described above, selectins and their ligands are responsible for the inital contact of neutrophils with the endothelium, and local inflammatory mediators stimulate Mac-1 and LFA-1 to mediate the firm adhesion of the neutrophil to the vessel wall [92, 93]. In contrast to these findings which seem to apply primarily to post-capillary venules, neutrophils relevant for liver injury accumulate predominantly in the sinusoids and not in post-sinusoidal venules [65]. Moreover, antibodies to the relevant adhesion molecules in the setting of post-capillary venules have no effect on the initial sequestration of neutrophils in sinusoids [68, 75, 82–84, 94].

Figure 4

General mechanisms of neutrophil (PMN) accumulation in sinusoids and venules of the liver. EC, endothelial cells; PC, parenchymal cells/hepatocytes; TNFα, tumor necrosis factor-α; IL-1, interleukin-1; IL-8, interleukin-8 and related chemokines; ICAM-1, intercellular adhesion molecule-1; VCAM-1, vascular cell adhesion molecule-1; ROS, reactive oxygen species; NF-κB, nuclear factor-κB; C_{5A}, chemotactic complement fragment from C5.

An adherence-independent mechanism seems to be involved. Due to their deformability, neutrophils can move rapidly through the narrow sinusoidal network of a normal liver, much as they do through the pulmonary capillary network of the alveolus [15]. However, during an inflammatory response in the liver, there is substantial swelling of sinusoidal lining cells [95]. In addition, vasoconstrictors such as endothelin-1 are generated [96], and they are not always completely compensated by release of vasodilators such as nitric oxide [97]. The resulting narrowing of sinusoids may contribute to neutrophil trapping. These microvascular changes in the liver are particularly significant in light of the fact that neutrophils develop reduced deformability after exposure to inflammatory mediators [98]. In fact, activated neutrophils accumulate even in a normal liver [99, 100]. Neutrophils apparently can be mechanically trapped in liver sinusoids under proinflammatory conditions.

Though sinusoidal neutrophils may appear to be primed [69, 101, 102], there is little evidence for reactive oxygen formation in sinusoids. Exposure to two independent stimulus conditions (e.g. ischemia/reperfusion and endotoxemia) can activate sinusoidal neutrophils to generate reactive oxygen in the vasculature [103, 104]. However, even under these circumstances, neutrophils fail to contribute to parenchymal cell injury [104]. The injury to endothelial cells [104, 105] and parenchymal cells is caused mainly by Kupffer cells [63, 104], which are also activated by complement factors [66, 103]. One apparent reason for the limited impact of sinusoidal phagocytes is the neutralization of cytotoxic mediators by glutathione release into the sinusoids [106–108]. Additional experiments have shown that loading the liver with primed neutrophils fails to significantly disturb the hepatic microcirculation or cause parenchymal cell injury [99, 100]. Stimulation with the non-physiological agonist phorbol myristate acetate results in tissue injury [99], though distinguishing between the effects of release of cytotoxic mediators and microcirculatory failure is problematic [99]. Thus, it appears that neutrophil accumulation in the hepatic vasculature is insufficient to cause irreversible parenchymal cell damage.

Transendothelial migration

In models where the sinusoidal endothelium is intact, neutrophils must emigrate to attack hepatocytes [57, 65, 109]. The pathophysiologically relevant transmigration in the liver occurs predominantly in sinusoids [65]. This situation is fundamentally different when compared with other organs such as the intestine or heart [53, 92]. The transmigration process in the liver is apparently dependent on CD18 integrins and ICAM-1 [68], and β1 integrins/VCAM-1 [82]. Though transcriptional up-regulation of ICAM-1 [68] and VCAM-1 [82] on sinusoidal endothelial cells is necessary, that alone is insufficient for emigration. Comparison of IL-1 and TNFα administration to galactosamine-sensitized animals showed that despite ICAM-1 induction and hepatic neutrophil sequestration in both groups, only TNF/galactosamine treatment resulted in neutrophil transmigration and injury [68]. A potential difference between the effect of IL-1 and TNFα is that only TNFα was found to up-regulate the Mac-1 (CD11b/CD18) on neutrophils [68], and Mac-1 has been shown to be critical for endotoxin-induced liver injury [57]. Recent evidence suggests that C-X-C chemokines (e.g. IL-8, CINC, KC/Gro, ENA-78) may play an important role in neutrophil extravasation. Overexpression of CINC by transfecting its gene into liver cells induced neutrophil sequestration and extravasation with significant parenchymal cell damage *in vivo* [70]. Endotoxin treatment of mice causes neutrophil sequestration in the hepatic vasculature, however, only animals with an additional injection of galactosamine showed neutrophil transmigration and injury [65]. In this model, parenchymal cell apoptosis proved to be the signal for extravasation of neutrophils and their attack on hepatocytes [110]. These observations point to the importance of transendothelial migration as a necessary step in the mechanisms of neutrophil-induced liver injury, and the generation of C-X-C chemokines is able to promote this step under certain conditions *in vivo*. Of particular interest and importance is the fact that hepatocytes can produce C-X-C chemokines *in vitro* in response to various cytokines [111, 112], and hepatocytes have been shown to produce the bulk of C-X-C chemokines in the liver *in vivo* [71, 73, 74]. Neutralizing antibodies to C-X-C chemokines have proved to be effective against neutrophil-induced liver injury during ischemia-reperfusion [74] and partial hepatectomy [73]. The transmigration step is largely circumvented if the sinusoidal lining cells are damaged or even removed, e.g. during severe ischemia-reperfusion injury [113–115]. Neutrophils can then find direct access to parenchymal cells.

Neutrophil adherence to hepatocytes

Neutrophils adherent to hepatocytes during endotoxemia have been observed by electron microscopy [109]. Though activated neutrophils can generate a brief oxidative burst in suspension when stimulated with chemotactic factors, adherence to cells or extracellular matrix proteins will substantially increase and prolong the release of reactive oxygen [116, 117]. The adherence-dependent oxidant burst depends on Mac-1 (CD11b/CD18) on neutrophils binding to a relevant counterligand (e.g. ICAM-1 or fibrinogen) [116]. This phenomenon has been observed with neutrophils adherent to parenchymal cells *in vitro* (e.g. cardiac myocytes [118] and hepatocytes [119]) Antibodies to Mac-1 and ICAM-1 were shown to reduce the adherence of stimulated neutrophils to *Listeria monocytogenes*-infected hepatocytes *in vitro*, and they attenuated reactive oxygen production [119].

This phenomenon may be applicable to interactions of neutrophils with hepatocytes in other inflammatory settings. Though hepatocytes do not constitutively express ICAM-1 [79–81, 84, 86], stimulation with cytokines such as TNFα, IL-1α, IL-1β, or interferon-γ (IFNγ) transcriptionally activates the ICAM-1 gene and increases the expression of ICAM-1 on rat, mouse, and human hepatocytes *in vitro* [80, 81, 86] and *in vivo* [68, 79, 84, 89–91, 94, 109]. Cytokine stimulation also leads to the release of a soluble form of ICAM-1 [85, 86, 120]. A recent, more detailed, evaluation of adhesion molecules involved in the adherence of neutrophils to hepatocytes *in vitro* indicated that unstimulated neutrophils adhere to cytokine-treated hepatocytes via the CD18- integrin, lymphocyte function-associated antigen (LFA-1; CD11a/CD18) and ICAM-1 [121]. The more relevant adhesion of activated neutrophils, i.e. after exposure to chemotactic stimuli such as IL-8 and N-formyl-1-methionyl-1-leucyl-1-phenylalanine (fMLP), to cytokine-treated hepatocytes revealed two independent adhesion mechanisms. An LFA-1/ICAM-1-dependent adhesion and a Mac-1-dependent adhesion that appears to be independent of ICAM-1 [121]. Because the cytotoxic potential of activated neutrophils depends on the adherence to parenchymal cells, these new *in vitro* data are consistent with *in vivo* results showing a reduced cytotoxicity of hepatic neutrophils in anti-Mac-1 antibody-treated animals [122] and significantly reduced parenchymal cell damage [57, 122, 123]. The beneficial effects of anti-ICAM-1 antibodies are more pronounced in models with intact sinusoidal lining cells [68] compared with models with direct access of the neutrophils to parenchymal cells [84]. This suggests that ICAM-1 may be more critical for transendothelial migration than for adherence and cytotoxicity of activated neutrophils to parenchymal cells.

Mechanisms of neutrophil-induced parenchymal cell injury

The molecular mechanism of neutrophil-induced target cell injury is still uncertain. Activated neutrophils generate two major cytotoxic mediators, i.e. reactive oxygen species and proteases. Although NADPH oxidase-derived superoxide and its dismutation product, hydrogen peroxide, are the primary reactive oxygen species formed by activated neutrophils, the concomitant release of myeloperoxidase results in formation of hypochlorous acid (HOCl) as the major oxidant. There is extensive evidence *in vivo* for priming and enhanced generation of reactive oxygen species [124] and hepatic lipid peroxidation [125–128] during a neutrophil-induced injury phase. Furthermore, antioxidants and other interventions directed toward detoxification of reactive oxygen species have been shown to attenuate inflammatory liver injury [104, 127–129]. In addition, neutrophils store various proteases in granules and can release these proteolytic enzymes during activation. Protease inhibitors have been shown to attenuate neutrophil-induced liver injury [130]. These data suggest a critical role for reactive oxygen species and proteases in the pathophysiology *in vivo*.

Experiments *in vitro* using coculture of neutrophils and hepatocytes have generally indicated that proteases, not reactive oxygen species, are involved in the injury mechanism [131–135]. In general, only neutrophils were stimulated in these *in vitro* experiments using physiologically relevant activators such as opsonized zymosan

[131], TNFα [134], and fMLP [135], as well as artificial activators such as phorbol myristate acetate [132, 133]. The proteases elastase and cathepsin G released by neutrophils are mainly responsible for the injury. This has been demonstrated by the hepatotoxic effect of isolated elastase and cathepsin G [131], use of specific inhibitors in coculture experiments [131, 133–135], and isolation of cytotoxic fractions of neutrophil supernatant [136]. Induction of an acute phase response in hepatocytes by turpentine, which increases the synthesis of antiproteases, was found to reduce the neutrophil-induced hepatocellular injury *in vitro* [137] and *in vivo* [67].

It appears that *in vitro* experiments performed thus far mimic only one aspect of a more complex pathophysiology. An explanation of the differences between *in vivo* and *in vitro* experiments may involve the following issues. For neutrophils to effectively kill their target *in vivo*, antiproteases of the plasma have to be prevented from neutralizing the proteases. Because these antiproteases are more susceptible to inactivation by oxidants, the neutrophil generates hypochlorous acid to provide an area where proteases are not disturbed by plasma antiproteases [138]. Thus, under *in vivo* conditions, reactive oxygen species are critical for a protease-mediated injury mechanism.

In addition to the described supportive role, reactive oxygen may be involved in the activation of transcription factors such as nuclear factor-κB (NF-κB) and AP-1, which provide the signal for activation of proinflammatory genes [139]. There is evidence for activation of NF-κB in all liver cell types including hepatocytes during endotoxemia [140] and the inhibitory effect of antioxidants on NF-κB activation, cytokine formation, and hepatocellular ICAM-1 up-regulation [141].

One controversial issue is the question of whether adhesion to hepatocytes is required for neutrophil-mediated injury. The fact that the supernatant of activated neutrophils can cause hepatocyte injury appears to argue against the requirement of direct neutrophil-hepatocyte contact [131, 135]. However, these experiments only demonstrate that maximally stimulated neutrophils release stable cytotoxic mediators that are able to cause parenchymal cell injury. In fact, proteases released by 200–1000 neutrophils per hepatocyte were used [131, 135]. Thus, the amount of proteases required to injure hepatocytes without cell-cell contact is much higher than the 5–20 neutrophils per hepatocyte used in the coculture systems. This indicates the higher cytotoxic efficiency of an adherent neutrophil that is not only due to the closer contact, i.e. higher concentration of cytotoxic mediators, but also due to the fact that adherence of neutrophils to a target cell further activates the phagocyte [116]. Moreover, the mediators used to activate neutrophils *in vitro* are known to be present *in vivo* to up-regulate Mac-1 on neutrophils [78, 86, 121]. In addition to the direct visual evidence for neutrophil adhesion to hepatocytes *in vivo* [109] and *in vitro* [132], antibodies against Mac-1 reduce adherence as well as the cytotoxic effect of neutrophils *in vitro* [119] and *in vivo* [57, 122]. These data together strongly underline the importance of neutrophil adhesion for the cytotoxicity toward hepatic parenchymal cells.

References

1   Hammerschmidt PE, Bowers TK, Kammi-Kepfe CJ, Jacob HS, Craddock PR (1980) Granulocyte aggregometry: a sensitive technique for the detection of C5a and complement activation. *Blood* 55: 898–902

2   Craddock PR, Fehr J, Brigham KL, Broenerberg RS, Jacob HS (1977) Complement and leukocyte-mediated pulmonary dysfunction in hemodialysis. *N Eng J Med* 296: 769–774

3   Craddock PR, Hammerschmidt DE, White JG, Dalmasso AP, Jacob HS (1977) Complement (C5a)-induced granulocyte aggregation *in vitro*: A possible mechanism of complement-mediated leukostasis and leukopenia. *J Clin Invest* 60: 260–274

4   Craddock PR, Hammerschmidt DE, Moldow CF, Yamada O, Jacob HS (1979) Granulocyte aggregation as a manifestation of membrane interactions with complement. Possible role in leukocyte margination, microvascular occlusion, and endothelial damage. *Seminars in Hematology* 16: 140–147

5   McDonagh PF, Wilson DS, Iwamura H, Smith CW, Williams SK, Copeland JG (1996) CD18 Antibody treatment limits early myocardial reperfusion injury after initial leukocyte deposition. *J Surg Res* 64: 139–149

6   Lehr H-A, Weyrich AS, Saetzler RK, Jurek A, Arfors KE, Zimmerman GA, Prescott SM, McIntyre TM (1997) Vitamin C blocks inflammatory platelet-activating factor mimetics created by cigarette smoking. *J Clin Invest* 99: 2358–2364

7   Engler RL, Dahlgren MD, Morris DD, Peterson MA, Schmid-Schonbein GW (1986) Role of leukocytes in response to acute myocardial ischemia and reflow in dogs. *Am J Physiol* 251: H314–323

8   Alon R, Fuhlbrigge RC, Finger EB, Springer TA (1996) Interactions through L-selectin between leukocytes and adherent leukocytes nucleate rolling adhesions on selectins and VCAM-1 in shear flow. *J Cell Biol* 135: 849–865

9   Walcheck B, Moore KL, McEver RP, Kishimoto TK (1996) Neutrophil-neutrophil interactions under hydrodynamic shear stress involve L-selectin and PSGL-1. A mechanism that amplifies initial leukocyte accumulation on P-selectin *in vitro*. *J Clin Invest* 98: 1081–1087

10   Walcheck B, Kahn J, Fisher JM, Wang BB, Fisk RS, Payan DG, Feehan C, Betageri R, Darlak K, Spatola AF et al (1996) Neutrophil rolling altered by inhibition of L-Selectin shedding *in vitro*. *Nature* 380: 720–723

11   Fuhlbrigge RC, Alon R, Puri KD, Lowe JB, Springer TA (1996) Sialylated, fucosylated ligands for L-selectin expressed on leukocytes mediate tethering and rolling adhesions in physiologic flow conditions. *J Cell Biol* 135: 837–848

12   Bongrand P, Capo C, Mege J-L, Benoliel A-M (1988) Use of hydrodynamic flows to study cell adhesion. In: Bongrand P (ed): *Physical basis of cell-cell adhesion*. CRC Press, Boca Raton, 125–156

13   Atherton A, Born GVR (1972) Quantitative investigations of the adhesiveness of circulating polymorphonuclear leukocytes to blood vessel walls. *J Physiol* 222: 447–474

14   Atherton A, Born GVR (1973) Relationship between the velocity of rolling granulocytes and that of the blood flow in venules. *J Physiol* 233: 157–165

15   Doerschuk CM, Allard MF, Hogg JC (1989) Neutrophil kinetics in rabbits during infusion of zymosan-activated plasma. *J Appl Physiol* 67: 88–95

16   Doerschuk CM, Winn RK, Harlan JM (1989) Mechanisms of neutrophil emigration. In: Springer TA, Anderson DC, Rosenthal AS, Rothlein R (eds): *Leukocyte adhesion molecules: Structure, function, and regulation.* Springer-Verlag, New York, 87–94

17   Kishimoto TK (1993) The selectins. In: Lipsky PE, Rothlein R, Kishimoto TK, Faanes RB, Smith CW (eds): *Structure, function, and regulation of moleucles involved in leukocyte adhesion.* Springer-Verlag, New York, 107–134

18   Kansas GS (1996) Selectins and their ligands: Current concepts and controversies. *Blood* 88: 3259–3287

19   Springer TA (1990) Adhesion receptors of the immune system. *Nature* 346: 425–434

20   Butcher EC (1991) Leukocyte-endothelial cell recognition: Three (or more) steps to specificity and diversity. *Cell* 67: 1033–1036

21   Smith CW, Marlin SD, Rothlein R, Toman C, Anderson DC (1989) Cooperative interactions of LFA-1 and Mac-1 with intercellular adhesion molecule-1 in facilitating adherence and transendothelial migration of human neutrophils *in vitro. J Clin Invest* 83: 2008–2017

22   Springer TA (1995) Traffic signals on endothelium for lymphocyte recirculation and leukocyte emigration. *Annu Rev Physiol* 57: 827–872

23   Miller LJ, Bainton DF, Borregaard N, Springer TA (1987) Stimulated mobilization of monocyte Mac-1 and p150, 95 adhesion proteins from an intracellular vesicular compartment to the cell surface. *J Clin Invest* 80: 535–544

24   Gardner SE, Anderson DC, Webb BJ, Stitzel AE, Edwards MS, Spitzer RE, Baker CJ (1982) Evaluation of *Streptococcus pneumonia* type XIV opsonins by phagocytosis-associated chemiluminescence and a bactericidal assay. *Infec Immun* 35: 800–808

25   Afzelius BA (1976) A human syndrome caused by immotile cilia. Science 193: 317–319

26   McGillin JJ, Phair JP (1979) Adherence, augmented adherence and aggregation of polymorphonuclear leukocytes. *J Infect Dis* 139: 69–73

27   Rochon YP, Frojmovic MM, Mills EL (1993) Comparative studies of microscopically determined aggregation degranulation, and light transmission after chemotactic activation of adult and newborn neutrophils. *Blood* 75: 2053–2060

28   Agget PJ, Harries JT, Harvey BAM (1979) An inherited defect of neutrophil mobility in Shwachman syndrome. *J Pediatr* 94: 391–394

29   Afzelius BA, Eliasson R, Johnsen O (1975) Lack of dynein arms in immotile human spermatozoa. *J Cell Biol* 66: 225–232

30   Abramson JS, Lewis JC, Lyles DS (1982) Inhibition of neutrophil lysosome-phagosome fusion associated with influenza virus infection *in vitro. J Clin Invest* 69: 1393–1397

31   Catovsky D, Galton DAG, Robinson J (1972) Myeloperoxidase-deficient neutrophils in acute myeloid leukaemia. *Scand J Haematol* 9: 142–148

32 Smoluchowski MV (1917) Versuch einer mathematischen Theorie der Koagulations-kinetik kolloider Lösungen. *Zeitschrift für Physikalische Chemie* 92: 129–168

33 Simon SI, Burns AR, Taylor AD, Gopalan PK, Lynam EB, Sklar LA, Smith CW (1995) L-Selectin (CD62L) crosslinking signals neutrophil adhesive functions via the Mac-1 (CD11b/CD18) β_2-integrin. *J Immunol* 155: 1502–1514

34 Taylor AD, Neelamegham S, Hellums JD, Smith CW, Simon SI (1996) Molecular dynamics of of the transition from L-selectin- to β_2-integrin-dependent neutrophil adhesion under defined hydrodynamic shear. *Biophys J* 71: 3488–3500

35 Neelamegham S, Taylor AD, Hellums JD, Dembo M, Smith CW, Simon SI (1997) Modeling the reversible kinetics of neutrophil aggregation under hydrodynamic shear. *Biophys J* 72: 1527–1540

36 Xia Z, Frojmovic MM (1994) Aggregation efficiency of activated normal or fixed platelets in a simple shear field: Effect of shear and fibrinogen occupancy. *Biophys J* 66: 2190–2201

37 Hoffstein ST, Friedman RS, Weissmann G (1982) Degranulation, membrane addition, and shape change during chemotactic factor-induced aggregation of human neutrophils. *J Cell Biol* 95: 234–241

38 Sklar LA, Omann GM, Painter RG (1985) Relationnship of actin polymerization and depolymerization to light scattering in human neutrophils: Dependence on receptor occupancy and intracellular Ca^{++}. *J Cell Biol* 101: 1161–1166

39 Anderson DC, Kishimoto TK, Smith CW (1995) Leukocyte adhesion deficiency and other disorders of leukocyte adherence and motility. In: Scriver CR, Beaudet AL, Sly WS, Valle D (eds): *The metabolic and molecular bases of inherited disease*. McGraw-Hill, Seventh, 3955–3994

40 Arnaout MA, Hakim RM, Todd III RF, Dana N, Colten HR (1985) Increased expression of an adhesion-promoting surface glycoprotein in the granulocytopenia of hemodialysis. *N Eng J Med* 312: 457–462

41 Schwartz BR, Ochs HD, Beatty PG, Harlan JM (1985) A monoclonal antibody-defined membrane antigen complex is required for neutrophil-neutrophil aggregation. *Blood* 65: 1553–1556

42 Simon SI, Chambers JD, Sklar LA (1990) Flow cytometric analysis and modeling of cell-cell adhesive interactions: The neutrophil as a model. *J Cell Biol* 111: 2747–2756

43 Guyer DA, Moore KL, Lynam EB, Schammel CMG, Rogelj S, McEver RP, Sklar LA (1996) P-selectin glycoprotein ligand-1 (PSGL-1) is a ligand for L-selectin in neutrophil aggregation. *Blood* 88: 2415–2421

44 Finger EB, Purl K, Alon R, Lawrence MB, von Andrian UH, Springer TA (1996) Adhesion through L-selectin requires a threshold hydrodynamic shear. *Nature* 379: 266–269

45 Lawrence MB, Kansas GS, Kunkel EJ, Ley K (1997) Threshold levels of fluid shear promote leukocyte adhesion through selectins (CD62L, P, E). *J Cell Biol* 136: 717–727

46 Simon SI, Taylor A, Neelamegham S, Hellums JD, Smith CW (1997) Neutrophil aggregation mediated by β_2-integrin and ICAM-3 at low hydrodynamic shear. *FASEB J* 11: A102(Abstract)

47   Campanero MR, del Pozo MA, Arroyo AG, Sanchez-Mateos P, Hernandez-Caselles T, Craig A, Pulido R, Sanchez-Madrid F (1993) ICAM-3 interacts with LFA-1 and regulates the LFA-1/ICAM-1 cell adhesion pathway. *J Cell Biol* 123: 1007–1016

47a Neelamegham S, Taylor AD, Burns AR, Smith CW, Simon SI (1998) Hydrodynamic shear reveals distinct roles for LPA-1 and Mac-1 in neutrophil adhesion to ICAM-1. *Blood; in press*

48   Tsang YTM, Neelamegham S, Hu Y, Berg EL, Burns AR, Smith CW, Simon SI (1997) Synergy between L-selectin signaling and chemotactic activation during neutrophil adhesion and transmigration. *J Immunol* 159: 4566–4577

49   Gopalan PK, Smith CW, Lu H, Berg EL, McIntire LV, Simon SI (1997) Neutrophil CD18-dependent arrest on ICAM-1 in shear flow can be activated through L-selectin. *J Immunol* 158: 367–375

50   Wong J, Johnston B, Lee SS, Bullard DC, Smith CW, Beaudet AL, Kubes P (1997) A minimal role for selectins in the recruitment of leukocytes into the inflamed liver microvasculature. *J Clin Invest* 99: 2782–2790

51   Gaboury JP, Kubes P (1994) Reductions in physiologic shear rates lead to CD11/CD18-dependent, selectin-independent leukocyte rolling *in vivo*. *Blood* 83: 345–350

52   Romson JL, Hook BG, Kunkel SL, Abrams GD, Schork MA, Lucchesi BR (1983) Reduction of the extent of ischemic myocardial injury by neutrophil depletion in the dog. *Circulation* 67: 1016–1023

53   Entman ML, Smith CW (1994) Post-reperfusion inflammation: A model of reaction to injury in cardiovascular disease. *Cardiovas Res* 28: 1301–1311

54   Jaeschke H, Farhood AI, Smith CW (1990) Neutrophils contribute to ischemia/reperfusion injury in rat liver *in vivo*. *FASEB J* 4: 3355–3359

55   Jaeschke H (1996) Preservation injury: Mechanisms, prevention and consequences. *J Hepatol* 25: 774–780

56   Hernandez LA, Grisham MB, Twohig B, Arfors KE, Harlan JM, Granger DN (1987) Role of neutrophils in ischemia-reperfusion-induced microvascular injury. *Am J Physiol* 238: H699–H703

57   Jaeschke H, Farhood AI, Smith CW (1991) Neutrophil-induced liver cell injury in endotoxin shock is a CD11b/CD18-dependent mechanism. *Am J Physiol* 261: G1051–G1056

58   Hewett JA, Schultze AE, VanCise S, Roth RA (1992) Neutrophil depletion protects against liver injury from bacterial endotoxin. *Lab Invest* 66: 347–361

59   Mulligan MS, Smith CW, Anderson DC, Todd III RF, Miyasaka M, Tamatani T, Issekutz TB, Ward PA (1993) Role of leukocyte adhesion molecules in complement-induced lung injury. *J Immunol* 150: 2401–2406

60   Bautista AP (1997) Chronic alcohol intoxication induces hepatic injury through enhanced macrophage inflammatory protein-2 production and intercellular adhesion molecule-1 expression in the liver. *Hepatol* 25: 335–342.

61   Mulligan MS, Wilson GP, Todd III RF, Smith CW, Anderson DC, Varani J, Issekutz T,

Miyasaka M, Tamatani T, Rusche JR et al (1993) Role of beta-1, beta-2 integrins and ICAM-1 in lung injury after deposition of IgG and IgA immune complexes. *J Immunol* 150: 2407–2417

62 Mulligan MS, Johnson KJ, Todd III RF, Issekutz TB, Miyasaka M, Tamatani T, Smith CW, Anderson DC, Ward PA (1993) Requirements for leukocyte adhesion molecules in nephrotoxic nephritis. *J Clin Invest* 91: 577–587

63 Jaeschke H, Farhood A (1991) Neutrophil and Kupffer cell-induced oxidant stress and ischemia-reperfusion injury in rat liver *in vivo*. *Am J Physiol* 260: G355–G362

64 Vollmar B, Menger MD, Glasz J, Leiderer R, Messmer K (1994) Impact of leuko-cyte-endothelial cell interaction in hepatic ischemia-reperfusion injury. *Am J Physiol* 267: G786–G793

65 Chosay JG, Essani NA, Dunn CJ, Jaeschke H (1997) Neutrophil margination and extravasation in sinusoids and venules of the liver during endotoxin-induced injury. *Am J Physiol* 272: G1195–G1200

66 Jaeschke H, Farhood A, Bautista AP, Spolarics Z, Spitzer JJ (1993) Complement acti-vates Kupffer cells and neutrophils during reperfusion after hepatic ischemia. *Am J Physiol* 264: G801–G809

67 Schlayer HJ, Laaff H, Peters T, Woort-Menker M, Estler HC, Karck U, Schaefer HE, Decker K (1988) Involvement of tumor necrosis factor in endotoxin-triggered neu-trophil adherence to sinusoidal endothelial cells of mouse liver and its modulation in acute phase. *J Hepatol* 7: 239–249

68 Essani NA, Fisher MA, Farhood A, Manning AM, Smith CW, Jaeschke H (1995) Cytokine-induced hepatic intercellular adhesion molecule-1 (ICAM-1) messenger RNA expression and its role in the pathophysiology of murine endotoxin shock and acute liver failure. *Hepatol* 21: 1632–1639

69 Bautista AP, Spitzer JJ (1992) Platelet activating factor stimulates and primes the liver, Kupffer cells and neutrophils to release superoxide anion. *Free Rad Res Commun* 17: 195–209

70 Maher JJ, Scott MK, Saito JM, Burton MC (1997) Adenovirus-mediated expression of cytokine-induced neutrophil chemoattractant in rat liver induces a neutrophilic hepati-tis. *Hepatol* 25: 624–630

71 Zhang P, Xie M, Zagorski J, Spitzer JA (1995) Attenuation of hepatic neutrophil seques-tration by anti-CINC antibody in endotoxic rats. *Shock* 4: 262–268

72 Simonet WS, Hughes TM, Nguyen HQ, Trebasky LD, Danilenko DM, Medlock ES (1994) Long-term impaired neutrophil migration in mice overexpressing human inter-leukin-8. *J Clin Invest* 94: 1310–1319

73 Colletti LM, Kunkel SL, Green M, Burdick MD, Strieter RM (1996) Hepatic inflam-mation following 70% hepatectomy may be related to upregulation of epithelial neu-trophil activating protein-78. *Shock* 6: 397–402

74 Colletti LM, Kunkel SL, Walz A, Burdick MD, Kunkel RG, Wilke CA, Strieter RM (1996) The role of cytokine networks in the local liver injury following hepatic ischemia/reperfusion in the rat. *Hepatol* 23: 506–514

75   Jaeschke H, Farhood A, Fisher MA, Smith CW (1996) Sequestration of neutrophils in the hepatic vasculature during endotoxemia is independent of β_2 integrins and intercellular adhesion molecule-1. *Shock* 6: 351–356

76   Hewett JA, Jean P, Kunkel SL, Roth RA (1993) Relationship between tumor necrosis factor-α and neutrophils in endotoxin-induced liver injury. *Am J Physiol* 265: G1011–G1015

77   Jaeschke H, Farhood A, Smith CW (1994) Contribution of complement-stimulated hepatic macrophages and neutrophils to endotoxin-induced liver injury in rats. *Hepatol* 19: 973–979

78   Witthaut R, Farhood A, Smith CW, Jaeschke H (1994) Complement and tumor necrosis factor-α contribute to MAC-1 (CD11b/CD18) upregulation and systemic neutrophil activation during endotoxemia *in vivo*. *J Leuko Biol* 55: 105–111

79   Essani NA, McGuire GM, Manning AM, Jaeschke H (1995) Differential induction for mRNA of ICAM-1 and selectins in hepatocytes, Kupffer cells and endothelial cells during endotoxemia. *Biochem Biophys Res Commun* 211: 74–82.

80   Kvale D, Brandtzaeg P (1993) Immune modulation of adhesion molecules ICAM-1 (CD54) and LFA-3 (CD58) in human hepatocytic cell lines. *Hepatol* 17: 347–352

81   Morita M, Watanabe Y, Akaike T (1994) Inflammatory cytokines up-regulate intercellular adhesion molecule-1 expression on primary cultured mouse hepatocytes and t-lymphocyte adhesion. *Hepatol* 19: 426–431

82   Essani NA, Bajt SL, Vonderfecht SL, Farhood A, Jaeschke H (1997) Transcriptional activation of vascular cell adhesion molecule-1 (VCAM-1) gene *in vivo* and its role in the pathophysiology of neutrophil-induced liver injury in murine endotoxin shock. *J Immunol* 158: 5941–5948

83   Essani NA, Fisher MA, Simmons, CA, Hoover JL, Farhood A, Jaeschke, H (1998) Increased P-selectin gene expression in the liver vasculature and its role in the pathophysioogy of neutrophil-induced liver injury in murine endotoxin shock. *J Leuko Biol* 63: 288–296

84   Farhood A, McGuire GM, Manning AM, Miyasaka M, Smith CW, Jaeschke H (1995) Intercellular adhesion molecule-1 (ICAM-1) expression and its role in neutrophil-induced ischemia-reperfusion injury in rat liver. *J Leuko Biol* 57: 368– 374

85   Jaeschke H, Essani N, Fisher MA, Vonderfecht SL, Farhood A, Smith CW (1996) Release of soluble intercellular adhesion molecule-1 into bile and serum in murine endotoxin shock. *Hepatol* 23: 530–536

86   Mickelson JK, Kukielka G, Bravenec JS, Mainolfi E, Rothlein R, Hawkins HK, Kelly JH, Smith CW (1995) Differential expression and release of CD54 induced by cytokines. *Hepatol* 22: 866–875

87   Hellerbrand C, Wang SC, Tsukamoto H, Brenner DA, Rippe RA (1996) Expression of intercellular adhesion molecule 1 by activated hepatic stellate cells. *Hepatol* 24: 670–676

88   Lou D, Vanderkerken K, Bouwens L, Kuppen PJK, Baekeland M, Seynaeve C, Wisse E

(1996) The role of adhesion molecules in the recruitment of hepatic natural killer cells (pit cells) in rat liver. *Hepatol* 24: 1475–1480

89   Steinhoff G, Behrend M, Schrader B, Duijvestijn AM, Wonigeit K (1993) Expression patterns of leukocyte adheison ligand molecules on human liver endothelia. Lack of ELAM-1 and CD62 inducibility on sinusoidal endothelia and distinct distribution of VCAM-1, ICAM-1, ICAM-2, and LFA-3. *Am J Pathol* 142: 481–488

90   Scoazec JY, Durand F, Degott C, Delautier D, Bernuau J, Belghiti J, Benhamou JP, Feldmann G (1994) Expression of cytokine-dependent adhesion molecules in postreperfusion biopsy specimens of liver allograft. *Gastroenterol* 107: 1094–1102

91   Volpes R, Van Den Oord J, Desmet VJ (1990) Immunohistochemical study of adhesion moleucles in liver inflammation. *Hepatol* 12: 59–65

92   Granger DN, Kubes P (1994) The microcirculation and inflammation: modulation of leukocyte-endothelial cell adhesion. *J Leuko Biol* 55: 662–675

93   Kishimoto TK, Rothlein R (1994) Integrins, ICAMs, and selectins: role and regulation of adhesion molecules in neutrophil recruitment to inflammatory sites. *Adv Pharmacol* 25: 117–169

94   Vollmar B, Glasz J, Menger MD, Messmer K (1995) Leukocytes contribute to hepatic ischemia/reperfusion injury via intercellular adhesion molecule-1-mediated venular adherence. *Surg* 117: 195–200

95   McCuskey RS (1993) Hepatic microvascular responses to endotoxemia and sepsis. *Prog Appl Microcirc* 19: 76–84

96   Bauer M, Zhang JX, Bauer I, Clemens MG (1994) Endothelin-1 induced alterations of hepatic microcirculation: sinusoidal and extrasinusoidal sites of action. *Am J Physiol* 267: G143–G149

97   Nishida J, McCuskey RS, McDonnell D, Fox ES (1994) Protective role of NO in hepatic microcirculatory dysfunction during endotoxemia. *Am J Physiol* 267: G1135–G1141

98   Worthen GS, Schwab III B, Elson EL, Downey GP (1989) Mechanics of stimulated neutrophils: Cell stiffening induces retention of capillaries. *Science* 245: 183–186

99   Zhang JX, Jones DV, Clemens MG (1994) Effect of activation on neutrophil-induced hepatic microvascular injury in isolated rat liver. Shock 1: 273–278

100 Bilzer M, Lauterburg BH (1994) Oxidant stress and potentiation of ischemia-reperfusion inury to the perfused rat liver by human polymorphonuclear leukocytes. *J Hepatol* 20: 473–477

101 Bautista AP, Meszaros K, Bojta J, Spitzer JJ (1990) Superoxide anion generation in the liver during the early stage of endotoxemia in rats. *J Leuk Biol* 48: 123–128

102 Jaeschke H, Bautista AP, Spolarics Z, Spitzer JJ (1991) Superoxide generation by Kupffer cells and priming of neutrophils during reperfusion after hepatic ischemia. *Free Rad Res Commun* 15: 277–284

103 Liu P, Vonderfecht SL, Fisher MA, McGuire GM, Jaeschke H (1994) Priming of phagocytes for reactive oxygen production during hepatic ischemia and reperfusion increases the susceptibility for endotoxin-induced liver injury. *Circ Shock* 43: 9–17

104 Liu P, McGuire GM, Fisher MA, Farhood A, Smith CW, Jaeschke H (1995) Activation

of Kupffer cells and neutrophils for reactive oxygen formation is responsible for endo-toxin-enhanced liver injury after hepatic ischemia. *Shock* 3: 56–62

105 Arai M, Mochida S, Ohno A, Ogata I, Fujiwara K (1993) Sinusoidal endothelial cell damage by activated macrophages in rat liver necrosis. Gastroenterol 104: 1466–1471

106 Jaeschke H (1991) Vascular oxidant stress and hepatic ischemia-reperfusion injury. *Free Rad Res Commun* 12–13: 737–743

107 Jaeschke H (1992) Enhanced sinusoidal glutathione efflux during endotoxin-induced oxidant stress *in vivo*. *Am J Physiol* 263: G60–G68

108 Liu P, Fisher MA, Farhood A, Smith CW, Jaeschke H (1994) Beneficial effect of extra-cellular glutathione against reactive oxygen-mediated reperfusion injury in the liver. *Circ Shock* 43: 64–70

109 Ohira H, Ueno T, Torimura T, Tanikawa K, Kasukawa R (1995) Leukocyte adhesion molecules in the liver and plasma cytokine levels in endotoxin-induced rat liver injury. *Scan J Gastro* 30: 1027–1035.

110 Jaeschke H, Fisher MA, Lawson JA, Simmons CA, Farhood A, Jones DA (1998) Acti-vation of caspase 3(CPP32)-like proteases is essential for TNFα induced hepatic parenchymal cell apoptosis and neutrophil-mediated necrosis in a murine endotoxin shock model. *J Immunol* 160: 3480–3486

111 Thornton AJ, Strieter RM, Lindley I, Baggiolini M, Kunkel SL (1990) Cytokine-induced gene expression of a neutrophil chemotactic factor/IL-8 in human hepatocytes. *J Immunol* 144: 2609–2613

112 Shiratori Y, Hikiba Y, Mawet E, Niwa Y, Matsumura M, Kato N, Shiina S, Tada M, Komatsu Y, Kawabe T, et al (1994) Modulation of KC/gro protein (interleukin-8 relat-ed protein in rodents) release from hepatocytes by biologically active mediators. *Biochem Biophys Res Commun* 203: 1398–1403

113 Fisher MA, Eversole RR, Beuving LJ, Jaeschke H (1997) Sinusoidal endothelial cell and parenchymal cell injury during endotoxemia and hepatic ischemia-reperfusion: protec-tion by the 21-aminosteroid tirilazad mesylate. *Int Hepatol Commun* 6: 121–129

114 McKeown CMB, Edwards V, Phillips MJ, Harvey PRC, Petrunka CN, Strasberg SM (1988) Sinusoidal lining cell damage: The critical injury in cold preservation of liver allo-grafts in the rat. *Transp* 46: 178–191

115 Caldwell-Kenkel JC, Currin RT, Tanaka Y, Thurman RG, Lemasters JJ (1989) Reperfu-sion injury to endothelial cells following cold ischemic storage of rat livers. *Hepatol* 10: 292–299

116 Shappell SB, Toman C, Anderson DC, Taylor AA, Entman ML, Smith CW (1990) Mac-1 (CD11b/CD18) mediates adherence-dependent hydrogen peroxide production by human and canine neutrophils. *J Immunol* 144: 2702–2711

117 Nathan CF, Srimal S, Farber C, Sanchez E, Kabbash L, Asch A, Gailit J, Wright SD (1989) Cytokine-induced respiratory burst of human neutrophils: Dependence on extra-cellular matrix proteins and CD11/CD18 integrins. *J Cell Biol* 109: 1341–1349

118 Entman ML, Youker KA, Shappell SB, Siegel C, Rothlein R, Dreyer WJ, Schmalstieg FC,

Smith CW (1990) Neutrophil adherence to isolated adult canine myocytes: Evidence for a CD18-dependent mechanism. *J Clin Invest* 85: 1497–1506

119 Maroushek-Boury NM, Czuprynski CJ (1995) Listeria monocytogenes infection increases neutrophil adhesion and damage to a murine hepatocyte cell line *in vitro*. *Immunol Lett* 46: 111–116

120 Adams DH, Mainolfi E, Elias E, Neuberger JM, Rothlein R (1993) Detection of circulating intercellular adhesion molecule-1 after liver transplantation-evidence of local release within the liver during graft rejection. *Transp* 55: 83–87

121 Nagendra AR, Mickelson JK, Smith CW (1997) CD18 integrin and CD54-depedent neutrophil adhesion to cytokine-stimulated human hepatocytes. *Am J Physiol* 272: G408–G416

122 Jaeschke H, Farhood A, Bautista AP, Spolarics Z, Spitzer JJ, Smith CW (1993) Functional inactivation of neutrophils with a Mac-1 (CD11b/CD18) monoclonal antibody protects against ischemia-reperfusion injury in rat liver. *Hepatol* 17: 915–923

123 Bauer C, Siaplaouras S, Soule HR, Moyle M, Marzi I (1995) A natural glycoprotein inhibitor (NIF) of CD11b/CD18 reduces leukocyte adhesion in the liver after hemorrhagic shock. Shock 4: 187–192

124 Jaeschke H, Bautista AP, Spolarics Z, Spitzer JJ (1992) Superoxide generation by neutrophils and Kupffer cells during *in vivo* reperfusion after hepatic ischemia in rats. *J Leuko Biol* 52: 377–382

125 Mathews WR, Guido DM, Fisher MA, Jaeschke H (1994) Lipid peroxidation as molecular mechanism of liver cell injury during reperfusion after ischemia. *Free Radical Biol Med* 16: 763–770

126 Walsh TR, Rao PN, Makowka L, Starzl TE (1990) Lipid peroxidation is a nonparenchymal cell event with reperfusion after prolonged liver ischemia. *J Surg Res* 49: 18–22

127 Jaeschke H (1991) Reactive oxygen and ischemia/reperfusion injury of the liver. *Chem Biol Int* 79: 115–136

128 Wu TW, Hashimoto N, Au J, Wu J, Mickle DAG, Carey D (1991) Trolox protects rat hepatocytes agains oxyradical damage and the ischemic rat liver from reperfusion injury. *Hepatol* 13: 575–580.

129 Marubayashi S, Dohi K, Ochi K, Kawasaki T (1986) Role of free radicals in ischemic rat liver cell injury: Prevention of damage by α-tocopherol administration. *Surg* 99: 184–192

130 Li XK, Matin AFM, Suzuki H, Uno T, Yamaguchi T, Harada Y (1993) Effect of protease inhibitor on ischemia-reperfusion injury of the rat liver. *Transp* 56: 1331–1336

131 Mavier P, Preaux A-M, Guigui B, Lecs MC, Zafrani ES, Dhumeaux D (1988) *In vitro* toxicity of polymorphonuclear neutrophils to rat hepatocytes: Evidence for a protease-mediated mechanism. *Hepatol* 8: 254–258

132 Guigui B, Rosenbaum J, Preaux A-M, Martin N, Zafrani ES, Dhumeaux D, Mavier P (1988) Toxicity of phorbol myristate acetate-stimulated polymorphonuclear neutrophils against rat hepatocytes. Demonstration and mechanism. *Lab Invest* 59: 831–837

133 Harbrecht BG, Billiar TR, Curran RD, Stadler J, Simmons RL (1993) Hepatocyte injury by activated neutrophils *in vitro* is mediated by proteases. *Ann Surg* 218: 120–128

134 Oka Y, Murata A, Nishijima J, Ogawa M, Mori T (1993) The mechanism of hepatic cellular injury in sepsis: an *in vitro* study of the implications of cytokines and neutrophils in its pathogenesis. *J Surg Res* 55: 1–8

135 Ganey PE, Bailie MB, VanCise S, Madhukar BV, Robinson JP, Roth RA (1994) Activated neutrophils from rat injured isolated hepatocytes. *Lab Invest* 70: 53–60

136 Ho JS, Buchweitz JP, Roth RA, Ganey PE (1996) Identification of factors from rat neutrophils responsible for cytotoxicity to isolated hepatocytes. *J Leuk Biol* 59: 716–724

137 Mavier P, Rosenbaum J, Preaux A-M, Malla A, Dhumeaux D (1990) Decreased toxicity of polymorphonuclear neutrophils toward hepatocytes isolated from rats with acute inflammatory reaction. *Hepatol* 12: 1337–1341

138 Weiss SJ (1989) Tissue destruction by neutrophils. *N Eng J Med* 320: 365–376

139 Baeuerle PA, Henkel T (1994) Function and activation of NF-κB in the immune system. *Annu Rev Immunol* 12: 141–179.

140 Essani NA, McGuire GM, Manning AM, Jaeschke H (1996) Endotoxin-induced activation of nuclear transcription factor-κB and expression of E-Selectin messenger RNA in hepatocytes, Kupffer cells and endothelial cells *in vivo*. *J Immunol* 156: 2956–2963

141 Essani NA, Fisher MA, Jaeschke H (1997) Inhibition of NF-κB activation by dimethyl sulfoxide correlates with suppression of TNF-α formation, reduced ICAM-1 gene transcription and protection against endotoxin-induced liver injury. *Shock* 7: 90–96

Cytokines, coagulation and fibrinolysis

C. Erik Hack

Central Laboratory of the Netherlands Red Cross Blood Transfusion Service, and Department of Internal Medicine, Free University Hospital, Plesmanlaan 125, NL-1066 CX Amsterdam, The Netherlands

Introduction

Sepsis/septic shock results from the excessive activation and release of a number of inflammatory mediators. Cytokines are generally considered to be key factors in this respect as these hormone-like proteins are released in excessive amounts during sepsis and are able to induce the release and activation of a number of secondary and tertiary mediators [1]. The main cytokines involved in the pathogenesis of sepsis are tumor necrosis factor-α (TNFα), interleukin-1α, -β (IL-1α/β) and interleukin-1-receptor antagonist (IL-1ra), IL-6, IL-8 and other chemokines, IL-10, IL-12, and interferon-gamma. Among the secondary mediators activated by cytokines are plasma cascade systems such as the coagulation, fibrinolytic and contact systems. These systems have in common that during activation proenzymes are converted into active serine proteinases in a waterfall or "cascade"-like fashion. In this chapter we will first discuss some aspects of the biochemistry and biology of these systems. Then we will elaborate on the role of cytokines in the activation of clotting and fibrinolysis, in particular during sepsis. Finally, we will summarize possible effects of clotting or fibrinolytic proteins on the release of cytokines.

The coagulation system

Central in the coagulation system is the conversion of fibrinogen into fibrin by the serine proteinase thrombin. Thrombin is generated from prothrombin by another serine proteinase, activated factor X (FXa), which, for optimal activity, requires the presence of a cofactor, activated factor V, and phospholipids (which serve as a surface on which to assemble the various clotting factors) as cofactors, and calcium ions. Traditionally, activation of factor X has been considered to occur via an extrinsic pathway (one of the components of this pathway, tissue factor, is not present in plasma) or an intrinsic pathway (all components are present in plasma). The intrinsic pathway consists of factor XII (FXII), prekallikrein (PK), high molecular weight

Cytokines in Severe Sepsis and Septic Shock, edited by H. Redl and G. Schlag†
© 1999 Birkhäuser Verlag Basel/Switzerland

kininogen (HK) and factors XI, IX and VIII, and becomes activated upon contact of blood with an artificial surface such as glass. The initial phase of this pathway (also known as the contact system) comprises activation of FXII and PK, and will be discussed below. FXIIa can activate FXI, which in turn activates FIX, which together with FVIII then activates FX. The extrinsic pathway consists of FVII and a transmembrane protein, tissue factor (TF). Under normal conditions TF is not exposed on endothelial cells, but is present on extravascular cells. Activation of this pathway occurs when the continous layer of the endothelium is disrupted and blood is exposed to these extravascular cells, or when TF is exposed by endothelial cells, as may occur upon stimulation with cytokines (see below). Upon contact with blood, TF binds and activates FVII, which then activates factor X. This process is inhibited by tissue factor pathway inhibitor (TFPI).

The traditional view of an intrinsic and extrinsic pathway of coagulation may be incorrect: *in vivo* extrinsic pathway activation likely encompasses more than factor VII and tissue factor, i.e. factors VIII and IX (which serve to amplify the tissue factor-factor VII pathway and which are both necessary for the rapid generation of a substantial amount of thrombin via the extrinsic pathway), and factor XI (which is thought to be activated *in vivo* by thrombin rather than by factor XII) [2–5]. In this view, FXI constitutes a second amplification loop necessary for very rapid generation of thrombin in particular when the initial activation of the extrinsic pathway is driven by limited amounts of tissue factor [6]. Activation of coagulation is counteracted by various mechanisms: the presence of inhibitors such as TFPI and antithrombin III (inhibits thrombin and various other activated clotting factors); and the protein C system. The central protein of the latter system is protein C (PC) which is activated by thrombin bound to the transmembrane protein thrombomodulin (TM). Thus, upon binding to TM, which under normal conditions is present on endothelial cells and contributes to the anti-coagulant properties of these cells, the specificity of thrombin is changed in that it activates protein C and no longer cleaves fibrinogen. In the presence of the cofactor protein S, activated PC counteracts coagulation by inactivating FVa and FVIIIa.

The contact system

The contact system consists of the proteins FXII (formerly known as Hageman factor), PK (Fletcher factor) and HK [7]. Via activation of factor XI, which in turn activates factor IX, contact activation may induce activation of factor X and prothrombin. It is, however, doubtful whether this contact system-dependent activation of factor XI is important for physiological hemostasis. Clinical studies reveal that only deficiency of factor XI, but not that of one of the other contact system proteins, results in a (mild) bleeding disorder. This, together with the lack of evidence that *in vivo* the contact system participates in the hemostatic process makes it doubtful whether factor XI should be considered as a contact system protein (see also above). Presumably, the contact system serves *in vivo* as an auxiliary fibrinolytic system [8, 9]. In agreement herewith, persons with a deficiency of factor XII are prone to develop thromboembolic disease, rather than a bleeding disorder [10]. Moreover, infusion of the vasopressin analogue 1-desamino-8-D-arginine-vasopressin (DDAVP; used to assess the capacity of the endothelium to release tissue-type plasminogen activator *in vivo*) induces activation of plasminogen [11], which in part is dependent on the presence of factor XII [12].

Contact activation yields bradykinin (released from HK by kallikrein), which can induce vasodilation, hypotension, an increase in vasopermeability and bronchoconstriction [13]. Bradykinin mediates its effects by binding to specific receptors on cells. Some of the biological effects of bradykinin are due to the induction of the formation of nitric oxide [14]. Several activation products of the contact system have inflammatory properties: kallikrein and factor XIIa have chemotactic and/or agonistic activity for neutrophils [15, 16], whereas β-factor XIIa is able to activate the complement system [17, 18].

The fibrinolytic system

Central in the fibrinolytic system is the conversion of the plasminogen into the fibrin-degrading enzyme plasmin [8]. Activation of the fibrinolytic system may occur via several pathways, i.e. via tissue-type plasminogen activator (tPA)- or urokinase-type plasminogen activator (uPA)-dependent pathways [8]. Both plasminogen activators are inhibited by plasminogen activator inhibitors (PAIs) [19]. In the circulation, PAI-1 is the most important inhibitor of tPA as well as of uPA [19, 20], whereas the activity of plasmin is rapidly inhibited by its inhibitor α2-antiplasmin (α2AP) [21]. In addition to the tPA- and the uPA-dependent pathways, there is evidence for a third, factor XII-dependent pathway of plasminogen activation [8], although the molecular aspects of this pathway are not exactly known.

Tumor necrosis factor and interleukin-1

The cytokines TNF and IL-1 are considered to be major endogenous mediators of sepsis [1]. Although they bind to different cellular receptors, TNF-receptors (TNF-R) or IL-1-receptors (IL1-R), and differ in their three-dimensional structure, both cytokines have multiple overlapping and synergistic activities [22, 23].

Both TNF and IL-1 have many cell-specific effects [22] and only those relevant for hemostasis are mentioned here. Interactions of TNF and IL-1 with endothelial cells are of major importance for inflammatory reactions, and may induce various effects on clotting and fibrinolysis: expression of tissue factor and downregulation of thrombomodulin, which reduces the anticoagulant properties and enhances the procoagulant activity of the endothelial surface [24–29]. The effects of TNF on the endothelial cells proceed mainly via triggering of TNF-R-p55 [30]. Both cytokines also induce the release of uPA as well as the synthesis of PAI-1 [31–36]. TNF and IL-1 also influence the inhibition of fibrinolysis in another way: either cytokine can induce the synthesis of a protein called TSG-6, which potentiates plasmin inhibition by activating inter-α–trypsin inhibitor [37].

Consistent with the procoagulant effects of TNF and IL-1 *in vitro* are histological studies in animals showing that local injection of TNF or IL-1 induces the activation of neutrophils and the deposition of fibrin [23, 37–44]. Systemic injection of TNF also induces activation of coagulation and fibrinolysis. Typically, coagulation proceeds for hours after injection of this cytokine whereas fibrinolysis is only shortly (approximately 60 min) activated and then inhibited, resulting in a so-called procoagulant state [45–48]. Such a procoagulant state can also be induced by a low dose of IL-1β (3 ng/kg of body weight) [49]. Notably, both TNF and IL-1 are able to induce the release of tPA into the circulation whereas, *in vitro*, both cytokines decrease the synthesis of tPA by endothelial cells. A possible explanation is that TNF and IL-1 induce the release of vasopressin [50] which, in turn, causes the release of tPA [11].

Activation of coagulation and fibrinolysis by TNF has also been studied in non-human primates. In baboons challenged with 100 μg of TNF per kg of body weight a significant rise in thrombin-antithrombin III complexes was not observed unless a monoclonal antibody that blocks PC was co-administered [51]. In this model, TNF-induced activation of clotting was enhanced by injection of phospholipid microvesicles. However, in another study in baboons, a similar dose of TNF did induce the generation of thrombin as well as the release of tPA and PAI-1 [52], and these effects were shown to result from triggering of TNF-R-p55.

Finally, observations in patients indicate that recombinant TNF is also able to activate the contact (as well as the complement) system [53].

The intravenous injection of a low dose of endotoxin elicits the release of TNF in human volunteers with peak levels at 90 minutes following the challenge [54]. Similarly, IL-1 increases, reaching peak levels at 2 to 3 h following the endotoxin challenge [55]. The coagulation and clotting systems are both activated during experimental human endotoxemia [56]. Fibrinolysis is only activated during the first two hours after the endotoxin challenge to become inhibited later on by increasing levels of PAI-1 whereas coagulation proceeds for hours [56, 57] resulting in a procoagulant state as has been found following TNF injection (see above). Attenuating the effects of TNF using recombinant dimeric TNF-R in low grade endotoxemia in humans resulted in a greatly reduced fibrinolytic response whereas the activation of coagulation was unaffected [58], pointing to a central role of TNF in the activation of fibrinolysis but not in that of coagulation in this condition. A similar model for experimental endotoxemia has been developed in chimpanzees [59]. In this model coagulation has been found to be completely dependent on the expression of tissue factor, but independent of TNF or IL-1 [60] (in agreement with observations in the human model). Thus, presumably the observed activation of coagulation during low grade experimental endotoxemia results from the direct effects of endotoxin on the endothelium or monocytes [61]. In contrast, the release of tPA, the formation of plasmin, and the increase in circulating PAI-1 in this model is completely inhibited by anti-TNF antibodies [60, 61], supporting the observations in the human model [58]. In agreement herewith, pentoxyfylline, which attenuates the release of TNF (and IL-6) during low grade endotoxemia, reduces the activation of fibrinolysis but has no effect on coagulation [61].

TNF and IL-1β are also released into the circulation following a (sub)lethal challenge with endotoxin or (live) bacteria, peak levels of TNF occurring approximately 1 to 2 h after the challenge whereas those of IL-1β reaching their summit one hour later. In these models both the fibrinolytic as well as the clotting system are activated with again fibrinolysis being inhibited a few hours after the challenge whereas coagulation proceeds for a longer period [62]. In contrast to low grade endotoxemia, in these more severe models for sepsis, inhibition of TNF does reduce activation of coagulation but has hardly any effect on fibrinolysis [63, 64]. Similarly, IL-1ra attenuates activation of coagulation in these models without affecting plasmin formation [65]. Sepsis in baboons by *E. coli* is also accompanied by a significant increase in circulating TM, which reaches peak levels at 8 h after the challenge. This increase can be almost prevented by the administration of anti-TNF [66].

In clinical sepsis there is, as far as we know, no evidence that TNF is directly involved in the clotting abnormalities observed in patients suffering from this disease. In a subgroup of 26 patients participating in the first large multicenter trial on the efficacy of IL-1-ra in clinical sepsis, IL-1-ra treatment was shown to reduce thrombin formation but had no effect on plasmin generation [67], findings consistent with the observations in baboons (see above).

Interleukin-6

Although there is abundant evidence that IL-6 is released during sepsis, the precise role of IL-6 in the pathogenesis of this condition is still not well established. Most likely it is the main inducer of the synthesis of acute phase proteins by the liver [68], although other related cytokines such as LIF may be involved as well [69]. We are not aware of *in vitro* studies showing a procoagulant effect of IL-6. Yet, *in vivo*, IL-6 seems to have a procoagulant effect, as was found in a study evaluating the effects of a neutralizing anti-IL-6 in a chimpanzee model for experimental low-grade endotoxemia [70]. This is consistent with observations in humans where IL-6 was shown to have a small effect on clotting and no effect on fibrinolysis [71]. In agreement with an effect of IL-6 on clotting is the observation in baboons that clotting times are prolonged upon administration of recombinant IL-6 subcutaneously at a dose of 100 µg per kg body weight [72]. Notably, in this latter study the most pronounced effects were seen at the time when levels of acute phase proteins were at their highest. Hence the decreased levels of clotting factors or their inhibitors may have been due to a decreased synthesis, e.g. because their synthesis is regulated like that of a negative phase protein [73, 74]. Consistent with this latter interpretation is that circulating levels of thrombin-antithrombin did not increase in the baboons receiving IL-6 [72].

Other cytokines

In addition to TNF, IL-1 and IL-6, various other cytokines are involved in the pathogenesis of sepsis. However, evidence that these cytokines may modulate activation of the coagulation or the fibrinolytic systems *in vivo* is at present not available. *In vitro*, the anti-inflammatory cytokine IL-10 can inhibit endotoxin-stimulated tissue factor expression and induction of procoagulant activity by monocytes [75, 76] whereas IL-4 is unable to do so [77].

Finally, for one cytokine not supposed to play a role in endotoxin-induced shock (though it likely plays a role in that induced by superantigens), IL-2, some data on its effects on clotting and fibrinolysis exist. In patients with cancer this cytokine can induce the activation of coagulation and fibrinolysis [78, 79] which likely results from the release of TNF.

Effects of clotting factors on cytokines

Thrombin can stimulate the release of chemokines by endothelial or monocyte cells via catalytic activation of the thrombin receptor [80, 81]. In addition, thrombin can induce monocytes to secrete IL-8 and the chemokine monocyte chemotactic protein (MCP)-1 indirectly by activating platelets, which in turn stimulate monocytes via P-selectin and P-selectin glycoprotein ligand-1 [82]. Also in a whole blood culture system thrombin was shown to be able to induce the release of IL-8 but not that of other pro-inflammatory cytokines [83]. Thrombin is also able to induce the production of IL-6 by fibroblasts or epithelial cells [84] whereas fibrin may enhance the expression of IL-1β by mononuclear cells [85]. Thus, these *in vitro* data show that activated clotting factors may modulate the production of cytokines by various cell populations.

Whether these effects of thrombin or other clotting factors occur *in vivo* has yet to be established. In low grade endotoxemia in primates, inhibition of factor VII has no effect on the release of cytokines [59], indicating that in this model activated clotting factors (at least activated via the extrinsic pathway) do not contribute to the induction or release of cytokines. On the other hand, administration of TFPI to animals suffering from lethal *E. coli* sepsis results in an attenuated IL-6 response without affecting the response of TNF [86, 87], suggesting that some activated clotting factors may contribute to the generation of IL-6 in this condition. Elucidating the mechanism via which TFPI affects IL-6 *in vivo* is important since TFPI reduces mortality in this model, even when administered after the challenge. One possibility is that the effect of TFPI on cytokines is related to the formation of thrombin since, at least *in vitro*, TFPI can affect thrombin-induced cytokine IL-8 release in whole blood cultures [83]. TFPI also greatly reduces the increase in IL-8 in baboons lethally challenged with *E. coli* (PM Jansen et al., submitted). Similar effects are exerted by high doses of antithrombin III in this model (CE Hack et al, unpublished observations). That activated clotting factors can contribute to the release of cytokines in this baboon model for sepsis was also demonstrated by a study whereby a neutralizing antibody against factor XII reduced the release of IL-6 [65].

Conclusions

It is clear from *in vitro* as well as *in vivo* studies that TNF and IL-1 can both induce activation of the clotting and the fibrinolytic systems. Studies with inhibitors of either cytokine indicate that in the mild models of sepsis, only the activation of the fibrinolytic system seems to be triggered by TNF whereas cytokines have no effect on the coagulative response. In the more severe models, both cytokines seems to be involved in the activation of the clotting system whereas the effects on the fibrinolytic system are only mild. To what extent these interactions between IL-1 and TNF with the clotting and the fibrinolytic systems occur in septic patients remains to be established. Under some conditions IL-6 may contribute to clotting activation as well, although the molecular mechanisms of this interaction are not known. Finally, some anti-coagulant agents have anti-inflammatory effects *in vivo* and are able to confer (partial) protection in lethal sepsis models. These protective effects are accompanied by reduced levels of circulating cytokines. The mechansims underlying these anti-inflammatory effects of some clotting inhibitors are not well understood.

References

1   Hack CE, Aarden LA,Thijs LG (1997) Role of cytokines in sepsis. *Adv Immunol* 66: 101–195

2   Naito K, Fujikawa K (1991) Activation of human blood coagulation factor XI independent of factor XII. *J Biol Chem* 266: 7353–7358

3   Gailani D, Broze GJ jr (1991) Factor XI activation in a revised model of blood coagulation. *Science* 253: 909–912

4   Broze GJ Jr (1992) The role of tissue factor pathway inhibitor in a revised coagulation cascade. *Seminars Hematology* 29: 159–169

5   Davie EW, Fujikawa K, Kisiel W (1991) The coagulation cascade: initiation, maintenance, and regulation. *Biochemistry* 30: 10363–10370

6   Borne PAKr von dem, Meijers JCM, Bouma BN (1995) Feedback activation of factor XI by thrombin in plasma results in additional formation of thrombin that protects fibrin clots from fibrinolysis. *Blood* 86: 3035–3042

7   Kaplan AP (1985) The intrinsic coagulation, fibrinolytic and kinin-forming pathways of man. In: Kelley WN, Harris ED, Ruddy S, Sledge CB (eds): *Textbook of rheumatology.* WB Saunders, Philadelphia, 95–114

8   Bachmann F (1987) Fibrinolysis. In: Verstraete M, Vermylen J, Lijnen R, Arnout J (eds): *Thrombosis and Haemostasis XIth Congress.* Leuven University Press, Leuven, 227–265

9   Kluft C, Dooijewaard G, Emeis JJ (1987) Role of the contact system in fibrinolysis. *Thromb Haemost* 13: 50–68

10 Ratnoff OD, Busse RJ Jr, Sheon RP (1968) The demise of John Hageman. *N Engl J Med* 279: 760–761

11 Levi M, De Boer JP, Roem D, Ten Cate JW, Hack CE (1992) Plasminogen activation *in vivo* upon intravenous infusion of DDAVP: quantitative assessment of plasmin-α2-antiplasmin complexes with a novel monoclonal antibody based radioimmunoassay. *Thromb Haemost* 67: 111–116

12 Levi M, Hack CE, De Boer JP, Brandjes DPM, Büller HR, ten Cate, WJ (1991) Reduction of contact activation related fibrinolytic activity in factor XII deficient patients. Further evidence for the role of the contact system in fibrinolysis *in vivo. J Clin Invest* 88: 1155–1160

13 Yamamoto T, Cochrane CG (1981) Guinea pig Hageman factor as a vascular permeability enhancement factor. *Am J Pathol* 105: 164–175

14 Vane JR, Anggård EE, Botting RM (1990) Regulatory functions of the vascular endothelium. *N Engl J Med* 323: 27–36

15 Colman RW, Wachtfogel YT, Kucich U, Weinbaum G, Hahn S, Pixley RA, Scott CF, De Agostini A, Burger D, Schapira M (1985) Effect of cleavage of the heavy chain of human plasma kallikrein and its functional properties. *Blood* 65: 311–318

16 Kaplan AP, Kay AB, Austen KF (1972) A prealbumin activator of prekallikrein. II. Appearance of chemotactic activity for neutrophils by the conversion of human prekallikrein to kallikrein. *J Exp Med* 135: 81–97

17 Ghebrehiwet B, Randazzo BP, Dunn JT (1983) Mechanisms of activation of the classical pathway of complement by Hageman Factor fragment. *J Clin Invest* 71: 1450–1455

18 Ghebrehiwet B, Silverberg M, Kaplan AP (1981) Activations of the classical pathway of complement by Hageman Factor fragment. *J Exp Med* 153: 665–676

19 Kruithof EKO (1988) Plasminogen Activator Inhibitor type 1: biochemical, biological and clinical aspects. *Fibrinolysis* 2: 59–70

20 Sprengers ED, Kluft C (1987) Plasminogen activator inhibitors. *Blood* 69: 381–387

21   Travis J, Salvesen GS (1983) Human plasma proteinase inhibitors. *Annu Rev Biochem* 52: 655–709

22   Le J, Vilçek J (1987) Biology of disease; tumor necrosis factor and interleukin 1: cytokines with multiple overlapping biological activities. *Lab Invest* 56: 234–248

23   Movat HZ, Burrowes CE, Cybulsky MI, Dinarello CA (1987) Acute inflammation and a Shwartzman-like reaction induced by interleukin-1 and tumor necrosis factor. *Am J Pathol* 129: 463–476

24   Bevilacqua MP, Pober JS, Majeau GR, Fiers W, Cotran RS, Gimbrone MA Jr (1986) Recombinant tumor necrosis factor induces procoagulant activity in cultured human vascular endothelium: characterization and comparison with the actions of interleukin 1. *Proc Natl Acad Sci USA* 83: 4533–4537

25   Nawroth PP, Stern DM (1986) Modulation of endothelial cell hemostatic properties by tumor necrosis factor. *J Exp Med* 163: 740–745

26   Lentz SR, Tsiang M, Sadler JE (1991) Regulation of thrombomodulin by tumor necrosis factor-α: Comparison of transcriptional and posttranscriptional mechanisms. *Blood* 77: 542–550

27   Pober JS, Gimbrone MA Jr, Lapierre LA, Mendrick DL, Fiers W, Rothlein R, Springer TA (1986) Overlapping patterns of activation of human endothelial cells by interleukin 1, tumor necrosis factor, and immune interferon. *J Immunol* 137: 1893–1896

28   Koga S, Morris S, Ogawa S, Liao H, Bilezikian JP, Chen G, Thompson WJ, Ashikaga T, Brett J, Stern DM (1995) TNF modulates endothelial properties by decreasing cAMP. *Am J Physiol* 268: 1104–1113

29   Parry GC, Mackmann N (1995) Transcriptional regulation of tissue factor expression in human endothelial cells. *Arterioscler Thromb Vasc Biol* 15: 612–621

30   Kirchhofer D, Tschopp TB, Hadvary P, Baumgartner HR (1994) Endothelial cells stimulated with tumor necrosis factor-alpha express varying amounts of tissue factor resulting in homogenous fibrin deposition in a native blood flow system. Effects of thrombin inhibitors. *J Clin Invest* 93: 2073–2083

31   Sawdey M, Podor TJ, Loskutoff DJ (1989) Regulation of type 1 plasminogen activator inhibitor gene expression in cultured bovine aortic endothelial cells. Induction by transforming growth factor-β, lipopolysaccharide, and tumor necrosis factor-α. *J Biol Chem* 264: 10396–10401

32   Nachman RL, Hajjar KA, Silverstein RL, Dinarello CA (1986) Interleukin 1 induces endothelial cell synthesis of plasminogen activator inhibitor. *J Exp Med* 163: 1595–1600

33   Schleef RR, Bevilacqua MP, Sawdey M, Gimbrone MA Jr, Loskutoff DJ (1988) Cytokine activation of vascular endothelium. *J Biol Chem* 263: 5797–5803

34   Van Hinsbergh VWM, van den Berg EA, Fiers W, Dooijewaard G (1990) Tumor necrosis factor induces the production of urokinase- type plasminogen activator by human endothelial cells. *Blood* 75: 1991–1998

35   Van Hinsbergh VWM, Kooistra T, van den Berg EA, Princen HMG, Fiers W, Emeis JJ (1988) Tumor necrosis factor increases the production of plasminogen activator inhibitor in human endothelial cells *in vitro* and rats *in vivo*. *Blood* 72: 1467–1473

36 Niedbala MJ, Picarella MS (1992) Tumor necrosis factor induction of endothelial cell urokinase- type plasminogen activator mediated proteolysis of extracellular matrix and its antagonism by gamma-interferon. *Blood* 79: 678–687

37 Wisniewski HG, Hua JC, Poppers DM, Naime D, Vilçek J, Cronstein BN (1996) TNF/IL-1-inducible protein TSG-6 potentiates plasmin inhibition by inter-α-inhibitor and exerts a strong anti-inflammatory effect *in vivo*. *J Immunol* 156: 1609–1615

38 Remick DG, Strieter RM, Eskandari MK, Nguyen DT, Genord MA, Raiford CL, Kunkel SL (1990) Role of tumor necrosis factor-alpha in lipopolysaccharide-induced pathologic alterations. *Am J Pathol* 136: 49–60

39 Piguet PF, Grau GE, Vassalli P (1990) Subcutaneous perfusion of tumor necrosis factor induces local proliferation of fibroblasts, capillaries, and epidermal cells, or massive tissue necrosis. *Am J Pathol* 136: 103–110

40 Remick DG, Kunkel RG, Larrick JW, Kunkel SL (1987) Acute *in vivo* effects of human recombinant tumor necrosis factor. *Lab Invest* 56: 583–590

41 Butler LD, Layman NK, Cain RL, Riedl PE, Mohler KM, Bobbitt JL, Belagajie R, Sharp J, Bendele AM (1989) Interleukin 1-induced pathophysiology: induction of cytokines, development of histopathologic changes, and immunopharmacologic intervention. *Clin Immunol Immunopathol* 53: 400–421

42 Okusawa S, Gelfland JA, Ikejima T, Connolly RJ, Dinarello CA (1988) Interleukin 1 induces a shock-like state in rabbits. *J Clin Invest* 81: 1162–1172

43 Johnson J, Brigham KL, Jesmok G, Meyrick B (1991) Morphologic changes in lungs of anesthetized sheep following intravenous infusion of recombinant tumor necrosis factor alpha. *Am Rev Respir Dis* 144: 179–186

44 Stephens KE, Ishizaka A, Larrick JW, Raffin TA (1988) Tumor necrosis factor causes increased pulmonary permeability and edema. Comparison to septic acute lung injury. *Am Rev Respir Dis* 137: 1364–1370

45 van der Poll T, Büller HR, ten Cate H, Wortel CH, Bauer KA, Van Deventer SJH, Hack CE, Sauerwein HP, Rosenberg RD, ten Cate JW (1990) Activation of coagulation after administration of tumor necrosis factor to normal subjects. *N Engl J Med* 322: 1622–1626

46 van der Poll T, Levi M, Buller HR, Van Deventer SJH, De Boer JP, Hack CE, ten Cate, JW (1991) Fibrinolytic response to tumor necrosis factor in healthy subjects. *J Exp Med* 174: 729–732

47 Bauer KA, ten Cate H, Barzegar S, Spriggs DR, Sherman ML, Rosenberg RD (1989) Tumor necrosis factor infusions have a procoagulant effect on hemostatic mechanism of humans. *Blood* 74: 165–172

48 Van Hinsbergh VWM, Bauer KA, Kooistra T, Kluft C, Dooijewaard G, Sherman ML, Nieuwenhuizen W (1990) Progress of fibrinolysis during tumor necrosis factor infusions in humans. Concomitant increase in tissue-type plasminogen activator, plasminogen activator inhibitor type-1, and fibrin(ogen) degradation products. *Blood* 76: 2284–2289

49 Ogilvie AC, Hack CE, Wagstaff J, Mierlo GJvan, Eerenberg AJM, Thomsen LL, Hoekman K, Rankin EM (1996) IL-1beta does not cause neutrophil degranulation but does

lead to IL-6, IL-8, and nitrite/nitrate release when used in patients with cancer. *J Immunol* 156: 389–394

50 Naito Y, Fukata J, Shindo K, Ebisui O, Murakami N, Tominaga T, Nakai Y, Mori K, Kasting NW, Imura H (1991) Effects of interleukins on plasma arginine vasopressin and oxytocin levels in conscious freely moving rats. *Biochem Biophys Res Commun* 174: 1189–1195

51 Taylor FB, He SE, Chang ACK, Box J, Ferrell G, Lee D, Lockhart M, Peer G, Esmon CT (1996) Infusion of phospholipid vesicles amplifies the local thrombotic response to TNF and anti-protein C into a consumptive response. *Thromb Haemost* 75: 578–584

52 Poll T van der, Jansen PM, Zee KJ van, Burress Welborn III M Jong I de, Hack CE Loetscher HR, Lesslauer W Lowry SF, Moldawer LL (1996) Tumor necrosis factor-α induces activation of coagulation and fibrinolysis in baboons through an exclusive effect on the p55 receptor. *Blood* 88: 922–927

53 Nurnberger W, Holthausen S, Schirlau K, Michelmann I, Burdach S, Gobel U (1993) Activation of the complement and contact system during rTNF-alpha/rIFN-gamma therapy. *Mol Immunol* 30 (suppl 1): 39

54 Michie HR, Manogue KR, Spriggs DR, Revhaug A, O'Dwyer S, Dinarello CA, Cerami A, Wolff SM, Wilmore DW (1988) Detection of circulating tumor necrosis factor after endotoxin administration. *N Engl J Med* 318: 1481–1486

55 Cannon JG, Tompkins RG, Gelfand JA, Michie HR, Stanford GG, Van der Meer JWM, Endres S, Lonnemann G, Corsetti J, Chernow B et al (1990) Circulating interleukin-1 and tumor necrosis factor in septic shock and experimental endotoxin fever. *J Infect Dis* 161: 79–84

56 Suffredini AF, Harpel PC, Parillo JE (1989) Promotion and subsequent inhibition of plasminogen activator after administation of intravenous endotoxin to normal subjects. *N Engl J Med* 18: 1165–1171

57 Van Deventer SJH, Büller HR, Ten Cate JW, Aarden LA, Hack CE Sturk A (1990) Experimental endotoxemia in humans: analysis of cytokine release and coagulation, fibrinolytic, and complement pathways. *Blood* 76: 2520–2526

58 van der Poll T, Coyle SM, Levi M, Jansen PM, Dentener M, Barbosa K, Buurman WA, Hack CE, ten Cate JW, Agosti JM et al (1997) Effect of a recombinant dimeric tumor necrosis factor receptor on inflammatory responses to intravenous endotoxin in normal humans. *Blood* 89: 3727–3734

59 Levi M, ten Cate H, Bauer KA, van der Poll T, Edgington TS, Buller HR, Van Deventer SJH, Hack CE, ten Cate JW, Rosenberg RD (1994) Inhibition of endotoxin-induced activation of coagulation and fibrinolysis by pentoxifylline or by a monoclonal anti-tissue factor antibody in chimpanzees. *J Clin Invest* 93: 114–120

60 van der Poll T, Levi M, Van Deventer SJH, ten Cate H, Haagmans BL, Biemond BJ, Buller HR, Hack CE, ten Cate JW (1994) Differential effects of anti-tumor necrosis factor monoclonal antibodies on systemic inflammatory responses in experimental endotoxemia in chimpanzees. *Blood* 83: 446–451

61 Biemond BJ, Levi M, Cate Hten, Poll Tvan der, Buller HR, Hack CE Cate, JWten (1995)

Plasminogen activator and plasminogen activator inhibitor I release during experimental endotoxaemia in chimpanzees: effect of interventions in the cytokine and coagulation cascades. *Clin Sci* 88: 587–594

62 De Boer JP, Creasey AA, Chang A, Roem D, Brouwer MC, Eerenberg AJM, Hack CE, Taylor FB Jr (1993) Activation patterns of coagulation and fibrinolysis in baboons following infusion with lethal or sublethal dose of *E. coli*. *Circ Shock* 39: 59–67

63 Poll T van der, Jansen PM, Zee KJ van, Hack CE, Oldenburg HA, Loetscher H, Lesslauer W, Lowry SF, Moldawer LL (1997) Pretreatment with a 55kDa tumor necrosis factor receptor-immunoglobulin fusion protein attenuates activation of coagulation, but not of fibrinolysis during lethal bacteremia in baboons. *J Infect Dis* 176: 296–299

64 Fiedler VB, Loof I, Sander E, Voehringer V, Galanos C, Fournel MA (1992) Monoclonal antibody to tumor necrosis factor-alpha prevents lethal endotoxin sepsis in adult rhesus monkeys. *J Lab Clin Med* 120: 574–588

65 Jansen PM, Boermeester MA, Fischer E, Jong IWde, Poll Tvan der, Moldawer LL, Hack CE, Lowry SF (1995) Contribution of interleukin-1 to activation of coagulation and fibrinolysis, neutrophil degranulation, and the release of secretory-type phospholipase A2 in sepsis: studies in nonhuman primates after interleukin-1α administration and during lethal bacteremia. *Blood* 86: 1027–1034

66 Martin SJ, Green DR, Cotter TG (1994) Dicing with death: dissecting the components of the apoptosis machinery. *Trends Biochem Sci* 19: 26–30

67 Boermeester MA, Leeuwen PAM van, Coyle SM, Wolbink GJ, Hack CE, Lowry SF (1995) Interleukin-1 blockade attenuates mediator release and dysregulation of the hemostatic mechanism during human sepsis. *Arch Surg* 130: 739–748

68 Gauldie J, Richards C, Harnish D, Lansdorp PM, Baumann, H (1987) Interferon β2/B-cell stimulatory factor type 2 shares identity with monocyte-derived hepatocyte-stimulating factor and regulates the major acute phase protein response in liver cells. *Proc Natl Acad Sci USA* 84: 7251–7255

69 Baumann H, Won K-A, Jahreis GP (1989) Human hepatocyte-stimulating factor-III and interleukin- 6 are structurally and immunologically distinct but regulate the production of the same acute phase plasma proteins. *J Biol Chem* 264: 8046–8051

70 van der Poll T, Levi M, Hack CE, ten Cate H, Van Deventer SJH, Eerenberg AJM, De Groot ER, Jansen J, Gallati H, Büller HR et al (1994) Elimination of interleukin 6 attenuates coagulation activation in experimental endotoxemia in chimpanzees. *J Exp Med* 179: 1253–1259

71 Stouthard JLM Levi M, Hack CE Veenhof, CH Romijn HA, Sauerwein HP, Poll T van der (1996) Interleukin-6 stimulates coagulation, not fibrinolysis, in humans. *Thromb Haemost* 76: 738–742

72 Mestries J-C, Kruithof EKO, Gascon M-P, Herodin F, Agay D, Ythier A (1994) *In vivo* modulation of coagulation and fibrinolysis by recombinant glycosylated human interleukin-6 in baboons. *Eur Cytokine Netw* 5: 275–281

73 Citarella F, Felici A, Brouwer M, Wagstaff J, Fantoni A, Hack CE (1997) Interleukin-6

downregulates factor XII production by human hepatoma cell line (HepG2). *Blood* 90: 1501–1507

74   Niessen RWLM, Lamping RJ, Jansen PM, Prins MH, Peters M, Taylor FB Jr, Vijlder J (1997) Antithrombin acts as a negative actue phase protein as established with studies on HepG2 cells and in baboons. *Thromb Haemost* 78: 1088–1092

75   Ramani M, Ollivier V, Khechai F, Vu T, Ternisien C, Bridey F, De Prost D (1993) Interleukin-10 inhibits endotoxin-induced tissue factor mRNA production by human monocytes. *FEBS Lett* 334: 114–116

76   Pradier O, Gerard C, Delvaux A, Lybin M, Abramowicz D, Capel P, Velu T, Goldman M (1993) Interleukin-10 inhibits the induction of monocyte procoagulant activity by bacterial lipopolysaccharide. *Eur J Immunol* 23: 2700–2703

77   Jungi TW, Brcic M, Eperon S, Albrecht S (1994) Transforming growth factor-beta and interleukin-10, but not interleukin-4, down regulate procoagulant activity and tissue factor expression in human monocyte-derived macrophages. *Thromb Res* 76: 463–474

78   Baars JW, De Boer JP, Wagstaff J, Roem D, Eerenberg AJM, Nauta J, Pinedo HM, Hack CE (1992) Interleukin-2 induces activation of coagulation and fibrinolysis: resemblance to the changes seen during experimental endotoxaemia. *Br J Haematol* 82: 295–301

79   Olksowics L, Strack M, Dutcher JP, Sussman I, Caliendo G, Sparano J, Wiernik PH (1994) A distinct coagulopathy associated with interleukin-2 therapy. *Br J Haematol* 88: 892–894

80   Murakami K, Ueno A, Yamanouchi K, Kondo T (1995) Thrombin induces GROalpha/MGSA production in human umbilical vein endothelial cells. *Thromb Res* 79: 387–394

81   Colotta F, Sciacca FL, Sironi M, Luini W, Rabiet MJ, Mantovani A (1994) Expression of monocyte chemotactic protein-1 by monocytes and endothelial cells exposed to thrombin. *Am J Pathol* 144: 975–985

82   Weyrich AS, Elstad MR, McEver RP, McIntyre TM, Moore KL, Morrissey JH, Prescott SM, Zimmerman GA (1996) Activated platelets signal chemokine synthesis by human monocytes. *J Clin Invest* 97: 1525–1534

83   Johnson K, Aarden L, Choi Y, Groot E, Creasey A (1996) The proinflammatory cytokine response to coagulation and endotoxin in whole blood. *Blood* 87: 5051–5060

84   Sower LE, Froelich CJ, Carney DH, Fenton JW, Klimpel GR (1995) Thrombin induces IL-6 production in fibroblasts and epithelial cells. Evidence for the involvement of the seven-transmembrane domain (STD) receptor for alpha-thrombin. *J Immunol* 155: 895–901

85   Perez RL, Roman J (1995) Fibrin enhances the expression of IL-1beta by human peripheral blood mononuclear cells. Implications for inflammation. *J Immunol* 154: 1879–1887

86   Creasey AA, Chang AC, Feigen L, Wun TC, Taylor FB Jr, Hinshaw LB (1993) Tissue factor pathway inhibitor reduces mortality from *Escherichia Coli* septic shock. *J Clin Invest* 91: 2850–2856

87   Carr C, Bild GS, Chang ACK, Peer GT, Palmier MO, Frazier RB, Gustafson ME, Wun

TC, Creasey AA, Hinshaw LB et al (1995) Recombinant E.coli derived tissue factor pathway inhibitor reduces coagulopathic and lethal effects in the baboon Gram-negative model of septic shock. *Circ Shock* 44: 126–135

Apoptosis: Its role in the systemic inflammatory response syndrome and the involvement of cytokines

R. William G. Watson

R. William G. Watson, Surgical Professorial Unit, Mater Hospital, University College Dublin, 47 Eccles Street, Dublin 7, Ireland

Introduction

Death, along with growth, is a critical part of the life cycle of all living things. The loss of leaves during the autumn, as a result of environmental changes during winter, is central to the survival and continued growth of a tree. Harmful levels of UV-radiation from the sun causes damage and death of keratinocytes and resulting sunburn. The death of cells is not always as a result of damage but may occur spontaneously to allow for further development and growth. For plants to conduct fluid, cells that form the xylem must die giving way to hollow tubes. In humans cell death is vital for embryonic development of fingers and toes. Homeostatic control of cell numbers is a result of the dynamic balance between cell proliferation and cell death and essential to maintain a steady volume [1]. Cancer cells have lost their ability to control this balance resulting in an accumulation of cells [2]. Thymocytes that fail to mature with functional receptors are induced to die, thereby limiting the release of none functional cells into the host and preventing autoimmune targeting of the host [3]. During inflammation there is an increased production and accumulation of lymphocytes, monocytes and neutrophils to overwhelm the invading foreign pathogen [4]. This production of inflammatory cells itself can be detrimental or "double edged" to the host due to the overproduction of anti-microbial agents causing tissue damage [5]. The resolution of an inflammatory response is thus important in preventing this host damage. The final step in resolving inflammation is the removal of the influxed cells from the inflammatory site. These must die *in situ* as they can not migrate from the site [6].

Cells die by one of two processes, necrosis or programmed cell death (apoptosis) [7–9]. Necrotic death occurs as a result of severe injury to the cell, in a sudden and uncontrolled process. It is characterized by the swelling and rupture of the cell due to uncontrolled regulation of fluids and ions (sodium and calcium). The release of the intracellular contents of the cell into the surrounding environment can worsen the injury that initiated the process. Programmed cell death or apoptosis, as the name suggests, is a controlled process resulting in the death of a cell and removal by

Cytokines in Severe Sepsis and Septic Shock, edited by H. Redl and G. Schlag[†]

surrounding phagocytes (mainly the macrophage) [10]. In the classical Greek Hippocratic corpus the word "apoptosis", a compound of the words "apo" (apart) and "ptosis" (falling), referred to the loss of flower petals, or leaves in the autumn [1]. The concept that death is programmed has been well recognized, the transformation of a caterpillar via a pupa into a butterfly requires cells to die and reorganize [11]. The tail of a tadpole is lost by the process of apoptosis as it develops into a frog. *Caenorhabditis elegans*, a 1 mm nematode, demonstrated changes in cell numbers, which has significantly helped in the understanding of apoptosis. This worm loses exactly 131 cells during its development [12]. All these processes are programmed and result in the process of apoptosis.

Definitions and characteristics of apoptosis

Cells undergoing apoptosis all demonstrate more or less the same characteristics, however, individual cell types differ in the extent to which they express these changes. A number of morphologically identifiable stages have been reported. These include nuclear changes, exuberant cell surface protrusion, and breaking-up of the nucleus to form multiple fragments and compacted chromatin. These changes are accompanied by flipping of phosphatidylserine from the inner plasma membrane to the cell surface which can be detected by the phosphatidylserine-binding protein, Annexin V. Finally, the cell surface protuberances separate to produce membrane-enclosed apoptotic bodies of varying size in which the closely packed cytoplasmic organelles remain well preserved [7, 8]. The nuclear collapse that is the hallmark of apoptosis has as its biochemical correlate the fragmentation of DNA by endonucleases, producing fragments in the range 300 to 50 kbp. The DNA cleavage continues with internucleosomal double-stranded cutting to produce the familiar ladder on agarose gel electrophoresis [9] (Fig. 1).

Regulation of apoptosis

Even though death is programmed in all cells to occur at specific times in the development of the organism, apoptosis may occur as the result of various triggers including environmental change or genetic alterations. Regulating signals can come from a number of sources. Extracellular matrix proteins send signals to epithelial cells preventing them from dying, remove these signals and the cell will undergo apoptosis [13]. Migration of inflammatory neutrophils through endothelial cells triggers $\beta2$ integrin-mediated delays in spontaneous apoptosis [14]. The most well known surface receptors that signal the induction of apoptosis are part of the tumor necrosis factor receptor family. TNFR1 and Fas initiate death signals through "death domains" in their receptors on interaction with the corresponding

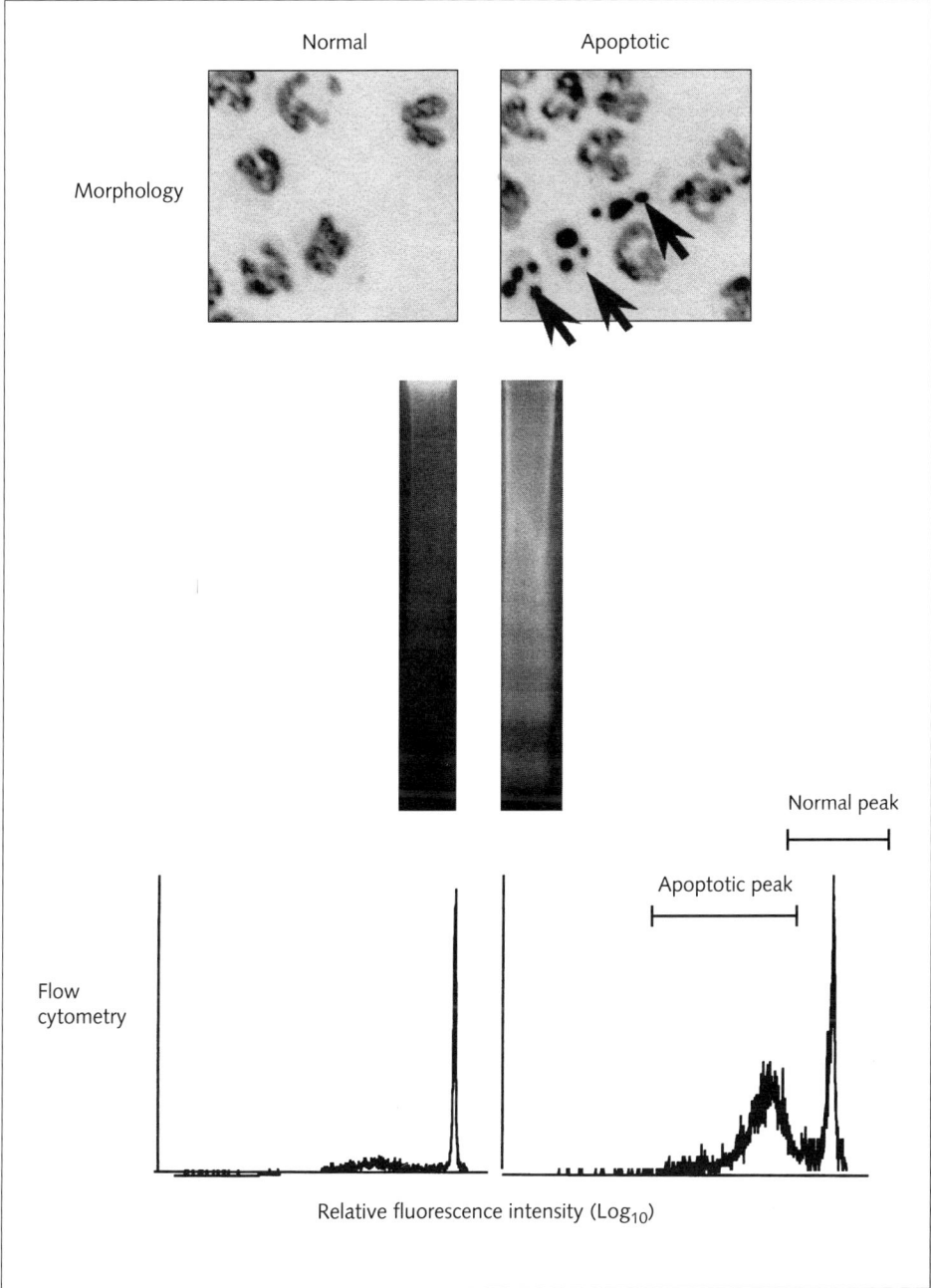

Figure 1
Characteristics of detectable features of apoptosis.

antigens TNFα and Fas ligand (Fas L), respectively [15–18]. The biological impor-tance of the Fas/FasL system has been extensively studied in T cells, where it plays a critical role in the clonal deletion of autoreactive T cells and activation-induced suicide of T cells [18, 19]. Fas L can function in either autocrine or paracrine path-ways to cell death [20]. A series of murine mutations in Fas (*lpr*) or in Fas L (*gld*) have provided a powerful means of demonstrating the involvement of this system in various apoptosis-activating pathways [21]. The Fas/Fas L system has also been implicated in "immune privilege" where several tissues in the body want to pro-tect themselves from autoimmunity [22]. These include certain cells of the testis [23], eye [24] and possibly the brain, which express high levels of Fas L. Interac-tion of Fas positive inflammatory cells, such as T cells or neutrophils [25, 26], induces an apoptotic response and prevents a potentially harmful inflammatory response.

The signaling mechanism by which Fas and TNFR1 induce cell death still remains unclear. However, ligation of Fas and TNFR1 results in the binding of MORT1 (or FADD) [27] and TRADD [28] proteins, respectively. These adapter proteins have been shown to then bind MACHα [29, 30], a novel ICE/CED-3 pro-teolytic enzyme, now called caspase [31]. This caspase family of proteases originat-ed from studies in *C. elegans*. During normal development, 131 of the total 1,090 cells of the worm die by apoptosis giving rise to the mature adult. Two genes, *ced-3* and *ced-4* are required for this programmed cell death [32]. The mammalian equivalent of these genes is interleukin 1β converting enzyme (caspase 1)[32] and CPP32 (caspase 3)[33]. Overexpression of these genes in transformed mammalian cells results in the induction of apoptosis. Likewise, inhibition of caspase activity by CrmA viral expression [34] or protease inhibitors block the expression of apoptosis [35]. These cysteine proteases are well conserved in animals and nematodes that would indicate that they are central to the processes of cell death. To date ten mem-bers make up the caspase family in human cells [31]. All are cysteine proteases with a common pentapeptide sequence -QACRG- that constitutes the active site of the molecule, and all cleave their target proteins at aspartic acid residues [36]. The cas-pases carry out their destruction of the cell through the cleavage of a number of sub-strates essential for cellular function. Interleukin 1β converting enzyme cleaves actin (which gives the cell its structure) resulting in cell shrinkage and blubbing [36]. CPP32 is specific for poly(ADP ribose) polymerase cleavage thus preventing the repair of the fragmented DNA, an important characteristic of apoptotic cell death [35].

The other gene identified from these worms was *ced-9*, which was shown to inhibit cell death of these 131 cells [36]. The mammalian equivalent of *ced-9* is Bcl-2, which when overexpressed in mammalian cells results in delayed apoptosis [36]. Again, similar to the caspase family, there is now a family of Bcl-2 like proteins including Bcl-x_L, Bax and Bad [37, 38]. Some of these proteins block apoptosis but other members of the family have been shown to induce it. The proportion of blockers to promoters determines if apoptosis can proceed. Transgenic mice with increased Bcl-2 expression result in the accumulation of follicular center B cells [39]. This effect is a result of decreased cell death rather than an effect on the rate of cell proliferation. Again, similar to *ced-3* and *-4*, Bcl-2 is able to function in cells from worms, insects, and mammals, blocking the activation of cell death; further implicating these genes as a central mechanism for cell death.

Reactive oxygen species have been shown to play a role in inducing apoptotic signals [40] as H_2O_2 [41] and radiation [42] both induce apoptosis in different cell systems. Antioxidants have also been shown to inhibit apoptosis induced by these treatments. Further studies have shown that Bcl-2 expression blocks apoptosis by protecting against oxidative stress [43]. Kane et al. [44] have shown that Bcl-2 blocks GT1-7 neural cell death brought on by depletion of glutathione. It is however believed that oxygen radicals are not directly responsible for the DNA degradation or the membrane damage seen during the final common pathway of apoptosis. Oxygen radicals may deplete thiols that could activate other enzymes responsible for cell death. The endogenous formation of reactive oxygen species and depletion of thiols could be a constitutive factor that tends to drive cells to apoptosis even in the absence of exogenous stimuli. Such a model of apoptosis is consistent with the view by Raff et al. [45] that the default state of cells is to die by programmed cell death unless kept alive by specific signals or anti-apoptotic agents.

Apoptosis and the systemic inflammatory response syndrome (SIRS)

It has been well established that the neutrophil plays an important role in the development of a number of inflammatory diseases ranging from rheumatoid arthritis [46] and myocardial reperfusion injury [47] to acute respiratory distress syndrome (ARDS) [48]. The removal of inflammatory neutrophils from the site of infection is an essential step in the resolution of this process.

Mature human neutrophils have the shortest life span and die rapidly via apoptosis *in vivo* and *in vitro*, resulting in the demise of the entire population within 72 h. As neutrophils proceed through apoptosis, functional activity declines. Apoptotic neutrophils lose CD16 (FcgRIII) [49] expression and demonstrate a reduced ability to degranulate, generate a respiratory burst, or undergo shape changes in response to external stimuli such as the chemotactic bacterial peptides [50]. Alterations in functional activity of these inflammatory cells induced by apoptosis may serve to render the cell functionally ineffective before removal by scavenger phagocytes. This state of ineffectiveness may benefit the host where resolution of the response is required. Prolonging neutrophil survival and hence causing the delay in their removal could potentially exacerbate the disease state and result in additional neutrophil-mediated tissue damage [5, 51] (Fig. 2).

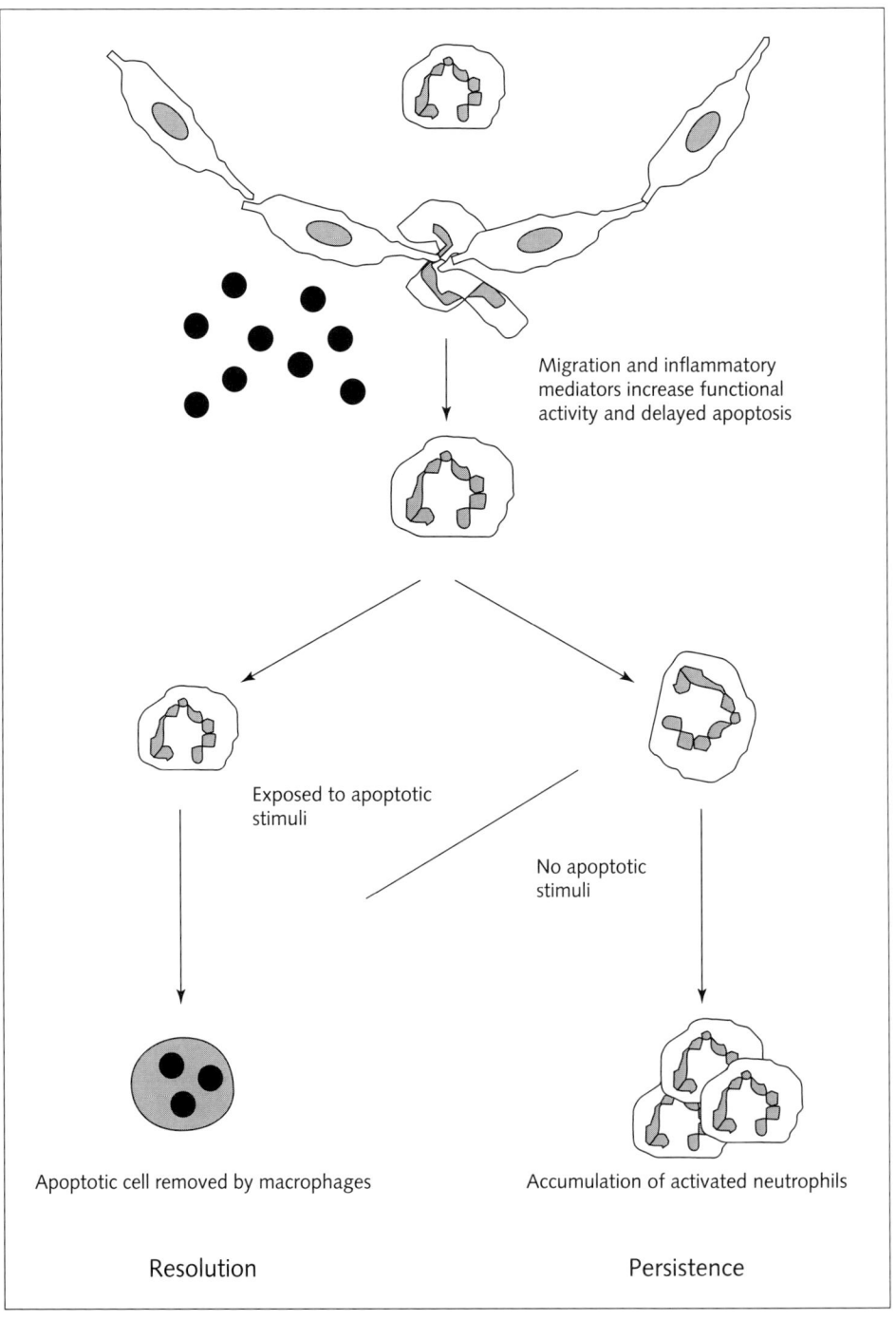

Migration and inflammatory mediators increase functional activity and delayed apoptosis

Exposed to apoptotic stimuli

No apoptotic stimuli

Apoptotic cell removed by macrophages

Accumulation of activated neutrophils

Resolution

Persistence

Modulation of neutrophil apoptosis

Although neutrophils appear to be committed to death via spontaneous apoptosis, it is clear that the life span and functional activity of mature neutrophils can be extended significantly by the inflammatory microenvironment. Proinflammatory cytokines, cell migration, and the neutrophil's state of activation have been shown to mediate neutrophil survival. The effect of a given mediator varies with the experimental circumstances and the cell population examined, however, C5a [50], granulocyte colony-stimulating factor (G-CSF) [52], granulocyte-macrophage colony-stimulating factor (GM-CSF) [50, 52], IFNγ [53], IL-6 [54], IL-2 [55], IL-1β [54] and bacterial products such as lipopolysaccharides (LPS) and formyl-methionyl-leucyl-phenylalanine (fMLP) [50], delay apoptosis. Recent studies have also demonstrated that the process of migration results in delayed apoptosis [56], this being mediated through β2 integrins [14]. Physiological activation is not solely responsible for suppression of neutrophil apoptosis. Anti-inflammatory glucocorticoids also exert a protective effect on neutrophil survival by delaying apoptosis [57].

Components of the inflammatory response do not, however, only delay the apoptotic process. The inflammatory mediators IL-6 [58], IL-10 [59], TNFα [60, 61] and anti-Fas antibodies [25, 26, 62] result in the induction of neutrophil cell death. IL-10 has been shown to prevent stimulated survival of neutrophils and results in apoptosis and clearance of an inflammatory response [59, 63]. Oxidative metabolites produced upon ingestion of bacteria have also been shown to induce apoptosis of both non-stimulated and inflammatory neutrophils [61]. Other oxidative stresses such as the sulfhydryl oxidation of neutrophil thiols also results in this effect [64]. This alteration in oxidative state of the cell may act as a signal to the neutrophil indicating that it has achieved its primary function of ingesting and killing bacteria and now must be removed from the inflammatory site (Tab. 1).

During inflammation there is evidence demonstrating that cellular susceptibility to Fas and TNFR1 can be lost [65]. This loss of susceptibility to cell death signals has been associated with decreased caspase 1 and caspase 3 protein expression. *In vitro* studies have demonstrated that elevations in intracellular anti-oxidants, GSH and NAC, may be involved in this process [26].

This regulation of neutrophil apoptosis by different components of the inflammatory response may play a critical role in the resolution of inflammation. Delayed apoptosis of these short-lived cells by inflammation is central to the fight against infection, however, the induction of apoptosis in functionally spent cells is central to their recognition by the surrounding local macrophages and removal from the site of inflammation (Fig. 2).

Figure 2
Requirement for the resolution or persistence of an inflammatory response.

Table 1 - Mediators involved in the regulation of neutrophil apoptosis

	Delay	**Induction**
Mediators	IL-1β	IL-6*
	IL-2	Il-10
	Il-6*	TNFα*
	G-CSF	Fas ligand
	GM-CSF	
	IFNγ	
	TNFα*	
	C5a	
	LPS	
	fMLP	
	Glucocorticoids	
Cellular process	β₂ integrins	Phagocytosis of opsonized
	Elevation in Ca²	*E. coli* and associated respiratory burst
		L-Selectin adhesion
		Reduced intracellular thios

*Conflicting evidence

Neutrophil apoptosis *in vivo*

The systemic inflammatory response syndrome (SIRS) denotes the generalized expression of a process that is normally localized to the site of an acute challenge [66]. Although apoptosis in critically ill patients has not been extensively studied, the available data show intriguing abnormalities.

Neutrophils harvested from burn patients show increased survival secondary to retarded neutrophil apoptosis. The apoptotic delay is mediated by a soluble serum factor whose activity can be blocked with a blocking antibody to GM-CSF [67], even though GM-CSF could not be measured in the serum. This suggests that the release of this endogenous mediator also modulates cell survival in the systemic circulation. Studies in a group of patients with SIRS have found that rates of spontaneous neutrophil apoptosis *in vitro* are reduced to approximately one quarter of those of control cells and that the altered responsiveness can be attributed to both cellular changes in patients' neutrophils, and to soluble factors in the serum. These studies are the first to demonstrate that delay in neutrophil apoptosis may account for the persistence of an inflammatory response and resulting detrimental tissue damage.

Apoptosis in multiple organ dysfunction syndrome

Liver

Hepatocyte injury can result from a number of mechanisms, including ischemia, free radical formation, and cytotoxicity mediated by bacteria or cytokines [68]. Apoptosis is a feature of various liver injuries, but its regulation/dysregulation remains poorly understood. The CD95 receptor system has been implicated in this process as hepatocytes are highly sensitive to TNF and Fas-mediated apoptosis [69]. TNF plays a pivotal role in sepsis, induced by endotoxin and other inflammatory mediators. Endotoxin-induced liver injury is TNF-mediated and apoptosis appears to be a decisive event in the prenecrotic phase of liver damage [70]. The cytotoxic effects of T and natural killer lymphocytes are mainly mediated through the initiation of apoptosis. The mechanism may involve an increased expression of receptors on hepatocytes and increased expression of ligands by T lymphocytes [71]. Neutrophils which also express Fas L may also play a role during their infiltration of the liver.

Lung

Neutrophils play a significant role in lung injury due to the release of a number of inflammatory mediators associated with their functional activity. Resolution of acute lung injury requires the removal of inflammatory neutrophils from the site via the process of apoptosis. These apoptotic bodies are then removed by the surrounding alveolar macrophages. Administration of LPS to the lung results in neutrophil infiltration, while high doses cause delayed neutrophil apoptosis and the development of acute lung injury [14]. Low doses of LPS cause neutrophil migration but these cells die by apoptosis within 72 h with no lung damage [72]. IL-10 has been shown to protect against acute lung injury by inducing neutrophil apoptosis and resolving the inflammatory response [58].

Conclusion

Controlling cell death is as important to the survival of living organisms as is the regulation of growth and development. Derangement of the normal process of apoptotic cell death is now recognized as playing a critical role in a variety of disease processes including autoimmunity, degenerative disorders, and cancer, and this recognition has opened the door to novel therapeutic possibilities directed at manipulation of apoptosis. An evolving understanding of the role of inflammatory cell apoptosis in the expression and termination of the host response to an acute life-

221

threatening stimulus should similarly provide us with new tools to modulate the inflammatory response for the ultimate benefit of the critically ill patients.

References

1   Kerr JFR, Wyllie AH, Currie AR (1972) Apoptosis: a basic biological phenomenon with wide-ranging implications in tissue kinetics *Br J Cancer* 26: 239–257

2   Carson DA, Ribeiro JM (1993) Apotosis and disease. *Lancet* 341: 1251–1254

3   Cohen JJ (1992) Apoptosis and programmed cell death in immunity. *Ann Rev Immunol* 10: 267–293

4   Weiss SJ (1989) Tissue destruction by neutrophils. *N Engl J Med* 320: 365–376

5   Smith JA (1994) Neutrophils, host defense and inflammation: a double-edged sword. *J Leukoc Biol* 56: 672–686

6   Haslett C (1992) Resolution of acute inflammation and the role of apoptosis in the tissue fate of granulocytes. *Clin Sci* 83: 639–648

7   Gerschenson LE, Rotello RJ (1992) Apoptosis: a different type of cell death *FASEB J* 6: 2450–2455

8   Kerr JFR, Winterford CM, Harmon BV (1994) Apoptosis: Its significance in cancer and cancer therapy. *Cancer* 73: 2013–2026

9   Cohen JJ (1993) Apoptosis. *Immunol Today* 14: 126–130

10   Savill JS, Wyllie AH, Henson JE, Walport MJ, Henson PM, Haslett C (1989) Macrophage phagocytosis of aging neutrophils in inflammation Programmed cell death in the neutrophil leads to its recognition by macrophages *J Clin Invest* 83: 865–875

11   Lockshin RA, Williams CM (1964) Programmed cell death II Endocrine potentiation of the breakdown of the intersegmental muscles of silkworms. *J Insect Physiol* 10, 643–649

12   Yuan J, Horvitz HR (1990) The Caenorhabditis elegans genes ced-3 and ced-4 act cell autonomously to cause programmed cell death. *Dev Biol* 138, 33–41

13   Boudreau N, Sympson CJ, Werb Z, Bissell MJ (1995) Suppression of ICE and apoptosis in mammary epithelial cells by extracellular matrix. *Science* 267: 891–893

14   Watson RWG, Rotstein OD, Nathens AB, Parodo J, Marshall J (1997) Neutrophil apoptosis is modulated by endothelial transmigration and adhesion molecule engagement. *J Immunol* 158: 945–953

15   Nagata S, Golstein P (1995) The Fas death factor. *Science* 267: 1449–1456

16   Suda T, Nagata S (1994) Purification and characterization of the Fas-ligand that induces apoptosis. *J Exp Med* 179: 873–879

17   Nagata S (1994) Fas and Fas ligand: a death factor and its receptor. *Adv Immunol* 57: 129–144

18   Vignaux F, Vivier E, Malissen B, Depraetere V, Nagata S, Golstein P (1995) TCR/CD3 coupling to Fas-based cytotoxicity. *J Exp Med* 181: 781–786

19   Alderson MR, Tough TW, Davis-Smith T, Braddy S, Falk B, Schooley KA, Goodwin RG,

Smith CA, Ramadell F, Lynch DH (1995) Fas ligand mediated activation-induced cell death in human T Lymphocytes. *J Exp Med* 181: 71–77

20   Dhein J, Walczak H, Baumler C, Debatin K, Krammer PH (1995) Autocrine T-cell suicide mediated by APO-1(Fas/CD95). *Nature* 373: 438–441

21   Nagata S, Takashi S (1995) Fas and Fas ligand: lpr and gld mutations. *Immunol Today* 16: 39–43

22   Griffith TS, Brunner T, Fletcher SM, Green DR, Ferguson FA (1995) Fas ligand-induced apoptosis as a mechanism of immune privilege. *Science* 270: 1189–92

23   Bellgrau D, Gold D, Selawry H, Moore J, Franzusoff A, Duke RC (1995) A role for CD95 ligand in preventing graft rejection. *Nature* 377: 630–632

24   Griffith TS, Yu X, Herndon JM, Green DR, Ferguson TA (1996) CD95-induced apoptosis of lymphocytes in an immune privileged site induced immunological tolerance. *Immunity* 5: 7–16

25   Liles WC, Kiener PA, Ledbetter JA, Aruffo A, Klebenoff SJ (1996) Differential expression of Fas (CD95) and Fas ligand on normal human phagocytes: Implications for the regulation of apoptosis in neutrophils. *J Exp Med* 184: 429–440

26   Watson RWG, Rotstein OD, Jimenez M, Parodo J, Marshall JC (1997) Augmented intracellular glutathione inhibits Fas-triggered apoptosis of activated human neutrophils. *Blood* 89: 4175–4181

27   Chinnaiyan AM, O'Rourke K, Tewari M, Dixit VM (1995) FADD, a novel death domain-containing protein, interacts with the death domain of Fas and initiates apoptosis. *Cell* 81: 505–512

28   Hsu H, Xiong J, Goeddel DV (1995) The TNF receptor 1-associated protein TRADD signals cell death and NK-κB activation. *Cell* 81: 495–504

29   Boldin MP, Goncharov TM, Goltsev YV, Wallach D (1996) Involvement of MACH, a novel MORT1/FADD-interacting protease, in Fas/APO-1- and TNF receptor-induced cell death. *Cell* 85: 803–815

30   Muzio M, Chinnaiyan AM, Kischkel FC, et al (1996) FLICE, a novel FADD-homologous ICE/CED-3-like protease, is recruited to the CD95 (Fas/APO-1) death-inducing signaling complex. *Cell* 85: 817–828

31   Alnemri ES, Livingston DJ, Nicholson DW, Salvesen G, Thornberry NA, Wong WW, and Yuan J (1996) Human ICE/CED-3 protease nomenclature. *Cell* 87: 171–176

32   Yuan J Shaham S, Ledoux S, Ellis HM, Horvitz HR (1993) The Celegans cell death gene ced-3 encodes a protein similar to mammalian interleukin-1β-converting enzyme. *Cell* 75: 641–652

33   Schlegel J, Peters I, Orrenius S, Miller DK, Thornberry NA, Yamin T-T, Nicholson DW (1996) CPP32/Apopain is a key interleukin-1 converting enzyme-like protease involved in Fas-mediated apoptosis. *J Biol Chem* 271: 1841–1844

34   Dbaibo GS, Perry DK, Gamard CJ, Platt R, Poirier GG, Obeid LM, Hannun YA (1997) Cytokine response modifier A (CrmA) inhibits ceramide formation in response to tumor necrosis factor (TNF)-α: CrmA and Bcl-2 target distinct components in the apoptotic pathway. *J Exp Med* 185: 481–490

35   Armstrong RC, Aja T, Xiang J, Gaur S, Krebs JF, Hoang K, Bai X, Korsmeyer SJ, Karanewsky DS, Fritz LC, Tomaselli KJ (1996) Fas-induced activation of the cell death-related protease CPP32 is inhibited by Bcl-2 and by ICE family protease inhibitors. *J Biol Chem* 271: 16850–16855

36   Hengartner MO, Horvitz HR (1994) Celegans cell survival gene ced-9 encodes a functional homolog of the mammalian proto-oncogene bcl-2. *Cell* 76: 665–676

37   Vaux DL (1993) Towards an understanding of the molecular mechanisms of physiological cell death. *Proc Am Nat Acad Sci* 90: 786–789

38   White E (1996) Life, death, and the pursuit of apoptosis. *Genes Dev* 10: 1–15

39   Strasser A, Harris AW, Bath ML, Cory S (1991) Novel primitive lymphoid tumours induced in transgenic mice by cooperation between myc and bcl-2. *Nature* 348: 331–333

40   Buttke TM, Sandstrom PA (1994) Oxidative stress as a mediator of apoptosis. *Immunol Today* 15: 7–10

41   Lennon SV, Martin SJ, Cotter TG (1991) Dose-dependent induction of apoptosis in human tumour cell lines by widely diverging stimuli. *Cell Prolif* 24: 203–214

42   Chang DJ, Ringold GM, Heller RA (1992) Cell killing and induction of manganous superoxide dismutase by tumor necrosis factor-alpha is mediated by lipoxygenase metabolites of arachidonic acid. *Biochem Biophys Res Commun* 188: 538–546

43   Hockenbery DM, Oltvai ZN, Yin XM et al (1993) Bcl-2 functions in an antioxidant pathway to prevent apoptosis. *Cell* 75: 241–251

44   Kane DJ, Sarafian TA, Anton R, Hahn H, Graalla EB, Valentine JS, Ord T, Bredesen DE (1993) Bcl-2 inhibition of neural death: decreased generation of reactive oxygen species. *Science* 262: 1274–1277

45   Barres BA, Hart IK, Coles HS, Burne JF, Voyvedic JT, Richartson WD, Raff MC (1992) Cell death and control of cell survival in the oligodendrocyte lineage. *Cell* 70: 31–46

46   Robinson J, Watson F, Bucknall RC, Edwards SW (1992) Activation of neutrophil reactive oxidant production by synovial fluid from patients with inflammatory joint disease: soluble and insoluble immunoglobulin aggregates activate different pathways in primed and unprimed. *Cells Biochem J* 286: 345–351

47   McCord JM (1987) Oxygen-derived radicals: a link between reperfusion injury and inflammation. *Fed Proc* 46: 2401–2406

48   Repine JE (1992) Scientific perspectives on adult respiratory distress syndrome. *Lancet* 339: 466–469

49   Homburg CHE, Haas M, von dem Borne AEG, Verhoeven AJ, Reutelingsperger CPM, Roos D (1995) Human neutrophils lose surface FcγRIII and acquire annexin V binding sites during apoptosis *in vitro*. *Blood* 85: 532–540

50   Lee A, Whyte MKB, Haslett C (1993) Inhibition of apoptosis and prolongation of neutrophil functional longevity by inflammatory mediators. *J Leukoc Biol* 54: 283–288

51   Malech HL, Gallin JI (1987) Neutrophils in human diseases. *N Engl J Med* 317: 687–694

52   Cox G, Gauldie J, Jordana M (1992) Bronchial epithelial cell-derived cytokines (G-CSF

and GM-CSF) promote the survival of peripheral blood neutrophils *in vitro*. *Am J Respir Cell Mol Biol* 7: 507–513

53   Colotta F, Re F, Polentarutti N, Sozzani S, Mantovani A (1992) Modulation of granulocyte survival and programmed cell death by cytokines and bacterial products. *Blood* 80: 2012–2020

54   Biffl WL, Moore EE, Moore FA, Barnett CC (1995) Interleukin-6 suppression of neutrophil apoptosis is neutrophil concentration dependent. *J Leukoc Biol* 58: 582–584

55   Pericle F, Liu JH, Diaz JI, Blanchard DK, Wei S, Forni G, Djeu JY (1994) Interleukin-2 prevention of apoptosis in human neutrophils. *Eur J Immunol* 24: 440–444

56   Tsuchida H, Takeda Y, Takei H, Shinzawa H, Takahashi T, Sendo F (1995) *in vivo* regulation of rat neutrophil apoptosis occurring spontaneously or induced with TNF-α or cycloheximide. *J Immunol* 154: 2403–2412

57   Liles C, Dale DC, Klebanoff SJ (1995) Glucocorticoids inhibits apoptosis of human neutrophils. *Blood* 86: 3181–3188

58   Afford SC, Pongracz J, Stockley RA, Crocker J, Burnett D (1992) The induction by human interleukin-6 of apoptosis in the promonocytic cell line U937 and human neutrophils. *J Biol Chem* 267: 21612–21616

59   Cox G (1996) Interleukin-10 enhances resolution of pulmonary inflammation *in vivo*, by promoting apoptosis of neutrophils. *Am J Physiol* 271: L566–L571

60   Takeda Y, Watanade H, Yonehara S, Yamashita T, Saito S, Sendo Fujiro (1993) Rapid acceleration of neutrophil apoptosis by tumor necrosis factor. *Internat Immunol* 5: 691–694

61   Watson RWG, Redmond HP, Wang JH, Bouchier-Hayes D (1996) Bacterial ingestion, tumor necrosis factor-alpha, and heat induced programmed cell death in activated neutrophils. *Shock* 5: 47–51

62   Liles WC, Klebanoff SJ (1995) Regulation of apoptosis in neutrophils-Fas track to death? *J Immunol* 155: 3289–3291

63   Watson RWG, Redmond HP, Wang JH, Condron C, Bouchier-Hayes D (1996) Neutrophils undergo apoptosis following ingestion of *Escherichia coli*. *J Immunol* 156: 3986–3992

64   Watson RWG, Rotstein OD, Nathens AB, Dackiw APB, Marshall JC (1996) Thiol-mediated redox regulation of neutrophil apoptosis. *Surgery* 120: 150–158

65   Watson RWG, Rotstein OD, Parodo J, Jimenez M, Soric I, Bitar R, Marshall JC (1997) Impaired apoptotic death signaling in inflammatory lung neutrophils is associated with decreased expression of interleukin 1β converting enzyme family proteases (Caspases). *Surg*ery 122: 163–172

66   Bone RC, Balk RA, Cerra FB, Dellinger RP, Fein AM, Knaus WA, Schein RMH, Sibbald WJ (1992) Definitions for sepsis and organ failure and guidelines for the use of innovative therapies in sepsis. *Chest* 101:1644–1655

67   Chitnis DC, Dickerson C, Munster AM, Winchurch RA (1996) Inhibition of apoptosis in polymorphonuclear neutrophils from burn patients. *J Leuk Biol* 59:835–839

68 Matuschak GM (ed) (1993) *Multiple systems organ failure: hepatic regulation of systemic host defense.* Marcel Dekker, New York
69 Galle PR, Hofmann WJ, Walczak H (1995) Involvement of the CD95 (APO-1/Fas) receptor and ligand in liver damage. *J Exp Med* 11: 1223–1230
70 Leist M Gantner F, Bohlinger I, et al (1995) Tumor necrosis factor-induced hepatocyte apoptosis precedes liver failure in experimental murine shock models. *Am J Pathol* 146: 1220–1234
71 Galle PR, Hofmann WJ, Walczak H, et al (1995) Involvement of the CD95 (APO-1/Fas) receptor and ligand in liver damage. *J Exp Med* 182: 1223–1230
72 Cox G, Cossley J, Xing Z (1995) Macrophage engulfment of apoptotic neutrophils contributes to the resolution of acute pulmonary inflammation *in vivo. Am J Respir Cell Mol Biol* 12: 232–237

Importance of cytokine metabolism for malnutrition, catabolism and endocrinological state in sepsis

Erich Roth and Michael Bergmann

Chirurgische Forschungslaboratorien, Universitätsklinik für Chirurgie, Währinger Gürtel 18–20, A-1090 Wien, Austria

Introduction

One of the most pronounced metabolic alterations found in the systemic immune response syndrome (SIRS) is the induction of catabolic reactions responsible for the loss of skeletal and fat tissue [1]. A prolonged catabolic state as found in patients with severe sepsis or severe burn injury may even cause death. This process was named autocannibalism of the human body [2], a reaction which cannot be stopped by nutrition and causes death due to nitrogen depletion. This lethal nitrogen depletion includes a deteriorating function of important body proteins, but also a diminished lung or heart function because of a reduced potency to maintain adequate organ functions. Experiments performed with the infusion of multiple "catabolic" hormones such as glucagon, glucocorticoids, and catecholamines revealed that these hormones are only partly responsible for the stimulated protein degradation as found in the catabolic state [3]. Therefore, the discovery that a so-called cytokine, namely cachectin or tumor necrosis factor-α (TNF, which turned out to be the same molecule), can stimulate catabolic processes has brought new hope into the field of metabolic research in SIRS [4]. In the meantime several experimental studies have confessed that TNF and other cytokines stimulate protein catabolism under experimental conditions, however, clinical trials have revealed that blockade of TNF by an antibody directed against TNF could neither reduce cachexia in animal models nor reduce mortality in septic patients. A recent publication even denies a direct effect of TNF on human muscle [5].

Recently H. R. Michie published a critical review about the importance of cytokines in catabolism, in which the author discussed the problems associated with studies involved in the administration of exogenous cytokines [6]. First, investigations about the mode of action of cytokines in most cases were performed by administrating pharmacological doses of cytokines mostly given by continuous infusion. According to these experiments, the catabolic or cachectic reaction of TNF was found during continuous infusion of pharmacological doses of the cytokine. However, we know from several clinical investigations that increased systemic levels of TNF are only found during a very short period of the disease. This is a typical example which shows the discrepancy between experimental settings and clinical reality. A continuous infusion causing permanent (and not transient) increases in plasma TNF is an artificial situation not found in most of the clinical situations with protein catabolism. Moreover, when measuring the potency of lipopolysaccharides (LPS) to stimulate TNF levels in whole blood (*ex vivo* assay) of septic patients, we had to learn that TNF stimulation by LPS in severe sepsis is markedly reduced [7]. This means that during the late sepsis-phase the cytokine reaction is different in comparison to the situation found in early sepsis, in hemorrhagic shock, in the immediate postoperative state, or in the phase of hypoxia/reperfusion injury. Therefore, the second problem we are faced with, is the fact that the severity of the cytokine reaction depends on the progression of the disease. This is further complicated by the fact that certain cytokines are found only in early sepsis, whereas others are elevated throughout the whole disease. Thus, there seems to be a kinetic reaction within the cytokine release. This already raises the third problem, the cytokine network. In sepsis we are confronted with a cytokine network, meaning that the release of a certain cytokine from a certain cell type evokes the stimulation of other cytokines. This situation is very hard to imitate in experimental conditions and therefore it is difficult to determine the metabolic effects of single cytokines. Fourth, most of our knowledge about cytokine action on human metabolism derives from results obtained by comparing plasma levels of cytokines with certain metabolic reactions. However, in contrast to hormones, cytokines act in an autocrine and paracrine manner. Therefore, cell to cell interactions are much more related to tissue concentrations and even to concentrations within the appropriate cells than to plasma levels. In this respect, we still have a lack of appropriate knowledge about the clinical relevance of altered systemic cytokine levels. To enlarge our knowledge in this respect will be an interesting focus of future studies.

The following chapter will concentrate on the impact of cytokines on protein catabolism in sepsis. We will correlate sepsis-related cachexia to cancer cachexia, since the immunological regulation of catabolism seems to be similar in both clinical situations. Further attention will be given to the effects of nutrients on cytokine metabolism and on the interplay of cytokines and hormones in the septic state.

Cytokines – modulators of protein catabolism, influence on glucose and fat metabolism

The molecular importance of cytokines in regulating body wasting and malnutrition was initially extensively investigated in cancer physiology. When the biological effect of TNF was published under the headline "Cachectin and tumor necrosis factor as two sides of the same biological coin" the close link between tumor cachexia and sepsis became obvious. The infusion of high levels of the tumor-derived factor TNF causes sepsis-related symptoms such as a hemodynamic shock, severe organ damage and the corresponding catabolic reaction. The examination of damaged organs revealed a severe interstitial pneumonitis, acute tubular necrosis and a disseminated intravascular coagulopathy with hemorrhagic lesions in the gastrointestinal tract, in the pancreas, and in the adrenals. The metabolic response was dominated by metabolic acidosis and hyperglycemia followed by hypoglycemia due to liver failure. Obviously the metabolic reactions observed in these experiments can also be explained by the severe organ damage. However, we still had to learn that cancer-related cytokines play a role in the induction of a septic shock and the hypothesis that cancer cachexia might be seen as a slow variation of the sepsis related autocannibalism was born.

Despite a now well documented role of TNF in catabolic metabolism, the initial enthusiasm for the role of TNF as a mediator of cancer cachexia is nowadays limited because plasma of cancer patients often lacks the activity of TNF. Subsequent studies have revealed that other cytokines such as IL-1, IL-6, INFγ, and leukemia inhibiting factor (LIF), might also contribute to the development of cachexia [9, 10, 11]. Administration of IL-6 antibody to cancer-bearing mice prevented the occurrence of cachexia in an experimental set-up [12]. Interestingly, even the administration of INFγ caused a transient cachexia. Immunization of mice bearing a Lewis lung adenocarcinoma with antibodies against INFγ reduced tumor growth, spared body protein, and improved food intake. However, it was unresolved whether part of the improvements in food intake and body weight were simply the result of reduced tumor burden [13]. The role of IL-1 in cancer cachexia is slightly uncertain because only sublethal administration of IL-1 to healthy animals could reproduce the host changes reminiscent of cachexia [14].

Recently a new cancer cachectic factor, which holds more promise than the above mentioned cytokines, has been detected. This lipid-mobilizing factor (LMF) was classified as a proteoglycan released by the tumor and is able to cause protein and fat catabolism. So despite initial draw-backs new hope has arisen to find an appropriate therapy for cancer cachexia [15].

Similar to cancer cachexia, our knowledge about the impact of cytokines on catabolism and cachexia in sepsis results from experimental studies. Lowry and coworker performed a study administrating an endotoxin bolus (20 U/kg) to healthy volunteers and measured the metabolic effects followed by endotoxin infusion [16]. The endotoxin infusion caused a cachectin and an IL-6 peak and only transient changes in epinephrine and cortisol, but no changes in circulating glucagon and insulin. In spite of these rather low alterations of plasma hormone levels, pronounced metabolic alterations were found. The endotoxin bolus produced increased energy expenditure, hyperglycemia, hypoaminoacidemia, and an increase in circulating free fatty acids. Organ-specific alterations were defined in the direction of increased peripheral output from amino acids, lactate and free fatty acids, along with an increased glucose uptake from skeletal muscle. Coordinately, there were increased splanchnic uptakes of lactate, amino acids, and free fatty acids and an increased splanchnic glucose output. In this study the influence of endotoxin on physiological parameters was also measured. Endotoxin caused a significant increase in body temperature (+2° C), heart rate (+60%), minute ventilation (+40%), splanchnic blood flow (+60%) and of splanchnic oxygen consumption (+70%). Therefore, nature reacts in a perfect manner toward an infection with invading microorganisms using endotoxin to perform a shift of the metabolism from the periphery (skeletal muscle) to central organs.

Jeejeebhoy and coworkers performed a similar study in an experimental rat model [17]. They determined body composition and metabolic rate in rat during a continuous infusion of TNF for ten days. Similar to the results described in humans by the group of Lowry, TNF-infused rats were hypermetabolic, hyperglycemic and had raised blood urea nitrogen. The rats were anorexic and had significant loss of muscle mass, especially in muscles with a predominance of type II fibers. However, the rats gained liver, heart, and lung mass. The gain in visceral mass was associated with an increase in organ DNA and protein content. Histological examinations showed that there was cell proliferation in the liver, heart, and kidneys.

These two studies clearly demonstrate that endotoxin, possibly via TNF, causes a shift of metabolic substrates from skeletal muscle to visceral organs which might even be necessary for survival of the organism. Therefore, therapeutic strategies in SIRS or severe sepsis must be evaluated in relation to endogenous life-saving reactions created already by nature during evolution. In this respect we should consider that therapeutic strategies such as antibodies against endotoxin, or cytokines, or the administration of growth hormone which prevent this teleological reaction may even harm the patient.

As might be anticipated, cytokine antagonists can interfere with the sepsis-induced catabolic state. This should be demonstrated here on two examples: the IL-1 receptor antagonist (ra) and IL-6 antibodies.

Vary and coworkers investigated the impact of infusion of IL-1 receptor antagonist (IL-1ra) on protein synthesis during an experimentally induced sepsis [18]. IL-1ra did not significantly alter hepatic protein metabolism in septic or control animals. In kidney, the protein content and rate of protein synthesis were both decreased by sepsis, and significantly ameliorated by the infusion of IL-1ra. Sepsis decreased the rate of protein synthesis in the small intestine. IL-1ra increased intestinal protein synthesis, however, the effects were localized to the seromuscular layer. The preservation of muscle protein by IL-1ra in sepsis did not adversely affect protein synthesis in any of the visceral tissue examined. The group also investigated the mechanism by which IL-1ra regulates protein synthesis in skeletal muscle during hypermetabolic sepsis [19]. Treatment of septic rats with IL-1ra prevented the sepsis-induced inhibition of protein synthesis and translational efficiency in gastrocnemius by maintaining peptide-chain initiation. The molecular mechanism was based on the fact that IL-1ra infusion maintained the ε-subunit of eukaryotic initiation factor (eIF) 1B.

Skeletal muscle contains multiple proteolytic systems: (i) a lysosomal pathway, which involves the proteases cathepsin B, H, L, and D, (ii) a cytosolic proteolytic pathway which involves ubiquitin, and (iii) μ, m, and muscle-specific calpains, which are Ca^{2+}-dependent proteases. Interestingly, the treatment of mice with anti-mouse IL-6 (mIL-6R) antibody prevented muscle atrophy in IL-6 transgenic mice [20]. mIL-6R decreased the enzymatic activities and mRNA levels of cathepsin (B and L) and mRNA levels of ubiquitin and increased the mRNA levels of muscle-specific calpain (calpain 3).

In summary, our knowledge of the influence of cytokines on protein, glucose and fat metabolism arises mostly from experimental studies where either endotoxin or single cytokines have been infused in animal models. From these studies we have learned that metabolic alterations as described in sepsis – increased protein breakdown, decreased glucose utilization, increased fat hydrolysis – are closely associated with alterations in the cytokine pattern. However, conclusions to which extent these experimental results are relevant for the clinical situation have to be drawn with caution.

Modulation of cytokines by nutrients

In an experimental study it was proven that the route of nutritional supply influences local and systemic responses to intraperitoneal bacterial challenge. In this study it was shown that the survival rate of rats was significantly higher (60% vs 22%) when rats received enteral nutrition (EN) instead of parenteral nutrition (PN) [21]. The authors of this study investigated the production of cytokines in peritoneal fluid, peritoneal exudative cells and bronchoalveolar lavage fluid and its dependence on the mode of nutrition. They documented that rats fed with EN had lowered TNF levels in the bronchoalveolar lavage fluid and in the peritoneal fluid, but higher INFγ levels in all measured compartments. In another experimental study the expression of intestinal and splenic cytokines on the mRNA levels was measured after PN [22]. PN significantly decreased the production of TNF and IL-6 in the spleen and increased the IL-6-specific mRNA in the Peyer's patches of the intestine.

The above mentioned studies clearly demonstrate that the production of cytokines is modulated by nutrition. A more specific immunomodulating effect has been proven for several nutrients including fatty acids and certain amino acids.

Fat

Endres et al. demonstrated that consumption of 15 g per day of eicosapentanaeoic acid (EPA), as fish oil, for a six week period, was sufficient to reduce the ability of monocytes from healthy subjects to produce IL-1 and TNF in response to an endo-toxin stimulus, by more that 30% [23]. The effect persisted for ten weeks after the subjects had returned to their normal diet. Opposite effects, however, were published in animal models. The administration of fish oils to mice led to a higher production of TNF and less PGE2 from macrophages in response to a challenge with lipopolysaccharide than macrophages from mice fed with other high-fat diets [24]. Supplementation of the diet with fish oil resulted in enhanced levels of TNF-specific mRNA and protein. Nuclear run-on assays demonstrated an increased transcription of TNF-specific mRNA by fish oil. A beneficial effect of fish oil was given in a burned animal model [25]. In this experiment mice were fed with diets containing 15% of energy from fish oil, safflower oil, or a 50:50 mixture. Survival was 84% in the fish oil group versus 36% in the safflower oil and only 25% or 20% in the control groups. The number of viable translocating bacteria was reduced in all tested organs in the fish oil group compared to the other groups. The authors concluded that diet enriched in fish oil has beneficial effects during gut-derived sepsis. In an *in vitro* study the effects of two lipid emulsions (with and without ω-3 fatty acids) upon proliferation of rat and human lymphocytes were investigated [26]. An emulsion containing ω-3 polyunsaturated fatty acids improved lymphocyte proliferation in comparison to a fat solution without ω-3 fatty acids. There are several other studies investigating the modulation of inflammation and cytokine production in dietary (ω-3) fatty acids (for review see [27]). To summarize this subject, the use of ω-3 fatty acids induces moderate clinical improvements in rheumatoid arthritis, psoriasis and colitis. Data on critically ill burn or postoperative cancer patients are still inconclusive. The ω-3 fatty acids markedly inhibited sterile inflammation in animal studies and improved survival in some experimental infections. Interestingly, ω-3 fatty acids decreased the production of pro-inflammatory cytokines in most human studies, but increased cytokine production capacity in mice. Differences in cytokine-producing cell types in studies may account for these paradoxical responses in humans and rodents.

Proteins

The influence of protein malnutrition (PM) or protein-calorie malnutrition (PCM) on immune and cytokine response was frequently investigated in animal models triggered with endotoxin. Already in 1982 Keenan et al. provided evidence that malnutrition suppresses the cytokine production [28]. The suppressed ability of PMN from malnourished subjects to produce leucocyte endogenous mediator was enhanced by feeding protein supplements. PM leads to a profound immunodeficiency, mostly related to decreased cell-mediated immunity, but humoral and non-specific immunity are also lowered. PCM is also associated with altered monocyte functions. It was shown in rats that PCM induces lower IL-1 secretion and consequently reduces the febrile responses to endotoxin. This may be an explanation for the frequent non-febrile infections observed in undernourished elderly subjects. In fact, all monocyte functions are reduced in PCM animals and patients, including monocyte phagocytosis and cytokine secretions such as IL-1β, TNF, and IL-6. By inducing lower monocyte secretion or an inappropriate response to monokine release, PCM is responsible for the lower acute-phase reaction and the lower lymphocyte stimulation. Consequently, the immune system stimulation is decreased during PCM, leading to increased risk of infection. Grimble and coworkers fed young rats a diet containing 8% casein, supplemented with isonitrogenous amounts of different amino acids such as alanine, glycine, serine, cysteine or taurine, prior to injection with TNF and investigated the effect of the diets on hepatic glutathione contents and the synthesis of acute-phase proteins [29]. In this paper it was shown that the possibility to respond to TNF is dependent on the composition of the diet. Cystein improved the response to TNF to maintain a high level of hepatic glutathione. On the other hand, Alexander et al studied the effect of overnutrition in guinea pigs exposed to *Plasmodium Berghei*, and found an increased mortality in overfed guinea pigs [30]. They hypothesized that alterations in TNF production may be partly responsible for this phenomenon.

Glutamine

Glutamine is of particular importance for the immune system. Glutamine is the most abundant free amino acid of the human body. In catabolic stress situations such as operations, trauma, and sepsis, there results an enhanced transport of glutamine to splanchnic organs and blood cells (for review see [31]). This stimulated glutamine release from skeletal muscle is accompanied by an intracellular glutamine deficiency, related to the prognosis of the patients [32]. Glutamine is an important metabolic substrate for cells cultivated under *in vitro* conditions and a precursor for purines, pyrimidines and phospholipids. Glutamine influences the expression of surface antigens on lymphocytes and monocytes (Fig. 1) and stimulates the production of IFNγ, TNF and IL-2 [33]. Glutamine is the most important energy substrate of the intestine. Intestinal glutamine extraction decreased in animals treated with IL-1 [34]. Concomitant with the above mentioned decrease in gut glutamine metabolism there was a 25% incidence of positive blood culture for Gram-negative organisms in IL-1 treated rats. In contrast to IL-1, TNF had no effects on the parameters of gut glutamine examined. These results indicate that IL-1 is a potential mediator of the alterations in gut glutamine metabolism observed in sepsis and endotoxemia. Recent results have indicated that glutamine is a modulator of reactive oxygen intermediate-mediated cytotoxicity of TNF in L929 fibrosarcoma cells [35]. When cultivating these cells by omission of glutamine from the medium, a desensitization of the cells to TNF cytotoxicity occurs. The authors explain this enhanced TNF cytotoxicity by

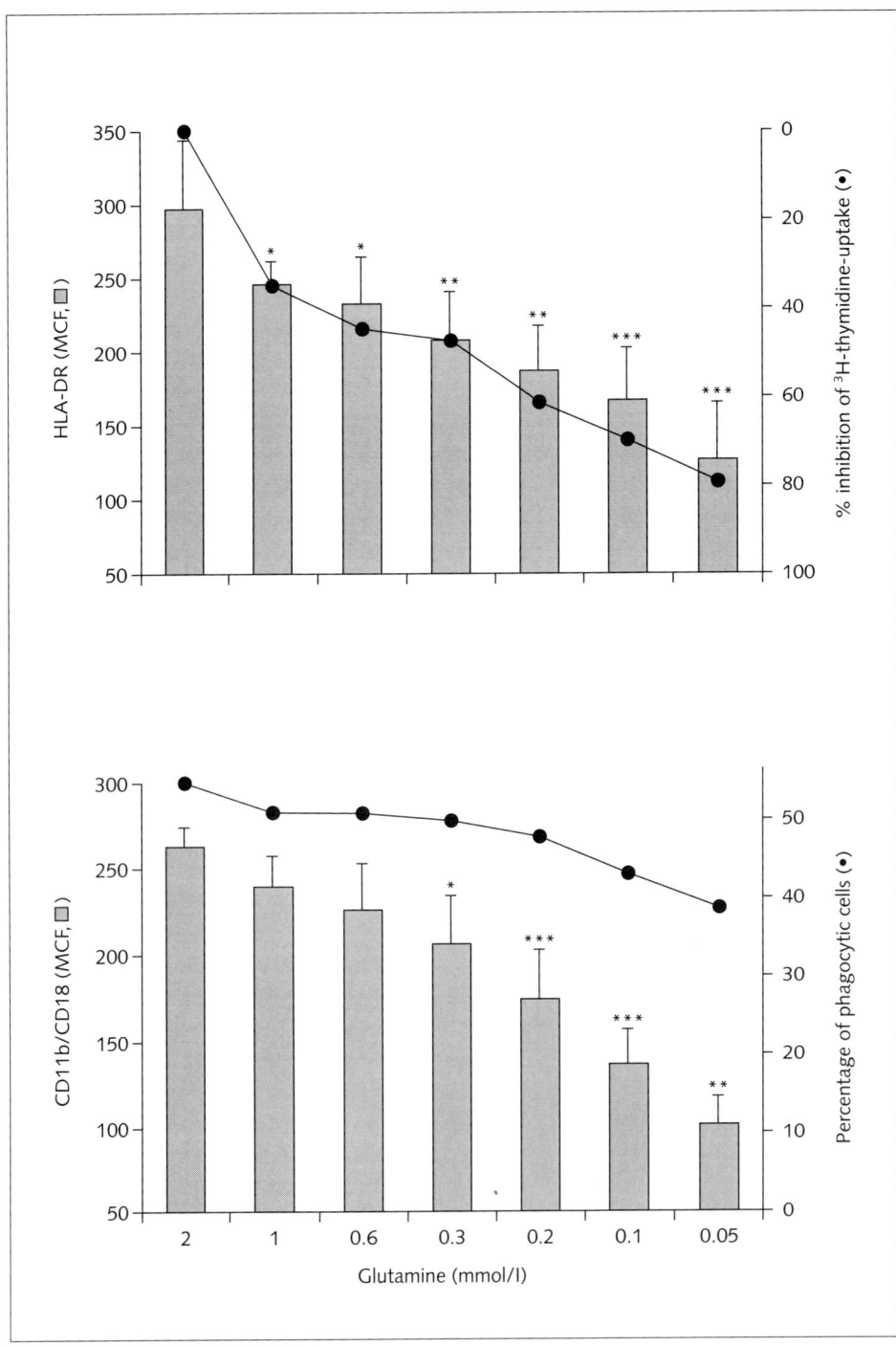

glutamine through a mechanism that renders the mitochondria more susceptible to TNF-induced mediators, resulting in enhanced production of reactive oxygen intermediates. However, it has to be mentioned that the administration of glutamine to cancer patients seems to be double-edged since glutamine is effective in modulating tumor cells in the direction of a lower state of differentiation [36]. Therefore, future studies in experimental carcinoma models must elucidate whether the immunostimulating properties of glutamine are advantageous in comparison to influencing cell modification to a lower degree of differentiation. In catabolic and septic patients the administration of glutamine seems to be advantageous and can even decrease mortality in severe sepsis.

Glycine

Glycine, a non-essential amino acid, has been shown to be protective against hypoxia, ischemia, and various cytotoxic substances in renal tubulus, hepatocytes, and in a low-flow liver perfusion model in the rat. Thurman and coworkers have found a pathomechanistic explanation for this protective effect of glycine [37]. When feeding endotoxin boostered rats with high doses of glycine, the survival of rats increases significantly. This reduced mortality was accompanied by reduced plasma levels of TNF (Fig. 2). Further experiments revealed that glycine blocked Ca^{2+} uptake of monocytes in cultured Kupffer cells, thereby minimizing toxic eicosanoid and cytokine production. We could confirm these results in human monocytes where the co-cultivation of monocytes with glycine also reduced the production of TNF. In later experiments Thurman could show that glycine may also prevent the nephrotoxicity of cyclosporin A by acting as an oxygen radical scavenger. Therefore, the administration of high amounts of glycine may indeed prevent metabolic reactions

Figure 1

Influence of glutamine on phagocytosis and antigen-presenting capacity of human monocytes.

Monocytes were cultured for seven days with the indicated concentrations of glutamine. The expression of HLA-DR-antigen (upper graph; mean channel fluorescence, MCF) was determined by a FACScan analysis. T cell proliferation was measured by a β counter and indicates the incorporation of ³H-thymidine in proliferating lymphocytes. The expression of CD11b/CD18 (lower graph; mean channel fluorescence, MCF) as well as the percentage of cells ingesting FITC-labelled E. coli were determined by FACScan analysis. Data with monocytes from four to six apparently healthy donors represent the mean ± SD. Statistically significant decrease in comparison to 2 mmol/l glutamine (GLN), Student's t-test: *p < 0.05, **p < 0.01, ***p < 0.001 [55].

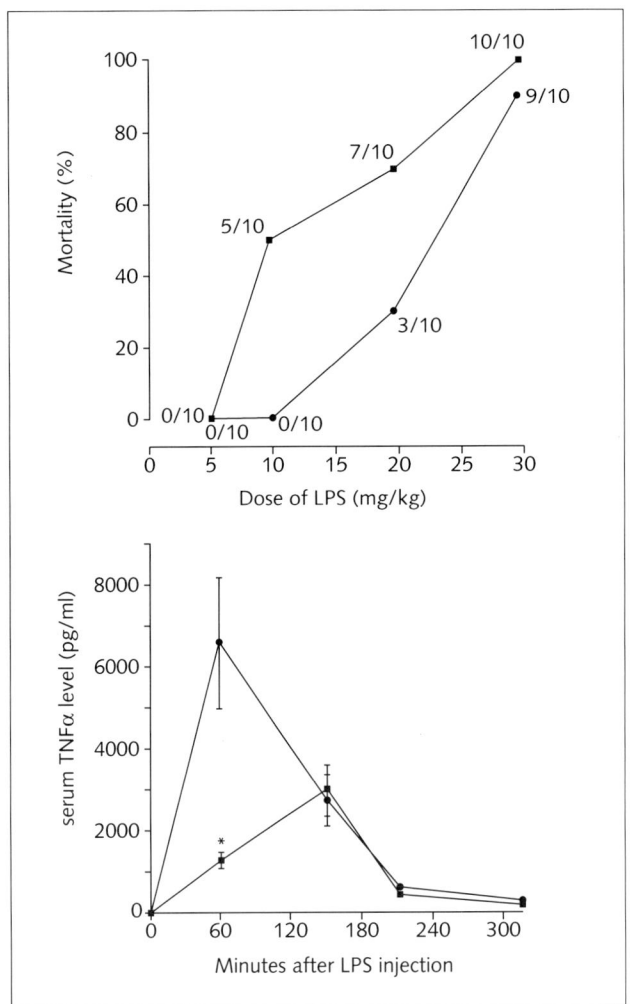

Figure 2

Effect of glycine on mortality and serum tumor necrosis factor-α (TNFα) levels after LPS injection.

Rats were fed control or glycine-containing diets for three days. Various amounts of LPS were injected via tail vein, and survival rates were monitored for 24 h (upper graph). Data represent percentage of dead animals after 24 h (n=10 for each point). c, glycine-fed group; p, control diet group. *p<0.05 with Fisher's test. Fractions represent survivors/total. To detect TNFα production, blood samples were collected before and at four time points after an injection of LPS (10 mg/kg) for up to 310 min (n = 4; lower graph). TNFα was measured by enzyme-linked immunosorbant assay. Data are means ± SE. *p<0.05 with Mann-Whitney's rank-sum test [37].

created during the ischemia/ reperfusion period, a pathophysiological situation also relevant in the septic state.

Interplay of cytokines and hormones

One of the main metabolic goals in sepsis is to concentrate the body energy resources on the production of acute phase proteins in the liver. This is achieved by hormones, cytokines and vasoactive substances. The latter provide the efficient blood supply to metabolically important organs such as the liver. Cytokines exert a profound direct influence on uptake and metabolism of glucose, amino acids and fat. However, the complex immunological and metabolic interaction in sepsis can only be understood if both the humoral and the cytokine network, and their interaction, are taken into account.

Despite the discrepancy between experimental models and the clinical situation, these models which are based on the application of single cytokines or hormones during endotoxemia have given some insight of how cytokines and hormones depend on each other. In a time course of endotoxemia it was observed that the peak of proinflammatory cytokines precedes the rise in sepsis-related catabolic hormones such as glucocorticoids, glucagon and epinephrine [38, 39]. Thus, it seemed likely that the acute inflammatory response cytokines contribute to the induction of this hormonal response [40, 41]. Sauerwein and coworkers demonstrated that IL-6 increased norepinephrine by 97%, cortisol by 45%, and glucagon by 15%. Obviously the induction of cortisol is partly mediated by the pituitary-adrenal axis, since IL-6, which can be produced in the pituitary gland in response to endotoxin, can induce the adrenocorticotropic hormone [42] . The high induction of norepinephrine by IL-6 in the acute inflammatory response serves two tasks. As a vasoactive substance it counter-regulates the sepsis-related vasoparalysis evoked by the induction of the inducible nitric oxide synthase and as a catabolic hormone it mobilizes energy resources for the hypermetabolic septic liver.

Interestingly, cytokines not only induce metabolic hormones but they also enhance the effect of some stress-related hormones on the production of acute phase proteins [43]. For example, catabolic hormone induces C-reactive protein (CRP) production. IL-6 further enhances this induction in a non-additive effect. Insulin on the contrary counteracts the IL-6 mediated synthesis of CRP. Dexamethasone alone has variable effects on the acute phase protein synthesis. In combination with IL-6 this hormone induces not only the production of CRP, but also of α-1-antichymotrypsin, α-1-acid glycoprotein, and haptoglobin. Despite the fact that not all catabolic hormones positively support the synthesis of all acute phase proteins, insulin obviously appears to counter-regulate the hepatic response to inflammation. This hormone enhances the production of albumin and transferrin and represses cytokine and glucocorticoid-stimulated acute phase protein expression [44]. The insulin-mediated suppression of the immediate hepatic response is exerted at the transcriptional level. The effect is mediated by at least two separate mechanisms. Insulin leads to an increase in the transcription of genes encoding the AP-1 components of JunA, JunB and c-Fos. On the other hand, it inhibits the transcriptional activation of CCAAT/enhancer-binding protein (C/EBP) beta.

According to the negative effect of insulin on the hepatic acute response reaction, the activity of this hormone is suppressed by proinflammatory cytokines. TNF can induce an insulin resistance. This was demonstrated in a variety of cell systems including adipocytes, muscle cells and hepatocytes. Recently the mechanism was elucidated. TNF increased serine phosphorylation of the insulin receptor substrate -1 (IRS-1) [45]. By this mechanism IRS-1 was converted to an inhibitor of the insulin receptor tyrosine kinase inhibitor. Furthermore, TNF induces the downregulation of the insulin-responsive glucose transporter GLUT-4 [46]. TNF-mediated insulin resistance might contribute to the impaired glucose utilization which is observed shortly after severe trauma. Furthermore, it might explain the enhanced insulin demand of patients in sepsis.

Interestingly, catabolic hormones, which are induced by proinflammatory cytokines, exert a negative feed-back mechanism in the sense that they downregulate those very cytokines. Initially the immunosuppressive effect of glucocorticoids on the acute inflammatory response was investigated [47]. However, glucocorticoids have been used for years to limit inflammatory responses in a variety of diseases. Therefore it was not surprising that these substances could also repress endotoxin-mediated upregulation of TNF, IL-6 and IL-1 beta. It should be noted that a systemic steroid therapy of septic shock patients did not improve the prognosis. Later, it became evident that catecholamines had also an immunosuppressive effect on these proinflammatory cytokines. The immunosuppressive effect involves LPS-stimulated expression of TNF, IL-6 and IL-1 beta, which is mediated at the mRNA level [48, 49]. The suppression correlates with an intracellular elevation of cAMP. Blockade of beta-1 receptors abrogated the immunosuppressive effect *in vitro*. The biological relevance of this mechanism for sepsis was demonstrated when Abraham and coworkers could increase cytokine expression in hemorrhagic shock by the beta-blocker propanolol in an animal model [50]. In human endotoxinemia the immunosuppressive effect could be reproduced [51]. Thus catecholamines, similar to corticosteroids, significantly contribute to the negative feed-back loop towards proinflammatory cytokines.

The immunomodulating effect of corticosteroids and catecholamines is further enhanced by the induction of IL-10 by the hormones [51, 52]. This could be demonstrated *in vitro* and *in vivo* in human endotoxinemia. IL-10 has an immunoenhancing effect on B-cells but causes a depression of monocyte function. It significantly attenuates TNF and IL-1 beta production at the transcriptional level. The peak of these cytokines in endotoxinemia models is 24 to 48 hours after the onset event. This means that IL-10 production is observed after the induction of catabolic hor-

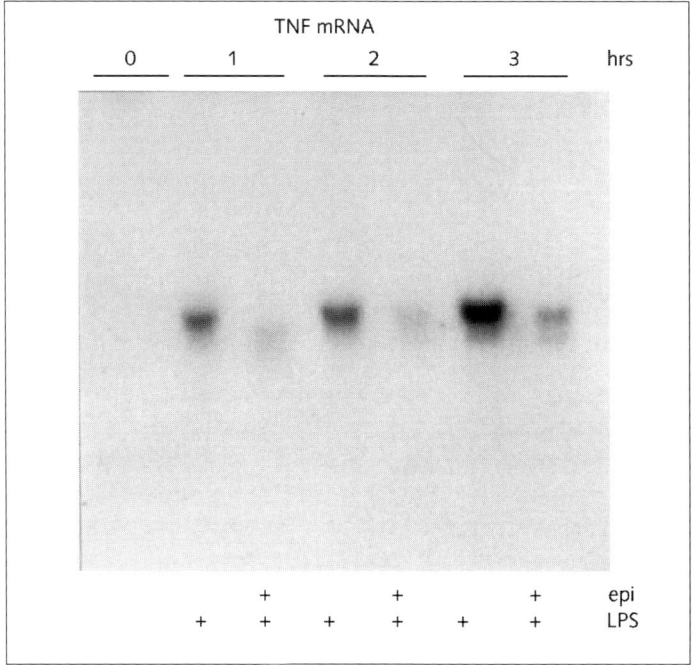

Figure 3
Effect of epinephrine on LPS-stimulated TNF-mRNA production.
Whole blood was stimulated with 1 µg/ml of E. coli-LPS for 3 h in the presence and absence
of 100 ng/ml of epinephrine. The total RNA was extracted and subjected to a Northern blot.
The blot was incubated with 32 P-labeled DNA probes, which were specific for the human
TNF gene. epi, epinephrine; LPS, lipopolysaccharide; hrs, hours post application of LPS [48].

mones in sepsis, which makes the induction of IL-10 by catecholamines and corti-costeroids a likely biologically relevant mechanism. In clinical sepsis IL-10 produc-tion is observed throughout the whole septic period, which corresponds to con-stantly elevated levels of catabolic hormones.

Two other mediators of the immunosuppressive effect of glucocorticoids are the IL-1 receptor antagonist and the soluble IL-1 receptor II. As observed for IL-10, these two substances rise in endotoxinemia models in the later phase of sepsis and contribute to the depression of the initially-overstimulated immunosystem [53].

In late sepsis these immunological side effects of catabolic hormones can have negative consequences for the organism. In this phase of the disease the immune sys-tem is in a state of immunological anergy or hyporesponsiveness. Further immuno-logical depression by glucocorticoids or catecholamines might be detrimental in fighting newly-acquired infections. However, we have observed that in late sepsis the immunodepressive effect of catecholamines is restricted to IL-1 beta, whereas LPS-stimulated levels of TNF, IL-6 and IL-10 are little affected [48] (Fig. 3). It should be noted that the glucocorticoid-mediated immunosuppression can be overcome by interferon gamma [54]. Thus, this cytokine which also appears later in the time course of an endotoxinemia model might counterregulate *in vivo* hormonally-induced immunosuppression.

It appears that in septic shock we have to expand the function of metabolic and vasoactive hormones. It seems obvious that these hormones have biologically significant immunological side effects. In this sense it might be possible that in septic shock the recruitment of immunosuppressive hormones serves also the task of limiting the exacerbated immune system.

References

1   Douglas W, Wilmore MD (1990) Catabolic illness. Strategies for enhancing recovery. *N Engl J Med* 325: 695–702

2   Cerra FB, Siegel JH,Coleman B, Border JR, McMenamy RR (1980) Septic auto cannibalism. *Ann Surg* 192: 570–580

3   Wernerman J, Brandt R, Strandell T, Allgén L-G, Vinnars E (1985) The effect of stress hormones on the interorgan flux of amino acids and on the concentration of free amino acids in skeletal muscle. *Clin Nutr* 4: 207–216

4   Beutler B, Cerami A (1986) Cachectin and tumour necrosis factor as two sides of the same biological coin. *Nature* 320: 584–588

5   De Blaauw I, Eggermont AMM, Deutz NEP, De Vries M, Buurman WA, Von Meyenfeldt MF (1997) TNF-α has no direct *in vivo* metabolic effect on human muscle. *Int J Cancer* 71:148–154

6   Michie HR (1996) Cytokines and the acute catabolic state. In: A Revhaug (ed): *Acute catabolic state*. Springer-Verlag Berlin, Heidelberg, 227–237

7   Ertel W, Kremer J-P, Kenney J, Steckholzer U, Jarrar D, Trentz O, Schildberg FW (1995) Downregulation of proinflammatory cytokine release in whole blood from septic patients. *Blood* 85: 1341–1347

8   Beutler B, Cerami A (1987) Cachectin: more than a tumor necrosis factor. *N Engl J Med* 316: 379–385

9   Moldawer LL, Rogy MA, Lowry SF (1992) The role of cytokines in cancer cachexia. *JPEN* 16: 43S–49S

10 Tisdale MJ (1997) Cancer cachexia: metabolic alterations and clinical manifestation. *Nutrition* 13: 1–7

11 Matthys P, Billiau A (1997) Cytokines and cachexia. *Nutrition* 13: 763–770

12 Oldenburg HSA, Rogy MA, Lazarus DD, Van Zee KJ, Keeler BP, Chizzonite RA, Lowry

SF, Moldawer LL (1993) Cachexia and the acute-phase protein response in inflammation are regulated by interleukin-6. *Eur J Immunol* 23: 1889–1894

13 Matthys P, Heremans H, Opdenakker G, Billiau A (1991) Anti-interferon γ antibody treatment, growth of Lewis lung tumors in mice and tumor associated cachexia. *Eur J Cancer* 27: 182–187

14 Otterness IG, Golden HW, Brissette WH, Seymour PA, Daumy GO (1989) Effects of continuously administered murine interleukin-1α: tolerance development and granuloma formation. *Infect Immun* 57: 2742–2750

15 Todorov P, Cariuk P, McDevitt T, Coles B, Fearon K, Tisdale M (1996) Characterization of a cancer chachectic factor. *Nature* 379: 739–742

16 Fong Y, Marano MA, Moldawer LL, Wei H, Calvano SE, Kenney JS, Allison AC, Cerami A, Thomas Shires G, Lowry SF (1990) The acute splanchnic and peripheral tissue metabolic response to endotoxin in humans. *J Clin Invest* 85: 1896–1904

17 Hoshino E, Pichard C, Greenwood CE, Kuo GC, Cameron RG, Kurian R, Kearns JP, Allard JP, Jeejeebhoy KN (1991) Body composition and metabolic rate in rat during a continuous infusion of cachectin. *Am J Physiol* 260: E27–E36

18 Cooney R, Owens E, Jurasinski C, Gray K, Vannice J, Vary T (1994) Interleukin-1 receptor antagonist prevents sepsis-induced inhibition of protein synthesis. *Am J Physiol* 267: E636–E641

19 Vary TC, Voisin L, Cooney RN (1996) Regulation of peptide-chain initiation in muscle during sepsis by interleukin-1 receptor antagonist. *Am J Physiol* 271: E513–E520

20 Tsujinaka T, Fujita J, Ebisui C, Yano M, Kominami E, Suzuki K,Tanaka K, Katsume A, Ohsugi Y, Shiozaki H et al (1996) Interleukin 6 receptor antibody inhibits muscle atrophy and modulates proteolytic systems in interleukin 6 transgenic mice. *J Clin Invest* 97: 244–249

21 Lin M-T, Saito H, Fukushima R, Inaba T, Fukats K, Inoue T, Furukawa S, Han I, Muto T (1996) Route of nutritional supply influences local, systemic, and remote organ responses to intraperitoneal bacterial challenge. *Ann Surg* 223: 84–93

22 Ogle CK, Zuo L, Mao JX, Alexander JW, Fischer JE, Nussbaum MS (1995) Differential expression of intestinal and splenic cytokines after parenteral nutrition. *Arch Surg* 130: 1301–1308

23 Endres S, Ghorbani R, Kelley VE, Georgilis K, Lonnemann G, van der Meer JWM, Cannon JG, Rogers TS, Klempner MS, Weber PC et al (1989) The effect of dietary supplementation with -3 polyunsaturated fatty acids on the synthesis of interleukin–1 and tumor necrosis factor by mononuclear cells. *N Engl J Med* 320: 265–271

24 Chang HR, Arsenijevic D, Vladoianu IR, Girardier L, Dulloo AG (1995) Fish oil enhances macrophage tumor necrosis factor-alpha mRNA expression at the transcriptional level. *Metabolism* 44: 800–805

25 Gianotti L, Alexander JW, Eaves-Pyles T, Fukushima R (1996) Dietary fatty acids modulate host bacteriocidal response, microbial translocation and survival following blood transfusion and thermal injury. *Clin Nutr* 15: 291–296

26 Calder PC, Sherrington EJ, Askanazi J, Newsholme EA (1994) Inhibition of lymphocyte

proliferation in vitro by two lipid emulsions with different fatty acid compositions. *Clin Nutr* 13: 69–74

27 Blok WL, Katan MB, van der Meer JWM (1996) Modulation of inflammation and cytokine production by dietary (ω-3) fatty acids. *J Nutr* 126: 1515–1533

28 Keenan RA, Moldawer LL, Yang RD, Kavamura I, Blackburn JL, Bistrian BR (1982) An altered response by peripheral leukocytes to synthesise or release leukocyte endogenous mediator in critically ill protein-malnourished patients. *J Lab Clin Med* 100: 844–857

29 Grimble RF (1993) New strategies for modulation of cytokine biology by nutrients. In: P Fürst (ed): *New strategies in clinical nutrition*. W. Zuckschwerdt Verlag, München, Bern, Wien, New York, 18–31

30 Alexander JW, Gonce SJ, Miskell PW, Peck MD, Sax H (1989) A new model for studying nutrition in peritonitis; adverse effect of overfeeding. *Ann Surg* 209: 334–340

31 Hall JC, Heel K, McCauley R (1996) Glutamine. *Br J Surg* 83: 305–312

32 Roth E, Funovics J, Mühlbacher F, Schemper M, Mauritz W, Sporn P, Fritsch A (1982) Metabolic disorders in severe abdominal sepsis: glutamine deficiency in skeletal muscle. *Clin Nutr* 1: 25–41

33 Rohde T, MacLean DA, Klarlund Pedersen B (1996) Glutamine, lymphocyte proliferation and cytokine production. *Scand J Immunol* 44: 648–650

34 Austgen TR, Chen MK, Dudrick PS, Copeland EM, Souba WW (1992) Cytokine regulation of intestinal glutamine utilization. *Am J Surg* 163: 174–180

35 Goossens V, Grooten J, Fiers W (1996) The oxidative metabolism of glutamine. *J Biol Chem* 271: 192–196

36 Spittler A, Oehler R, Goetzinger P, Holzer S, Reissner CM, Leutmezer F, Rath V, Wrba F, Fuegger R, Boltz-Nitulescu G (1997) Low glutamine concentrations induce phenotypical and functional differentiation of U937 myelomonocytic cells. *J Nutr* 127: 2151–2157

37 Ikejima K, Iimuro Y, Forman DT, Thurman RG (1996) A diet containing glycine improves survival in endotoxin shock in the rat. *Am J Physiol* 271: G97–G103

38 Byerley LO, Alcock NW, Starnes HF Jr (1992) Sepsis-induced cascade of cytokine mRNA expression: correlation with metabolic changes. *Am J Physiology* 262: E728–735

39 Chensue SW, Terebuh PD, Remick DG, Scales WE, Kunkel SL (1991) *In vivo* biologic and immunohistochemical analysis of interleukin-1 alpha, beta and tumor necrosis factor during experimental endotoxemia. Kinetics, Kupffer cell expression, and glucocorticoid effects. *Am J Path* 139: 395–402

40 Van der Poll T, Romijn JA, Endert E, Borm JJJ, Buller HR, Sauerwein HP (1991) Tumor necrosis factor mimics the metabolic response to acute infections in healthy humans. *Am J Physiol* 261: E457–E463

41 Stouthard JML, Romijn JA, van der Poll T et al (1995) Endocrine and metabolic effects of interleukin-6 in humans. *Am J Physiol* 331: E813–820

42 Tsigos C, Papanicolaou DA, Defensor R, Mitsiadis CS, Kyrou I, Chrousos GP (1997)

Dose effects of recombinant human IL-6 on pituitary hormone secretion and energy expenditure. *Neuroendocrinology* 66: 54–62

43 O'Riordain MG, Ross JA, Fearon KCH, Maingay J, Farouk M, Garden OJ, Carter DC (1995) Insulin and counterregulatory hormones influence acute-phase protein production in human hepatocytes. *Am J Physiol* 269: E323–E330

44 Campos SP, Baumann H (1992) Insulin is a prominent modulator of the cytokine-stimulated expression of acute-phase plasma protein genes. *Mol Cell Biology* 12: 1789–1797

45 Hotamisligil GS, Peraldi P, Budavari A, Ellis R, White MF, Spiegelmann BM (1996) IRS-1 mediated inhibition of insulin receptor tyrosine kinase activity in TNF-alpha and obesity induced insulin resistance. *Science* 271: 665–668

46 Stephens JM, Lee J, Pilch PF (1997) Tumor necrosis factor-alpha-induced insulin resistance in 3T3.L1 adipocytes is accompanied by a loss of insulin receptor substrate-1 and GLUT-4 expression without a loss of insulin receptor-mediated signal transduction. *J Biol Chem* 272: 971–976

47 Barber AE, Coyle SM, Marano MA, Fisher E, Calvano SE, Fong Y, Moldawer LL, Lowry SF (1993) Glucocorticoid therapy alters humoral and cytokine response to endotoxin in man. *J Immunol* 150: 1999–2006

48 Bergmann M, Gornikiewicz A, Sautner T, Gmeiner T, Mittelbäck M, Roth E, Függer R. *submitted*

49 Van der Poll T, Jansen J, Endert E, Sauerwein HP, Van Deventer SJH (1994) Noradrenaline inhibits lipopolysaccharide-induced tumor necrosis factor and interleukin 6 production in human whole blood. *Infect Immun* 62: 2046–2050

50 Le Tulzo Y, Shenkar R, Kaneko D, Moine P, Fantuzzi G, Dinarello CA, Abraham E (1997) Hemorrhage increases cytokine expression in lung mononuclear cells in mice: involvement of catecholamines in nuclear factor-kappaB regulation and cytokine expression. *J Clin Invest* 99: 1516–1524

51 Van der Poll T, Berber A, Coyle SM, Lowry SF (1996) Hypercortisolemia increases plasma interleukin-10 concentrations during human endotoxinemia – a clinical research center study. *J Clin Endocrinol Metab* 81: 3604–3606

52 Van der Poll T, Coyle SM, Barbosa K, Braxton CC, Lowry SF (1996) Epinephrine inhibits tumor necrosis factor- and potentiates interleukin 10 production during human endotoxemia. *J Clin Invest* 97: 713–719

53 Brown EA, Dare HA, Marsh CB Wewers MD (1996) The combination of endotoxin and dexamethasone induces type II interleukin 1 receptor (IL-1r) in monocytes: a comparison to interleukin 1 ß (IL–1 ß) and interleukin 1 receptor antagonist (IL-1ra). *Cytokine* 8: 828–836.

54 Luedka CE, A Cerami (1990) Interferon-gamma overcomes glucocorticoid suppression of cachectin/tumor necrosis factor biosynthesis by murine macrophages. *J Clin Invest* 86: 1234–1240

55 Spittler A, Winkler S, Götzinger P, Oehler R, Willheim M, Tempfer C, Weigel G, Függer R, Boltz-Nitulescu G, Roth E (1995) Influence of glutamine on the phenotype and function of human monocytes. *Blood* 86: 1564–1569

Therapy

Endotoxin scavengers as a therapeutic strategy for sepsis

Steven M. Opal

Infectious Disease Division, Brown University School of Medicine, Memorial Hospital of Rhode Island, 111 Brewster Street, Pawtucket, RI 02860, USA

Introduction

Bacterial endotoxin remains an important therapeutic target for the treatment of serious infections from Gram-negative bacterial pathogens. Despite recent failures in past clinical trials with novel anti-endotoxin therapies for septic shock [1–6], a critical need remains to improve the unacceptably high mortality rate associated with systemic infections from Gram-negative organisms. Endotoxin remains a viable target for innovative treatment regimens as endotoxin constitutes the most important microbially-derived mediator in septic shock.

Endotoxin, a complex, amphiphilic macromolecule, is an essential component of the outer cell wall of pathogenic Gram-negative bacteria [7]. It is released from the cell membrane of bacteria during normal growth and during bacteriolysis from exposure to complement, antibodies, antibiotics or neutrophils. Endotoxin is a highly toxic molecule in human plasma or tissues. If accidentally or intentionally introduced into the systemic circulation, endotoxin will produce a sudden and dramatic pathophysiological state which mimics bacteremic, Gram-negative septic shock [8, 9].

The endotoxin molecule itself is not intrinsically toxic. It can be viewed as an alarm signal that alerts the vertebrate host that a pathogenic Gram-negative bacterium has breached the integument or mucosal surface barriers of the host. This physiological defense mechanism is a highly advantageous response that evolved as a survival strategy against microbial invaders. This endotoxin response serves to localize, contain, and eradicate invading bacterial pathogens. Unfortunately, the same immunological responses that protect the host in the presence of localized infections may precipitate a potentially fatal systemic inflammatory process in the presence of Gram-negative bacteremia [10, 11].

Endotoxin induces septic shock through the systemic activation of a network of host-derived inflammatory mediators including: (1) the proinflammatory cytokines and chemokines; (2) neutrophil, monocyte, and endothelial cell activation; (3) the complement system; (4) the coagulation cascade and the fibrinolytic system; (5)

Cytokines in Severe Sepsis and Septic Shock, edited by H. Redl and G. Schlag[†]
© 1999 Birkhäuser Verlag Basel/Switzerland

platelet activating factor; (6) bradykinin; (7) the prostaglandins and leukotrienes; (8) reactive oxygen intermediates; (9) nitric oxide; and probably other host-derived mediators [10–12]. These inflammatory mediators combine to precipitate endotoxic shock. Therapeutic interventions which interfere with the recognition of endotoxin in the circulation or contribute to its removal may prove beneficial in the prevention and treatment of septic shock.

Using sensitive assays of endotoxin detection, it is evident that endotoxin is measurable in the majority of patients with septic shock. Our group has measured elevated plasma endotoxin levels in 79% of cases in a study of over 700 patients with severe sepsis and/or septic shock [13]. Patients with the highest levels of endotoxin were more likely to be in profound shock and were less likely to survive over the next 28 days than patients with lesser amounts of circulating endotoxin. Other studies have also found an association with systemic hypotension and endotoxemia [14, 15]. A curious yet consistent finding in these studies [13–15] is the frequent presence of endotoxin in the plasma of septic patients with Gram-positive bacterial infections and fungal infections. This has been attributed to the presence of an unrecognized Gram-negative bacterial infection (perhaps related to the presence of inhibitory antimicrobial agents) or excess translocation of enteric bacteria and/or endotoxin itself as a consequence of increased intestinal permeability. The splanchnic circulation may be inadequate in the presence of systemic hypotension regardless of the precipitating of shock [16]. This allows uptake of potentially injurious microbial components (including endotoxin) from the intestinal lumen during periods of prolonged systemic hypotension. This may account for the frequent presence of endotoxemia observed in the course of septic shock from Gram-positive organisms.

A great deal of recent information about the metabolic fate of endotoxin in human tissues has rekindled interest in anti-endotoxin therapies in the management of septic shock [17–23]. Despite recent disappointments with anti-endotoxin antibodies, it is clear that agents with much greater endotoxin neutralizing capacity might be efficacious where less active agents might have failed. A summary of the advantages and disadvantages of anti-endotoxin strategies is given in Table 1.

Numerous anti-endotoxin strategies are in various stages of preclinical and clinical development at the present time. Those agents that function to remove endotoxin from the systemic circulation will be the focus of this paper. The basic mechanisms by which endotoxin mediates its pathological effects and the potential sites of intervention with endotoxin scavengers are outlined in Figure 1.

Anti-endotoxin treatments have an advantage over most experimental anti-mediator therapies under investigation for sepsis. LPS is an unwanted microbial toxin which can be completely eliminated without potential harm to the patient. This may not be the case with treatments directed against host-derived inflammatory mediators [24, 25].

Key elements of inflammation, such as TNFα and IL-1β are physiological components of the host defense mechanisms which have evolved to effectively eliminate

Table 1 - Endotoxin as a target for new treatment strategies against sepsis

Advantages	Disadvantages
Principal mediator in Gram-negative sepsis	Endotoxin rapidly cleared from the circulation and difficult to measure
Shares little homology with human structures	May not benefit patients with pure Gram-positive sepsis
Inhibitors should not adversely affect the host immune response	Other components of Gram-negative bacteria and toxins contribute to sepsis
Humans are exquisitely susceptible to endotoxin	Relative frequency of Gram-negative pathogens as a cause of sepsis is decreasing
Prophylactic agents feasible	

microbial pathogens. Inhibitors of these cytokines may place the patient at risk from overwhelming infection from the very same invading microorganisms which initially precipitated the septic event. This has been shown to be potentially deleterious in some experimental animal systems [26]. Anti-endotoxin therapies do not jeopardize endogenous host defense mechanisms. This should allow their use as preventative agents or treatment interventions in the early phases of sepsis where therapeutic agents are most likely to be effective.

Specific anti-endotoxin strategies

Anti-endotoxin core glycolipid antibodies

Anti-endotoxin monoclonal antibodies (mAbs) have been studied recently in several large clinical trials. Antibodies directed toward the highly conserved, core glycolipid structure of endotoxin (lipid A and a short sequence of core oligosaccharides) were expected to provide broad cross-protection against endotoxins from a variety of pathogenic Gram-negative organisms [27]. The clinical trials with both E5 [3, 4] and HA-1A [2] anti-lipid A mAbs were largely unsuccessful. Several potential explanations may account for the failure of these anti-core glycolipid antibodies to protect patients from the lethal consequences of Gram-negative bacterial sepsis [1, 3, 28].

Unfortunately, other anti-endotoxin compounds with greater intrinsic activity may be difficult to develop following the disappointing results with the monoclonal antibodies E5 and HA-1A. These antibodies had rather low intrinsic binding

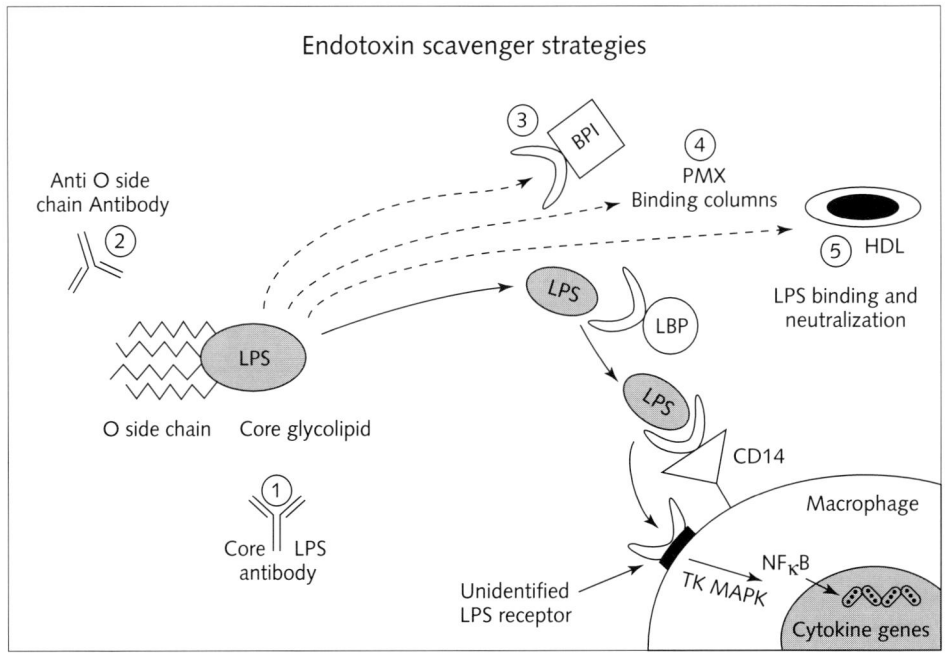

Figure 1

The pathophysiological sequence of events that result in endotoxin-mediated activation of inflammatory mediators in human sepsis. Highlighted areas where endotoxin scavengers may prove to be useful clinically are numbered in the figure. LPS-lipopolysaccharide; BPI-bactericidal/permeability-increasing protein; PMX-polymyxin; HDL-high density lipoprotein; LBP-lipopolysaccharide binding protein; TK-tyrosine kinase; MAPK-mitogen activated protein kinase; NFκB-nuclear factor in kappa B cells.

affinities to the lipid A component of bacterial endotoxin [28, 29]. HA-1A reacts with self antigens found on human B cells and red blood cells [30] and was shown to be detrimental in a canine peritonitis model of bacterial sepsis [31]. Despite some evidence of activity in meningococcal sepsis and other patient subgroups, clinical development of both of these antibodies has now been discontinued.

Interestingly, recent laboratory and clinical findings tend to substantiate the hypothesis that anti-core glycolipid antibodies may provide significant protection to patients in a variety of clinical settings. Goldie et al. [32] found that septic patients with pre-existing IgM anti-core glycolipid antibodies in the circulation have improved outcomes. Patients undergoing major surgery were less likely to succumb to sepsis if they maintained high levels of endogenous anti-core glycolipid antibodies [33]. Post-operative complications after major vascular surgical procedures were significantly less likely to occur in those patients with high titer antibodies against the core structure of LPS [34].

Rietschel and coworkers [11] have carefully studied the physicochemical properties of LPS and the immunodominant epitopes within the lipid A core structure and the oligosaccharide components of the highly conserved elements of bacterial endotoxin. They have described the relevant core glycolipid epitopes which are recognized by the human immune system in the presence of serotype specific O-side chains of polysaccharides on the outer part of the LPS molecule (known as complete or smooth LPS). This work is of critical importance since most bloodstream isolates of Gram-negative bacilli in human sepsis have complete LPS with O-polysaccharide side groups attached to the core structure. These side chains may serve to sequester core glycolipid epitopes from immune recognition and sterically inhibit antibody binding in virulent microbial pathogens. Outer core oligosaccharide epitopes on Rc mutants of *E. coli* have been identified which react with antibodies in the presence or absence of O-polysaccharide side chains of LPS. These reactive epitopes may be exploitable as a vaccine target in the development of vaccines against bacterial endotoxin [35].

Antibodies have been isolated and developed which bind with high affinity to endotoxin from a variety of Gram-negative bacterial pathogens. A chimeric IgG_1 monoclonal antibody known as SDZ 219-800 [36] has been developed which may prove to be an effective therapeutic agent in human endotoxemia. It is not clear if this antibody or similar anti-core glycolipid antibodies will ever be tested for efficacy in large scale clinical trials.

Active immunization with vaccines to raise endogenous anti-endotoxin antibodies against the conserved core glycolipid regions of bacterial endotoxin is another potential preventative or treatment strategy. Recent chemical formulations have yielded a vaccine preparation which appears to be promising. A detoxified LPS vaccine (using deacylated LPS from the *E. coli* J5 *gal*E mutant) combined with an outer membrane protein from group B meningococcus has been shown to be highly immunogenic and well tolerated in experimental animal systems [37]. Polyclonal antibodies produced in vaccine recipients bind to the inner core regions of LPS molecules (Rc region) from a number of common pathogenic Gram-negative bacilli and protect animals from lethal endotoxin challenge and invasive Gram-negative infections [37].

An active immunization strategy has several theoretical advantages. Among these are low production costs, avoidance of human blood products and recombinant protein production difficulties, ability to generate high titer endogenous antibodies in recipients, and the opportunity to use the vaccine as a preventative agent [7, 10, 37]. Prophylactic anti-endotoxin approaches are favored over delayed treatment strategies as humans respond precipitously to systemic endotoxin release with a complex array of host-derived inflammatory mediators. It is difficult at the bed-side to detect the early signs of endotoxemia in critically ill patients. Timely inter-vention with specific anti-endotoxin therapy after sepsis has begun may not be able to reverse the injurious systemic inflammatory response. A vaccine would induce the formation of anti-endotoxin antibodies before and during an episode of systemic endotoxin release and perhaps protect vaccine recipients at the critical phase of early Gram-negative sepsis [6, 10, 11].

Antibodies to O-specific polysaccharide antigens of LPS

Another potential anti-endotoxin antibody strategy would be the development of polyclonal antibodies directed against O-specific polysaccharide side chain antigens of LPS. Despite the fact that hundreds of serotype-specific polysaccharide antigens exist in the LPS structures of pathogenic Gram-negative organisms, a limited num-ber of common Gram-negative bacterial serotypes cause the majority of human blood stream infections. Cross et al. [38] have prepared a polyclonal hyperimmune human serum treatment against common strains of *Klebsiella* and *Pseudomonas* species. Clinical trials with this polyvalent antisera have met with limited success in selected patients but did not significantly benefit the entire study population.

Immunization of critically injured patients with a vaccine composed of polysac-charide antigens from bacterial LPS has been shown to raise significant serotype-specific antibody titers against O-side chain epitopes [39]. It may be possible to immunize acutely ill patients with such vaccines and offer protection against bacte-rial LPS molecules by active immunization. This approach to bacterial vaccine strategies has yet to be tested in a large clinical trial but it offers an opportunity to focus preventive efforts for anti-endotoxin vaccines on patient populations at great-est risk of endotoxin-mediated injury.

Bactericidal/permeability-increasing protein (BPI)

BPI is an endogenous human protein found in the azurophilic granules within neu-trophils. This 456 amino acid cationic protein attaches to the outer membrane of Gram-negative bacteria and disrupts the cell wall permeability characteristics of bacteria [40]. This antibacterial activity is accompanied by an ability to bind to the lipid A component of endotoxin [41, 42]. The high affinity binding results in the inactivation of endotoxin's ability to activate CD14-bearing immune effector cells (e.g. PMNs, and monocyte/macrophage cell lines).

BPI bears considerable structural homology with another important endotoxin binding protein, LPS binding protein (LBP) [43]. Both proteins bind with high affin-ity to the lipid portion of LPS. However, these two endotoxin binding proteins dif-

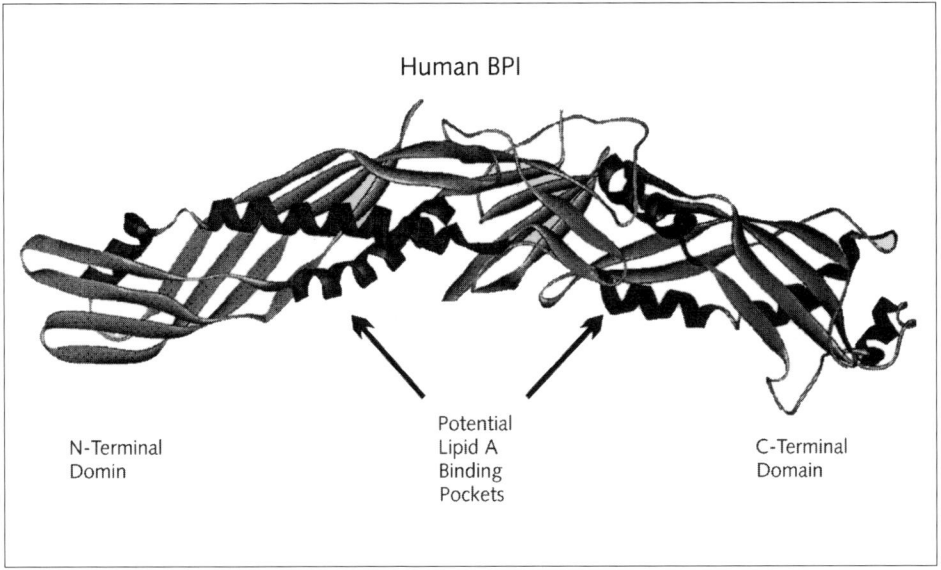

Human BPI

N-Terminal
Domin

Potential
Lipid A
Binding
Pockets

C-Terminal
Domain

Figure 2
Three dimensional model of bactericidal/permeability-increasing protein (BPI). Note two potential lipid A binding pockets along the under surface of the amino-terminus domain and the carboxyl-terminus domain. Figure obtained from the Brookhaven National Laboratory (Weblab Viewerlite, Molecular Simulations Inc.) (derived from work published from [46]).

fer functionally in that BPI inhibits LPS activation of CD14-bearing myeloid cells while LBP promotes LPS activity in these immune effector cells. BPI and LBP may act as molecular antagonists in biological fluids which compete with each other for LPS binding [44]. The net physiological effects of endotoxin release may depend upon the relative tissue concentrations of these two endotoxin binding proteins. LBP predominates in the systemic circulation as it is a hepatic acute phase protein [43–45]. BPI predominates in abscess cavities as neutrophils degranulate and release their intracellular contents into a site of inflammation [45].

The three dimensional structure of BPI has recently been determined by crystallographic analysis [46] (see Fig. 2). It forms a V-shaped molecule with planar symmetry between the amino-terminus domain and the carboxyl-terminus domains. Multiple amino acids converge to form a hydrophobic pocket along the inner surface of both the N-terminal and C-terminal domain of BPI. This hydrophobic region of the molecule appears to be the site into which the Lipid A portion of the LPS molecule fits. BPI binds to endotoxin with high affinity and effectively removes endotoxin from the circulation. The recombinant 55kDa holoprotein and the 23kDa amino terminal portion of BPI have both proven to be remarkably successful in endotoxin challenge experiments in experimental animals [42, 47] and human volunteer studies [48]. The protein also has some antibacterial properties as it increases the permeability of Gram-negative bacterial outer membranes which may be lethal to many enteric bacteria [40]. This provides the appealing opportunity of treatment with an endogenous human peptide that functions as an antibiotic as well as an endotoxin-neutralizing molecule.

The N-terminal domain of human recombinant BPI is now in extensive clinical trials in meningococcal sepsis, hemorrhagic states, and in partial hepatectomy. Initial clinical trials in children with meningococcal infections with septic shock were very encouraging in that the mortality rate in treated children was considerably lower than what would be predicted for this severely ill population [49]. A practical problem with recombinant BPI is its short serum half life (about two minutes). This necessitates administration of high doses of BPI by a continuous intravenous infusion. Recombinant derivatives of BPI with more favorable pharmacokinetic properties are available if current BPI products prove to be successful in ongoing clinical investigations [47].

Endotoxin binding by polymyxin B conjugates or filtration columns

Polymyxin B was discovered over 50 years ago as an antibiotic which inhibited Gram-negative bacilli including *Pseudomonas aeruginosa* [50]. It has largely been relegated to a drug of historical interest only as newer and less toxic antibiotics replaced polymyxin as the standard treatment for serious infections by *P. aeruginosa* [51]. However, its remarkable ability to bind to bacterial endotoxin has continued to interest investigators as a potential treatment for endotoxemia.

It is a cyclic and highly cationic peptide antibiotic which shares some structural characteristics with BPI and the Limulus endotoxin neutralizing protein [52]. Electrostatic and hydrophobic interactions with the lipid A structure of LPS account for its endotoxin neutralizing effects [53]. Polymyxin B has been administered to patients with endotoxemia with some evidence of potential benefit [54]. A conjugated form of polymyxin linked with dextran has been developed in an effort to maintain its endotoxin binding properties yet limit the nephrotoxicity of polymyxin itself. This polymyxin B-dextran conjugated material has been effective as an endotoxin scavenger in tissue culture systems [55], in a canine model of endotoxic shock [56], and in D-galactosamine-treated mice challenged with *E. coli* and antimicrobial agents [57].

A strategy which utilizes polymyxin B as a means of removing circulating endotoxin from the blood of septic patients has been described by Kodama et al [58, 59]. These Japanese investigators have used a hemoperfusion column fused with polymyxin to adsorb LPS from the systemic circulation. Preliminary experience with this endotoxin removal column has been promising and is under more extensive clinical investigation at the present time [58–60].

Reconstituted high density lipoprotein

High density lipoprotein (HDL) and other serum proteins such as low density lipoprotein will bind to endotoxin as it is released into the systemic circulation [61]. High density lipoprotein has a remarkable capacity for binding bacterial endotoxin with high affinity. LPS adsorption onto HDL particles forms a stable complex. This effectively removes LPS from the circulation as the HDL particle is cleared by hepatic uptake and excretion mechanisms [62]. HDL may have a physiological role as an endogenous LPS clearance system that limits the possible deleterious effects of systemic endotoxin release. LPS can be delivered to HDL carried by LPS binding protein or by soluble CD14 which can shuttle LPS to HDL. HDL serves as a systemic reservoir which takes up and eliminates LPS as it enters the circulation [62, 63].

The endotoxin neutralizing activity of HDL may prove to be a therapeutically viable treatment for human endotoxemia. Transgenic mice which express increased quantities of human apolipoprotein-A1(the principal protein component in HDL) are protected from the lethal effects of endotoxin challenge. Conversely, apolipoprotein-A1 knockout mice are highly susceptible to the toxic effects of endotoxin challenge [64]. It should be noted that critically ill patients frequently have diminished circulating levels of HDL. This may place such patients at greater risk from the deleterious effects of systemic endotoxin release [63].

It has been hypothesized that the administration of HDL to septic patients might replenish this physiological LPS clearance system and benefit patients with Gramnegative infections. In a phase I trial with LPS challenge in human volunteers, a reconstituted form of HDL from blood donors was effective in blocking the activation of proinflammatory cytokines and coagulation factors [65]. A Phase II clinical trial with reconstituted HDL in patients with peritonitis is planned in the near future.

Conclusions

Despite early disappointments with anti-endotoxin monoclonal antibodies, treatment strategies directed towards removal of systemic levels of bacterial endotoxin in septic patients remains a viable therapeutic approach. Efforts to remove bacterial endotoxin have the advantage of targeting a potentially lethal microbial mediator of sepsis. This approach obviates the legitimate concerns over disruption of the host defenses by anti-cytokine strategies and other anti-inflammatory treatments. Investigative efforts continue on a number experimental approaches directed against bacterial endotoxin. This research with endotoxin scavengers promises to lead to improvements in the outlook for septic patients in the future.

References

1   Cross AS, Opal SM (1994) Therapeutic intervention in sepsis with antibody to endotoxin: is there a future? *J Endo Res* 1: 57–69

2   McCloskey RV, Straube RC, Sanders C, Smith SM, Smith CR (1994) Treatment of septic shock with human monoclonal antibody HA-1A: a randomized, double-blind, placebo-controlled trial. *Ann Intern Med* 23: 994–1006

3   Cross AS (1994) Antiendotoxin antibodies: a dead end? *Ann Intern Med* 187: 464–477

4   Zeigler EJ, Fisher CJ Jr, Sprung CL, Straube RC, Sadoff J, Foulke GE, Wortel CH, Fink MP, Dellinger RP, Teng NNH et al (1991) Treatment of gram-negative bacteremia in septic shock with HA-1A human monoclonal antibody against endotoxin. *N Engl J Med* 324: 429–438

5   Greenman RL, Schein RMH, Martin MA, Wenzel RP, MacIntyre NR, Emmanuel G Chmel H, Kohler RB, McCarthy M, Plouffee J, Russell JA (1991) A controlled clinical trial of E5 murine monoclonal IgM antibody to endotoxin in the treatment of gram-negative sepsis. *JAMA* 266: 1097–1102

6   Opal SM (1995) Lessons learned from clinical trials of sepsis. *J Endotoxin Res* 2: 1–6

7   Rietschel ET, Kirikae T, Schade FU, Mamat U, Schmidt G, Loppnow H, Ulmer AJ, Zahringer U, Seyel U, Di Padova F et al (1994) Bacterial endotoxin: molecular mechanisms of structure to activity and function. *FASEB J* 218: 217–225

8   Suffredini AF, Fromm RE, Parker MM, Brenner M, Kovacs JA, Wesley RA, Parillo JE (1989) The cardiovascular response of normal humans to the administration of endotoxin. *N Engl J Med* 321: 280–287

9   Taveira da Silva AM, Kaulbach HC, Chuidian FS, Lambert DR, Suffredini AF, Danner RL (1993) Shock and multiple-organ dysfunction after self-administration of Salmonella endotoxin. *N Engl J Med* 328: 1457–1460

10 Horn DL, Opal SM, Lomastro E (1996) Antibiotics, cytokines, and endotoxin: a complex and evolving relationship in Gram-negative sepsis. *Scand J Infect Dis* 101: 9–13

11 Rietschel ET, Brade H, Holst O, Brade L, Muller-Loennies S, Mamat U, Zahringer U, Beckmann F, Seydel U, Bradenburg K et al (1996) Bacterial endotoxin: chemical composition, biological recognition, host response, and immunological detoxification. *Curr Topics Microbiol Immunol* 216: 39–81

12 Morrison DC, Ryan JL (1987) Endotoxins and disease mechanisms. *Ann Rev Med* 38: 417–432

13 Opal SM, Palardy JE, Parejo N, Dubin P, Fisher CJ, Vincent JL (1995) Endotoxemia in sepsis: Therapeutic and prognostic implications. *35th Interscience Conference of antimicrobial agents and chemotherapy*. San Francisco CA (abstract # G–88)

14 Danner RL, Elin RJ, Hosseini JM, Wesley JM, Reilly JM, Parillo JE (1991) Endotoxemia in human septic shock. *Chest* 99: 169–175

15 Casey LC, Balk RA, Bone RC (1993) Plasma cytokine and endotoxin levels correlate with survival in patients with the sepsis syndrome. *Ann Intern Med* 119: 771–778

16 Marshall JC, Sweeney D (1990) Microbial infection and the septic response in critical surgical illness: sepsis, not infection, determines outcome. *Arch Surg* 123: 1465–1469

17 Arditi M, Zhou J, Dorio R, Rong GW, Goyert SM, Kim KS (1993) Endotoxin-mediated endothelial cell injury and activation: role of soluble CD14. *Infect Immun* 61: 3149–3156

18 Pugin J, Heumann D, Tomasz A, Kravchenko VV, Akamatsu Y, Nishijima M,Glauser MP,Tobias PS, Ulevitch RJ (1994) CD14 as a pattern recognition receptor. *Immunity* 1: 509–516

19 Ge Y, Ezzell RM, Clark BD, Loiselle PM, Amato SF, Warren HS (1997) Relationship of tissue and cellular interleukin-1 and lipopolysaccharide after endotoxemia and bacteremia. *J Infect Dis* 176: 1313–1321

20 Wright SD (1995) CD14 and innate recognition of bacteria. *J Immunol* 155: 6–8

21 Ulevitch RJ, Tobias PS (1994) Recognition of endotoxin by cells leading to transmembrane signalling. *Current Opin Immunol* 6: 125–130

22 Ulevitch RJ, Tobias PS (1995) Receptor-dependent mechanisms of cell stimulation by bacterial endotoxin. *Ann Rev Immunol* 13: 437–457

23 Ge Y, Ezzell RM, Tompkins RG, Warren HS (1994) Cellular distribution of endotoxin after injection of chemically purified lipopolysaccharide differs from that after injection of live bacteria. *J Infect Dis* 169: 95–104

24 Zeni F, Freeman B, Natanson C (1997) Anti-inflammatory therapies to treat sepsis and septic shock: a reassessment. *Crit Care Med* 25: 1097–1100

25 Fisher CJ Jr., Agosti J, Opal SM, Lowry S, Sadoff J, Balk R, Abraham E, Schein R, Benjamin E (1996) Treatment of septic shock with tumor necrosis factor receptor: Fc Fusion protein. *New Engl J Med* 334: 1697–1702

26 Opal SM, Cross AS, Jhung J, Palardy JE, Parejo N (1996) Potential hazards of combination immunotherapy in the treatment of experimental sepsis. *J Infect Dis* 173: 1415–1421

27 Zeigler EJ, McCutchan JA, Douglas H, Braude AI (1975) Prevention of lethal Pseudomonas bacteremia with epimerase-deficient *E. coli* antiserum. *Trans Assoc Am Phys* 88: 101–108

28 Baumgartner J-D, Heumann D, Gerain J, Weinbreck P, Grau GE, Glauser MP (1990) Association between protective efficacy of anti-lipopolysaccharide (LPS) antibodies and suppression of LPS-induced tumor necrosis factor alpha and interleukin-6: comparison of O-side chain specific antibodies with core LPS antibodies. *J Exp Med* 171: 889–896

29 Warren HS, Amato SF, Fitting C, Black KM, Loiselle PM, Pasternack MS, Cavaillon J-M (1993) Assessment of ability of murine and human anti-lipid A monoclonal antibodies to bind and neutralize lipopolysaccharide. *J Exp Med* 177: 89–97

30 Bhart NM, Bieber MM, Chapman CJ (1993) Human anti-lipid A monoclonal antibod-

ies bind to human B cells and i-antigen on core red blood cells. *J Immunol* 151: 5011–5021

31 Quezado ZMM, Natanson C, Alling DW, Banks SM, Koev CA, Elin RJ, Hosseini JM, Bacher JD, Danner RL, Hoffman WD (1993) A controlled trial of HA-1A in a canine model of gram-negative septic shock. *JAMA* 269: 2221–2227

32 Goldie AS, Fearon KCH, Ross JA, Barclay GR, Jackson RE, Grant IS, Ramsay G, Blyth AS, Howie JC (1995) Natural cytokine and endogenous antiendotoxin core antibodies in sepsis syndrome. *JAMA* 274: 172–177

33 Nys M, Damas P, Joassin L, Lamy M (1993) Sequential anti-core glycolipid immunoglobulin antibody activities with and without septic shock and their relation to outcome. *Ann Surg* 217: 300–306

34 Bennett-Guerrero E, Ayuso L, Hamilton-Davies C, White HD, Barclay GR, Smith PK, King SA, Muhlbaier LH, Newman MF, Mythen MG (1997) Relationship of preoperative antiendotoxin core antibodies and adverse outcomes following cardiac surgery. *JAMA* 277: 646–650

35 Bhattercharjee AK, Opal SM, Palardy JE, Drabick JJ, Collins H, Taylor R Colton A, Cross AS (1994) Affinity purified E. coli J5 LPS-specific IgG protects neutropenic rats against gram-negative sepsis. *J Infect Dis* 170: 622–629

36 DiPadova FE, Gram H, Barclay GR, Poxton IR, Liehl E, Rietshel ET (1996) Monoclonal antibodies to endotoxin as a new approach in endotoxemia therapy. In: DL Morrison, JL Ryan (eds): *Novel therapeutic strategies in the treatment of sepsis*. Marcel Dekker, New York, 13–32

37 Bhattercharjee AK, Opal SM, Taylor R, Naso R, Semenuk M, Zollinger W, Moran EE, Young L, Hammack C, Sadoff J, Cross AS (1996) A non-covalent complex vaccine prepared with detoxified E. coli J5 LPS and Neisseria meningitidis group B outer membrane protein produces protective antibodies against gram-negative bacteria. *J Infect Dis* 173: 1157–1162

38 Donta ST, Peduzzi P, Cross AS, Sadoff J, Haakenson C, Gafford G, Elliston D, Beam TR, John JF, Riber B et al (1996) Immunoprophylaxis against *Klebsiella* and *Pseudomonas aeruginosa* infections. *J Infect Dis* 174: 537–543

39 Campbell WN, Hendrix E, Cryz S Jr. Cross AS (1996) Immunogenicity of a 24-valent Klebsiella capsular polysaccharide vaccine and as eight-valent Pseudomonas O-polysaccharide conjugate vaccine administered to victims of severe trauma. *Clin Infect Dis* 23: 179–181

40 Elsbach P, Weiss J (1993) Bactericidal/permeability-increasing protein and host defense against gram-negative bacteria in endotoxin. *Curr Opin Immunol* 5: 103–107

41 Marra MN, Wilde CG, Griffith JE, Snable JL, Scott RW (1990) Bactericidal/permeability-increasing protein has endotoxin-neutralizing ability. *J Immunol* 144: 662–666

42 Marra MN, Wilde CG, Collins MS, Snable JL, Thornton MB, Scott RW (1992) The role of bactericidal/permeability-increasing protein as a natural inhibitor of bacterial endotoxin. *J Immunol* 148: 532–537

43   Schumann RR, Leong SR, Flaggs GW (1992) Structure and function of lipopolysaccha-
      ride-binding protein. *Science* 49: 1431–1433
44   Heumann D, Gallay P, Betz-Corradin S, Barras C, Baumgartner J-D, Glauser MP (1993)
      Competition between bactericidal/permeability-increasing protein and lipopolysaccha-
      ride-binding protein for lipopolysaccaride binding to monocytes. *J Infect Dis* 167:
      1351– 1357
45   Opal SM, Marra MN, McKelligan B, Fisher CJ, Palardy JE, Scott R (1994) Relative con-
      centrations of endotoxin-binding proteins in body fluids during infection. *Lancet* 344:
      429–431
46   Beamer LJ, Carroll SF, Eisenberg D (1997) Crystal structure of human BPI and two
      bound phospholipids at 4.5 angstrom resolution. *Science* 276: 1861–1864
47   Opal SM, Palardy JE, Jhung JW, Donsky C, Romulo RLC, Parejo N, Marra MN (1995)
      Activity of lipopolysaccharide-binding protein-bactericidal/permeability increasing pro-
      tein fusion peptide in an experimental model of *Pseudomonas* sepsis. *Antimicrob Agents
      Chemother* 39: 2813–2815
48   Von der Mohlen MAM, Kimmings AN, Wedel NI, Mevissan, MLCM, Jansen J, Freid-
      mann N, Lorenz TJ, Nelson BJ, White M, Bauer R, et al (1995) Inhibition of endotox-
      in-induced cytokine release and neutrophil activation in humans using recombinant bac-
      tericidal/permeability-increasing protein (rBPI$_{23}$). *J Infect Dis* 172: 144–151
49   Giroir B, Carroll S, Scannon P (1997) *Phase I/II trial of rBPI$_{21}$ in children with severe
      meningococcemia*. Infectious Disease Society of America Annual Meeting, San Francis-
      co, CA Abstract # 414
50   Stansly PG, Shepard RG, White PJ (1947) Polymyxin: a new chemotherapeutic agent.
      Bull Johns Hopkins Hosp 81: 43
51   Horton J, Pankey GA (1982) Polymyxin B, Colistin, and sodium colistimethate. *Med
      Clin NA* 66: 135–142
52   Hoess A, Watson S, Siber GR, Liddington R (1993) Crystal structure of an endotoxin-
      neutralizing protein from the horseshoe crab, Limulus anti-LPS factor, at 1.5A resolu-
      tion. *EMBO J* 12: 3351–3356
53   Fukuoka S, Karube I (1994) Influence of cationic antibiotics on phase behavior of rough
      form lipopolysaccharide. *Appl Biochem Biotechnol* 49: 1–9
54   Endo S, Inada K, Kikuchi M (1994) Clinical effects of intramuscular administration of
      a small dose of polymyxin B to patients with endotoxemia. *Res Commun Chem Pathol
      Pharmacol* 83: 223–235
55   Coyne GP, Moritz JT, Fenwick BW (1994) Inhibition of lipopolysaccharide-induced
      TNF-α production by synthetic polymyxin B conjugated dextran. *Biotechnol Ther* 5:
      137–162
56   Lonegan JM Orlowski JP, Sato T, McHugh MJ, Zborowski M (1994) Extracorporeal
      endotoxin removal in a canine model of septic shock. *ASAIO J* 40: M654–657
57   Bucklin SE, Lake P, Logdberg L, Morrison DC (1995) Therapeutic efficacy of a
      polymyxin B-dextran conjugate in an experimental model of endotoxemia. *Antimicrob
      Agents Chemother* 39: 1462–1466

58 Kodama M, Tani T, Hanasawa K (1997) Extracorporeal removal of endotoxin in the septic patients by toraymyxin-Clinical results in a phase II and III study in Japan. *Shock* (suppl) 7: 6 abstr 22

59 Kodama M, Tani T, Maekawa K (1997) Endotoxin eliminating therapy in patients with severe sepsis-direct hemoperfusion using polymyxin B immobilized fiber column. *J Endotoxin Res; in press*

60 Aoki H, Kodama M, Tani T, Hanasawa K (1994) Treatment of sepsis by extracorporeal elimination of endotoxin using polymyxin B-immobilized fiber. *Am J Surg* 167: 412–417

61 Flegel WA, Baumstark MW, Weinstock C, Berg A, Northoff H (1993) Prevention of endotoxin induced monokine release by low-and high-density lipoproteins and by apolipoprotein A-1. *Infect Immun* 57: 2237–2245

62 Wurfel MM, Hailman E, Wright SD (1995) Soluble CD14 acts as a shuttle in the neutralization of lipopolysaccharide (LPS) by LPS-binding protein and reconstituted high density lipoprotein. *J Exp Med* 181: 1743–1754

63 Lerch PG, Fortsch V, Hodler G, Bolli R (1996) Production and characterization of a reconstituted high density lipoprotein (rHDL) for therapeutic application. *Vox Sang* 71: 155–164

64 Levine DM, Parker TS, Donnelly TM, Walsh AM, Rubin AL (1993) *In vivo* protection against endotoxin by plasma high density lipoprotein. *Proc Nat Acad Sci USA* 90: 12040–12044

65 Pajkrt D, Doran JE, Coster F, Lerch PG, Arnet B, van de Poll T, ten Cate JW, van Deventer SJH (1996) Anti-inflammatory affects of reconstituted high-density lipoprotein during human endotoxemia. *J Exp Med* 184: 1601–1608

Interfering with the production of cytokines in sepsis

Peter Zabel[1] and Soheyl Bahrami[2]

[1]Forschungszentrum Borstel, Zentrum für Medizin und Biowissenschaften, Parkallee 35, D-23845 Borstel, Germany
[2]Ludwig Boltzmann Institute for Experimental and Clinical Traumatology, Donaueschingenstr. 13, A-1200 Vienna, Austria

Introduction

During septic shock the host produces several proinflammatory cytokines which have been implicated as playing a critical role in the pathogenesis of the disease. The cytokines which contribute to pathological changes in septic shock are not unique to infection. Multiple trauma, ischemia-reperfusion injury, acute transplant rejection, antigen-specific immune responses, and various acute inflammatory states (pancreatitis) initiate the same cytokine cascade and result in both systemic and local inflammatory processes. However, septic shock is a special case, since no other disease is associated with such high mortality, despite our ability to provide patients with appropriate antibiotics and supportive therapy. Gene deletion, neutralizing antibody studies, and specific receptor blockade of cytokines have been shown to have a pivotal role in the pathogenesis of septic shock, at least in animal studies. Normally, cytokine response is regulated by the intricate network of proinflammatory and anti-inflammatory mediators. The inflammatory response is kept in check by down-regulating production and counteracting the effects of cytokines already produced.

The picture that emerges from analysis of data from patients with sepsis is that a complex mixture of pro- and anti-inflammatory molecules may be present [1, 2] (Tab. 1). These mediators initiate overlapping processes that directly influence endothelial, cardiovascular, hemodynamic, and coagulation mechanisms. The duration of illness may also alter the mix of mediators, leading to a state of metabolic disorder in which the body has no control over its own inflammatory response. If balance cannot be established and homeostasis is not restored, a massive proinflammatory reaction (SIRS) or a compensatory anti-inflammatory reaction (CARS) will ensue [3]. The preexisting status of the patient may affect the nature of the pro- and anti-inflammatory cytokine response. Genetic factors as well as gender play an important role in this balance. In infectious diseases the microorganism induces a cytokine profile which is distinct from that induced during a response to foreign-tissue antigens. For example, during bacterial infections there is little or no production of interferon (IFN)-γ or interleukin (IL)-2, whereas these cytokines are prominent

Table 1 - Partial list of proinflammatory and antiinflammatory cytokines

Proinflammatory molecules	Antiinflammatory molecules
TNF	TNF-Rc I +II
IL-1β	IL-1-Ra
IL-2	IL-4
IL-8	(IL-6)
IL-12	IL-10
IL-15	IL-13
IFNγ	TGFβ
MCPI/II	

components of the cytokine profile during transplant rejection and immune-mediated diseases. In both situations IL-1 and TNF are produced and function primarily as proinflammatory cytokines.

A distinction is made between the local effects of TNF and IL-1 and the consequences of their systemic levels. If the function of the host defense is the elimination of the invading organism or destruction of foreign tissue, inflammation is the price which is paid for an effective defense. In systemic inflammation, large amounts of TNF and IL-1 are released into the circulation. Many of the biological effects of TNF and IL-1 are similar to those observed during a septic event, and recent studies in humans have confirmed data from animal experiments. Therefore, it is well established that TNF and IL-1 play a critical role in sepsis. However, TNF has also been shown to be necessary in the host defense during experimental peritonitis. A comparative animal model study [4] showed clearly that blockade of TNF reduced endotoxemia mortality, but not mortality from cecal ligation and puncture (CLP). In other words, the TNF molecule exerts beneficial as well as harmful properties depending on its local or systemic concentration, "death from too much of a good thing" [5].

The consequences of IL-1 infusion into humans are similar to those observed for TNF except that induction of a coagulation cascade and an initial leukopenia [6] has not been observed in humans injected with IL-1. Systemic administration of intravenous IL-1 at doses of 1–10 ng/kg body weight produces fever, sleepiness, anorexia, generalized myalgias, arthralgias, and headache. The most dramatic biological response to IL-1 is observed at doses of 100 ng/kg or higher; at these levels a rapid fall in blood pressure takes place [7], indicating that also IL-1 is able to exert harmful effects in humans dose-dependently. The synergism between TNF and IL-1 is highly consistent and a frequently reported phenomenon also observed *in vivo* [8]. Efforts to understand how TNF and IL-1 manifest so many different biological properties can be focused on relatively few mechanistic pathways, mostly those

involving changes in constitutive and inducible gene expression or numbers of surface receptors for biologically active molecules. For example, inducible phospholipase A2 (PLA2), cyclooxygenase (COX), and inducible nitric oxide (NO) synthase,
genes controlling increased synthesis of inflammatory leukotrienes (LTs) and
prostaglandins (PGs), are highly relevant to understanding the multiple effects of
TNF and IL-1.

The best correlation of plasma cytokine levels with mortality from septic shock
– far better than that for TNF – has been found for IL-6 [9]. It is important to
emphasize that, unlike TNF and IL-1, there is no evidence that IL-6 is itself an
inflammatory cytokine except that elimination of IL-6 attenuates coagulation activation in experimental endotoxemia in chimpanzees [10]. In some models the production of IL-6 appears to be under the strict control of TNF and IL-1, and therefore one can conclude that elevated levels of IL-6 in patients with septic shock represent the net effect of biologically active TNF and IL-1, which are nearly impossible
to measure because plasma contains large concentrations of natural inhibitors for
TNF and IL-1.

In summary, there is strong evidence for a physiopathological role of an overwhelming production of TNF and IL-1 in the early state of septic shock, at least in
a subgroup of patients which has to be defined. Therefore, it is reasonable to
attempt to interfere induction by reducing production of TNF and IL-1.

Reducing production of IL-1 and TNF

In addition to the interference with induction (see chapter by S. Opal, this volume),
anti-TNF and anti-IL-1 agents can be classified according to the stage of production
of cytokine activity they inhibit. Synthesis can be inhibited by anti-inflammatory
cytokines, other endogenous mediators and synthetic drugs. Processing of the
cytokine pro-protein can be inhibited by specific inhibitors of the metalloprotease.
Finally, the effects of released cytokines can be antagonized by soluble receptors or
anti-cytokine antibodies (see chapter by E. Abraham, this volume). Inhibition of
TNF and IL-1 synthesis can be achieved by several means: (i) inhibition of transcription, (ii) decrease of the mRNA half-life, (iii) inhibition of translation, and (iiii)
inhibition of processing. Although some substances act on more than one level there
are at least preferential modes of action (see Tab. 2).

Reduction of transcription

At the transcriptional level, synthesis can be inhibited by anti-inflammatory
cytokines, increase of intracellular cAMP, antisense oligonucleotides, cytokine-suppressing anti-inflammatory drugs, or decrease of mRNA stability (Fig. 1).

Table 2 - Agents that inhibit tumor necrosis factor α (TNF)

Inhibition of TNF synthesis	
Cytokines	IL-4
	IL-10
	IL-13
	TGFβ
Other endogenous mediators	Corticosteroids
	Prostanoids
	Adenosine
	Histamine
	Nitric oxide
	ω-3 fatty acids
Synthetic drugs	Pentoxifylline
	Cyclosporin A
	Chlorpromazine
	Thalidomide
	Antisense oligonucleotides

Inhibition of TNF processing

Inhibitors of the TNF metalloprotease
Cytokine-suppressing antiinflammatory drugs

Inhibition of TNF effects

Anti-TNF antibodies
Soluble TNF receptors

modified from [33]

Anti-inflammatory cytokines
Only recently has the extent and complexity of the anti-inflammatory cytokine network been investigated. The evidence that anti-inflammatory cytokines do in fact play a role in down-regulating inflammation comes from (a) experiments in which neutralizing antibodies to certain cytokines worsen the inflammation and (b) gene deletion studies in mice which reveal a role for a particular cytokine as an anti-inflammatory agent. For example, antibodies to IL-1-receptor antagonist (IL-1-ra) worsen colitis, and mice deficient in IL-10 develop spontaneous inflammatory bowel disease [11].

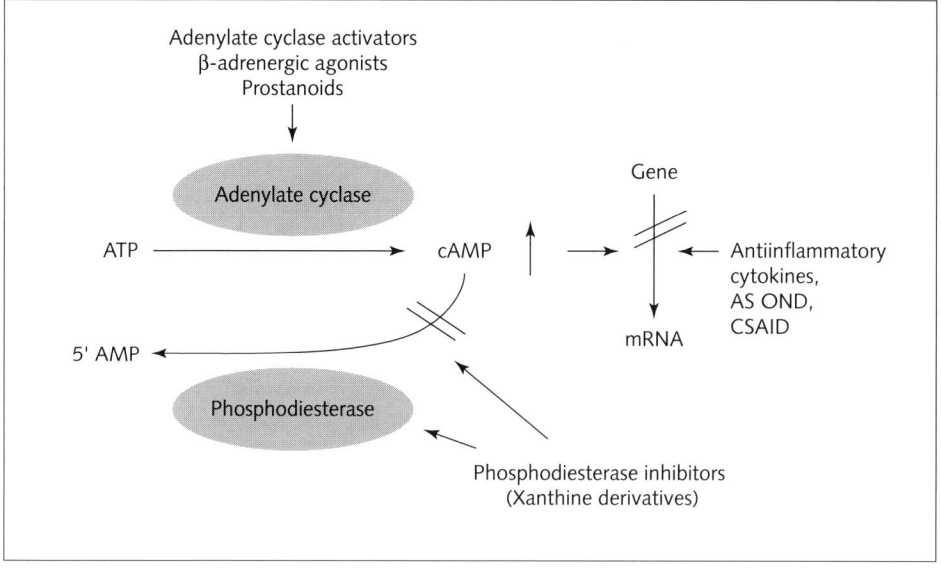

Figure 1
Inhibition of cytokine formation at the transcriptional level. AS OND, antisense oligonu-cleotide; CSAID, cytokine-suppressing antiinflammatory drug

IL-4, IL-10, IL-13, and transforming growth factor (TGF)-β each suppress gene expression and synthesis of IL-1, TNF, and other cytokines. *In vitro*, these cytokines can reduce endotoxin-induced gene expression and synthesis of IL-1 and TNF by as much as 90% and, when given to mice or rats, can reduce lethal endotoxemia. As such they might be potentially usefull in some clinical situations. IL-10 appears to be particularly useful because, unlike IL-4 and TGFβ, it has no clinical side effects. A randomized, double-blind, placebo-controlled trial (phase I) in healthy human volunteers demonstrated the absence of clinical toxicity and also investigated the effect of a single intravenous injection of IL-10 on cytokine production [12]. Blood was removed before and 3, 6, 24, and 48 h after the injection and incubated *in vitro* with endotoxin, and the amounts of IL-1β, TNF, IL-6, IL-8, IL-1-ra, and soluble TNF receptor- (sTNFR) p55 were measured. At doses of 10 and 25 μg/kg there was a 90% reduction in IL-1β, TNF, and IL-6 production in blood taken 3 and 6 h after injection; at 25 μg/kg a 50% reduction of IL-1β, TNF, and IL-6 production was present after 24 and 48 h. In contrast, there was no suppression of IL-1-ra or sTNFR-p55. A 40–60% reduction in circulating lymphocytes expressing CD4, CD8, and CD3 was observed after infusion of IL-10 [12]. The proliferative response to the mitogen phytohemagglutinin was suppressed in peripheral blood mononuclear cells (PBMC) from volunteers given 10 or 25 μg/kg IL-10 and was not reversed by using higher concentrations of the mitogen. These human studies confirm the *in vitro* effects of IL-10 and suggest IL-10 may be useful in suppressing inflammatory cytokine production in selected diseases.

IL-4 and IL-13 also suppress LPS-induced IL-1 and TNF gene expression and synthesis. In addition, they increase IL-1-ra production [13]. IL-4 and IL-13 share the same receptor complex on monocytes, and hence similar biological effects for both cytokines are often observed. There are, however, few if any receptors for IL-13 on T-lymphocytes, and hence the immunological suppressive effects of IL-4 and IL-10 on lymphocytes are not observed for IL-13. Similarly to IL-4, IL-10 and IL-13, TGFβ suppress gene expression and synthesis of IL-1 and TNF and also increase IL-1-ra production [14]. However, TGFβ, which has profound immunosuppressive effects, is a growth factor for normal and neoplastic cells.

Increased Intracellular cAMP Levels

The most studied class of agents that inhibit cytokine formation at the level of gene transcription contains those agents that increase the intracellular concentration of cyclic adenosine monophosphate (cAMP); among them are phosphodiesterase (PDE) inhibitors, adenylate cyclase activator, and β-agonists (Fig. 1). In general, the degree of intracellular cAMP closely correlates with the degree of cytokine inhibtion.

Phosphodiesterase inhibitors

The effect of PDE inhibitors on gene induction has been extensively studied. Theophylline [15], pentoxifylline (PTX) [15], rolipram [16], and amrinone [17] are among the PDE inhibitors shown to inhibit TNF mRNA accumulation. Published reports on the effect of PDE inhibitors, however, on synthesis of IL-1β are conflicting [18–22]. At the level of gene expression, cAMP-increasing agents markedly reduce TNFα mRNA but not IL-1β mRNA [23]. The PDE inhibitors theophylline, PTX, and 3-isobutyl-1-methylxanthine selectively block LPS-induced synthesis of TNFα in human mononuclear cells without affecting production of IL-1β [18]. Moreover, cAMP increase by enhanced formation via prostaglandin (PG) E2 leads to suppression of TNFα production with no effect on IL-1β [18]. Similarly, cAMP increase by the PDE inhibitor PTX reduces TNFα but not IL-6 levels [24, 25], suggesting that cyclic nucleotides differentially regulate the synthesis of cytokines.

PTX and the related xanthines that comprise the PDE inhibitors have been of considerable interest due to their recently characterized immunomodulatory properties. Originally developed for the treatment of vascular diseases, but used in many therapeutic applications, the pharmacokinetic and pharmacodynamic properties of PTX have been extensively characterized and indicate it to be a safe drug [26]. The modulation of several cytokines has been analyzed *in vitro* and *in vivo*. Importantly, PTX reduces production of the monokine TNF without affecting IL-1, IL-6 or

IL-8 [27–29]. Furthermore, IL-12 [4] as well as TH1-derived lymphokines like IFNγ and IL-2 are dose-dependently inhibited by PTX [30], whereas TH2-derived lymphokines like IL-4 are not influenced [31].

Since suppression of TNF and other cytokines by PTX *in vitro* can be mimicked by membrane-penetrating dibutyryl cAMP [29, 32] and is significantly correlated with the potential to inhibit phosphodiesterase activity [16], it can be assumed that the elevation of intracellular cAMP is the central mechanism for inhibiting cytokine formation, as has been previously described for TNF [15]. Increased levels of cAMP activate cAMP-dependent protein kinase A, resulting in phosphorylation of target proteins such as cAMP-responsive element (CRE)-binding proteins. These transcription factors bind to specific sequences of the promotor region of certain genes. Such a CRE-specific sequence has been reported in the 5'-flanking region of the TNF gene [33]. Three mechanisms are mostly involved in the PTX-induced increase in intracellular cAMP: (i) inhibition of phosphodiesterase activity, (ii) induction of PGs (e.g. PGE2 and PGI2) with subsequent stimulation of endogenous adenylate cyclase [34], and (iii) interaction with extracellular adenosine receptors [35]. The inhibition of phosphodiesterase activity might be the central mechanism in the inhibitory activity of PTX in mononuclear cells; however, endogenous PG production with activation of adenylate cyclase may contribute to the mode of action of PTX, as demonstrated by experiments involving the combination of PTX with cyclooxygenase inhibitors [34]. Nevertheless, it remains to be determined to what extent each of the above-mentioned mechanisms contributes to the action of PTX on different cell types. PTX reduces TNF production by inhibiting TNF-specific mRNA formation without affecting translation [15], which is an essential difference from the action of corticosteroids [36]. Importantly, this mechanism of action is also different from that of thalidomide (see below), which acts by enhancing the degradation of TNF mRNA [37].

Various *in vivo* studies in experimental animals as well as in humans support the concept that PTX-mediated immunological effects have profound influences on various diseases. With regard to septic shock, PTX treatment resulted in an increased survival rate in models of endotoxic shock [38] and, most importantly, also in the model of cecal ligation and puncture (CLP) [39], an animal model of sepsis in which blockade of TNF activity by neutralizing TNF antibodies failed to improve survival [4]. It has already been shown in clinical situations that PTX reduces the endotoxin-induced [24] and anti-CD₃-antibodies (OKT3)-induced [40] endogenous TNF formation as well as TNF-dependent cachexia in patients with advanced AIDS [41] and cancer [42]. Additionally, PTX exerts beneficial effects in sarcoidosis, a TH1-lymphokine-mediated disease [43]. In patients with septic shock PTX is able to decrease serum TNF but not IL-6 or IL-8 concentration [44]. In a clinical study (prospective, randomized, double-blind, placebo-controlled) in patients with severe sepsis, 90% of whom had septic shock, treatment with continuous intravenous administration of PTX significantly improved cardiopulmonary dysfunction and tended to improve survival without any adverse effect [45]. In a more recent study, supplemental PTX treatment significantly reduced the incidence of multiple organ failure in patients at risk of inflammatory respose syndrome after cardiac surgery [46].

The clinical efficacy of PTX in terms of organ dysfunction, survival, and mediator response, however, has to be evaluated in further studies, especially with regard to dose-dependency. PTX may have potential in immunotherapy, especially since it is superior to other xanthine derivatives with respect to therapeutic implications. Theophylline suppresses TNF production only weakly, and other recently developed xanthine derivatives have the disadvantage of not being fully characterized with regard to their relative toxicities, despite their pharmacological potential in suppressing TNF production [16, 47].

Although PTX is the most widely studied agent which inhibits PDE and thereby increases cAMP, it is rapidly metabolized systemically (liver first-path effect), with peak plasma concentrations being reached at 1.05 h by an elimination half-life of 0.8 h, respectively [26]. The intra- and interindividual variability in the first-path effect make it difficult to standardize dosage regimens clinically. Thus , efforts have been made to develop more stable xanthine derivatives, such as albifylline (HWA 138) with similar bioactivities to PTX but improved pharmacokinetics [48].

HWA 138 has been reported to attenuate acute lung injury in experimental animals [49, 50], decrease cytokine formation, ameliorate coagulation disturbances, and reduce mortality induced by endotoxin in rats [51]. Similarly, in a model of bacteremia in primates HWA 138 significantly inhibited TNFα formation [52]. Furthermore, HWA 138 was found to prevent lung injury induced by mediators released by endotoxin [53]. Compared with other xanthine derivatives, HWA was found (a) to be more potent in abrogation of the proinflammatory effects of TNF on granulocytes chemotaxis, adhesion, and toxic radical production *in vitro* [54] and (b) to counteract LPS-induced leukopenia more effectively [34]. However, the inhibition of cytokine formation *ex vivo* was similar to that by PTX [55]. HWA 138 and PTX show similar potency and efficacy in inhibiting LPS-induced TNF formation both *in vitro* and *in vivo* [56]. The similar effect of these two xanthine derivatives on cytokine formation and coagulation disturbances indicates that, at least to a substantial degree, other mechanisms may account for the significant protection against endotoxin-induced mortality by HWA only [56].

Nevertheless, inhibitors of TNF formation have been shown to exert differential effects in lethal endotoxemia and in infection with live microorganisms [57]. PTX, thalidomide, and chlorpromazine (CPZ) were tested in lethal endotoxemia in sensitized mice. Although both PTX and CPZ significantly reduced endotoxin-induced TNFα plasma levels, only CPZ significantly improved survival. Thus, it is clear that reduction in plasma TNF levels can not account alone for the protective effect of CPZ in lethal endotoxemia. CPZ, in contrast to PTX, significantly reduced postendotoxin IL-1β levels as well as plasma levels of sTNFR-p75. The anticytokine effect of CPZ may, therefore, be counteracted by decreased concentrations of circulating TNF-receptor (sTNFR-p75). No drug, however, improved survival in *Klebsiella pneumoniae*-infected mice, despite significantly reduced circulating TNFα concentrations in both PTX- and CPZ-treated animals [57]. Thus, it is important to note that there are substantial differences between the efficacy of different drugs in endotoxemia and in infection with live organisms.

Adenylate cyclase activators

Another approach to increasing intracellular cAMP is to activate the adenylate cyclase (Fig. 1). Forskolin, a well-known adenylate cyclase activator, has been shown to improve intracellular cAMP. Forskolin exerts beneficial effects against LPS-induced endothelial cytotoxicity by increasing intracellular cAMP [32]. Recently, it has been reported that increasing cAMP by means of forskolin inhibits NO formation and the expression of iNOS induced by endotoxin or cytokines in rat primary astrocytes and C6 glial cells, while compounds that decrease cAMP stimulate the production of NO [58].

β-adrenergic agonists

In general, catecholamines are used to treat the hemodynamic cosequences in patients with severe septic shock. β-adrenergic agonists exert many of their effects by elevation of intracellular cAMP concentration. In addition to their hemodynamic actions, β-adrenergic compounds may also exert beneficial effects by modulation of inflammatory response. Isoproterenol pretreatment has been shown to reduce endotoxin-induced TNF and NO formation and to increase the production of both IL-10 and IL-6 in rats [59]. The β-agonists procaterol, clenbuterol, fenoterol, and terbutaline were found to inhibit the induction of TNF and IL-1β by elevating intracellular cAMP levels, but with no effect on IL-8 formation [60]. Clinically relevant concentrations of inotropes, such as amrinone and dopamine, which increase cAMP, inhibited the IL-1α induced increase in human umbilical vein endothelial cell adhesion molecule concentrations [61]. In human endotoxemia, epinephrine, which also increases cAMP levels, not only influences bio-availability of TNF by an effect on the production of this proinflammatory cytokine, but also modulates the expression of its receptors in monocytes and granulocytes [62]. Further studies are necessary to investigate the mechanisms of these effects and to determine the efficacy of inotropes as anti-inflammatory agents.

Prostanoids

Many changes induced by IL-1 and TNF are mediated by PGs, particularly PGE2. In fact, the use of cyclooxygenase (COX) inhibitors for a variety of inflammatory conditions is often a therapeutic strategy to reduce IL-1- and TNF-induced PGE2. Humans injected with endotoxin, IL-1, or TNF experience fever, headache, myalgias, and arthralgias [24], each of which is reduced by coadministration of cyclooxygenase inhibitors [63]. One of the more universal activities of IL-1 and TNF is the induction of gene expression for type 2 PLA2 and COX-2. IL-1 and TNF induce transcription of COX-2, and neither cytokine increases production of COX-1. COX-2 production is elevated for several hours, and large amounts of PGE2 are produced. Furthermore, IL-1 and TNF preferentially stimulate new transcripts for the inducible form of PLA2 [64], which cleaves the fatty acid in the number 2 position of cell membrane phospholipids, e.g. arachidonic acid. The release of arachidonic acid is the rate-limiting step in the synthesis of PGs and LTs.

Cyclooxygenase inhibitors
Despite several studies there is no clear answer as to whether PGs suppress IL-1 production in cultured PBMC *in vitro*. This is probably due to the type of stimulant used and to the contribution of endogenous IL-1 production (IL-1 induced IL-1) to the total IL-1 synthesized [65]. In general, adding cyclooxygenase inhibitors to LPS-stimulated PBMC can suppress, augment, or have no effect on IL-1 production [66]. On the other hand, under the same culture conditions, LPS-induced TNF gene expression and synthesis is extensively sensitive to suppression by PGE2 and PGI2. In humans injected with LPS and pretreated with oral cyclooxygenase inhibitors, the circulating levels of TNF and IL-6 are higher than in controls not given cyclooxygenase inhibitors [63]. This observation is consistent with the mechanism that PGE2/PGI2-induced TNF suppression is via elevation in cAMP [18]. Consequently, the prostacyclin analogue iloprost has been shown to inhibit TNF production effectively by augmenting intracellular cAMP via activation of adenylate cyclase [67].

In patients with sepsis, the production of arachidonic acid metabolites by cyclooxygenase increases, but the physiopathological role of these prostanoids is unclear. In animal models, inhibition of cyclooxygenase by prophylactic administration of ibuprofen before the onset of sepsis reduces physiological abnormalities and improves survival [8, 68]. In pilot studies of patients with sepsis, treatment with ibuprofen led to improvements in gas exchange and airway mechanics [69]. In a randomized, double-blind, placebo-controlled trial of intravenous ibuprofen in 455 patients with severe sepsis, however, treatment with ibuprofen did not reduce the incidence or duration of shock or the acute respiratory distress syndrome and did not improve the rate of survival at 30 days [70].

Lipoxygenase inhibitors
Inhibitors of 13-lipoxygenase [71], but not 5-lipoxygenase [72], reduce TNF and Il-1β transcription. Earlier studies had implicated leukotrien (LT) B4 as the lipoxygenase product triggering IL-1 and TNF-synthesis. However, using specific inhibitors of 5-lipoxygenase, an important role of LTB4 in the production of

cytokines is unlikely. Nevertheless, a role of lipoxygenase products in stimulating IL-1 and TNF production is supported by several controlled studies in humans consuming dietary supplements of eicosapentaenoic (ω-3) fatty acids or a diet rich in these fatty acids. When ω-3 fatty acids are incorporated into cell membranes, the cyclooxygenase and lipoxygenase products following phospholipase-mediated hydrolysis of membrane phospholipids are not PGE2 and LTB4 but rather PGE3 and LTB5. This change alters the signal transduction pathway induced by exogenous stimulants and results in an attenuation in the synthesis of proinflammatory cytokines. Several clinical trials have demonstrated a beneficial effect of dietary supplementation, and controlled studies have consistently shown a 50–60% decrease in IL-1, IL-6, and TNF production in PBMC of subjects ingesting ω-3 fatty acid supplements compared to PBMC taken before this dietary intervention. This phenomenon can also be demonstrated by measuring cytokine production in whole blood (reviewed in [73]).

Antisense oligonucleotides

The regulation of expression of genetic information by complementary pairing of sense and antisense nucleic acid strands has been termed "antisense" (AS), a mechanism used throughout nature to control gene expression. A selective blockade of a specific gene responsible for a certain inflammatory disease is an attractive target for intervention. AS oligonucleotides (ONDs) are short (15–20 bases), single-stranded DNA fragments, which are directed to a specific mRNA. In addition, these DNA fragments can also be targeted against a genomic DNA sequence; this is termed antigene therapy. In general, three mechanisms of action have been reported for ONDs (Fig. 2). (1) ONDs can complementarily (antisense) hybridize in a base pair fashion to their target (sense) mRNA and thus block translation. (2) They can also bind to the genomic DNA in the nucleus, blocking transcription. (3) A non-specific binding of the ONDs to a target protein is another mechanism of action, which has been referred to as aptamer binding. In order to improve AS efficiency, chemical modifications have been developed and improvement of OND uptake achieved with different systems of vectorization, including liposomes, nanoparticles, or covalent attachment of carrier.

Therapeutic application of AS has been suggested by inhibition of inflammatory cytokines. However, as many of the targeted proteins are ubiquitously expressed, the systemic application of AS ONDs might also harm cells which are not the target of therapeutic intervention. There are also reports that widely used systemic applications to improve cellular OND uptake might be toxic or might trigger undesired immune resposes in humans (for mechanism of toxicity see [74]). In general, the AS OND approach is applicable to a wide variety of signal-transduction systems. Therapeutic application of AS ONDs has been suggested for inhibition of inflammatory cytokines [75]. The following examples demonstrate the diversity of

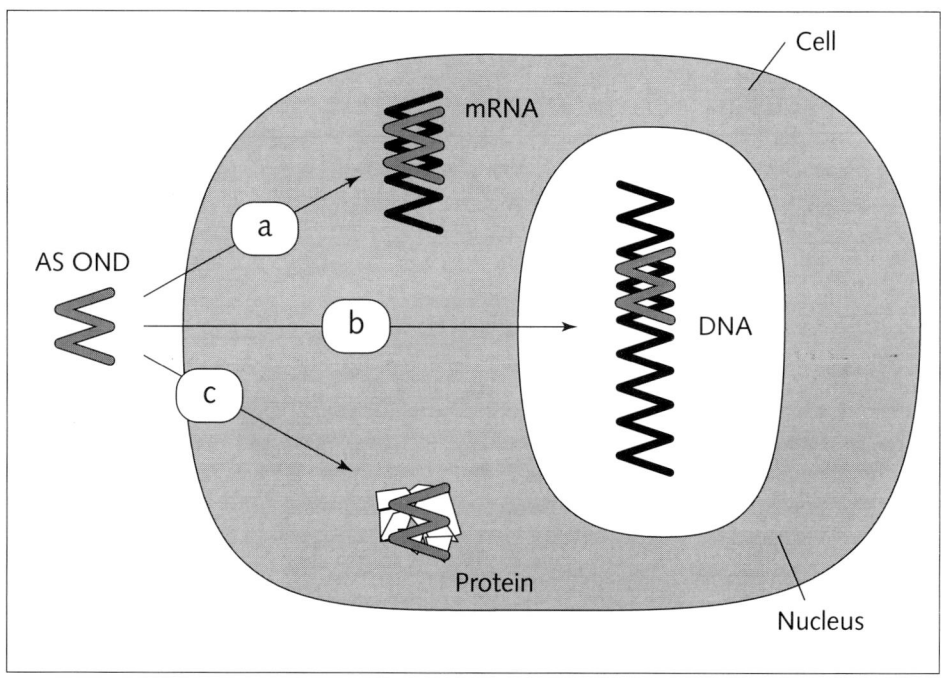

Figure 2
Cytokine regulation by antisense oligonucleotide (AS OND): (a) AS OND hybridization to mRNA (antisense therapy), (b) AS OND binding to DNA in the nucleus (antigene therapy), and (c) AS OND interaction with protein (aptamer binding).

questions that might be answered by the use of AS OND techniques and results that could have clinical relevance.

Interferons (IFN) are cytokines that play an important and complex role in the host response to pathogens. While IFNα and IFNβ are secreted by virus-infected cells, IFNγ is secreted by thymus-derived (T) cells under certain conditions. Several IFNγ-regulated genes are themselves components of transcription factors. AS ONDs that inhibit the expression of Raf kinase, an important intracellular mediator in T cell signaling, have a significant effect on a human Th1-like T cell clone, inhibiting antiCD3-induced secretion of IFNγ, with no effect on secretion of IL-2 (Th1, Th2 cells), IL-4 and IL-5 (Th2 cells) [76].

An AS OND knockdown strategy for inhibition of iNOS resulted in significant reduction of LPS- and IFNγ-induced iNOS mRNA and protein expression [77]. It also inhibited NO and cGMP production in a dose-dependent manner, indicating the efficacy and specify of AS ONDs in therapeutic approaches. AS ONDs, targeted against specific transforming growth factor β (TGFβ), a growth-regulatory and immunomodulatory cytokine, have been reported to reduce TGFβ mRNA levels and TGFβ secretion in malignant mesothelioma cell lines [78].

The binding of TNFα to TNF receptor type I (TNFRI) is considered the initial step for some of the multiple biological functions mediated by TNF. Thus TNFRI AS ONDs have been identified which specifically inhibited TNFRI mRNA and subsequently inhibited the functions of TNF mediated by TNFRI in a cellular assay [79]. The gene-specific AS inhibition occurred in a dose-dependent manner and correlated with the binding affinity of the OND for the target mRNA, reducing levels of TNF mRNA [79].

Despite the encouraging biological effects seen in numerous reports of apparent AS inhibition of gene expression in cells *ex vivo* as well as *in vivo*, only in a few cases has specific inhibition been rigorously demonstrated [80–84]. Thus there is a need for further studies in order to make a critical evaluation of the effectiveness of AS ONDs *in vivo*. Such studies could eventually lead to the developement of improved methods in AS therapy for human diseases.

Cytokine-suppressing anti-inflammatory drugs (CSAIDs)

Proinflammatory cytokines such as TNFα and IL-1 are secreted proteins produced by monocytes/macrophages and other cell types in response to many inflammatory stimuli by activation of protein kinase cascades that lead to gene expression. The signaling pathway in mammalian cells has been shown to be mediated via mitogen-activated protein kinases (MAP kinases) belonging to different phosphorylation cascades, each responding to different extracellular stimuli. Among them, a novel MAP kinase (p38) has been identified that was tyrosine phosphorylated in response to LPS [85]. The p38 MAP kinase signal-transduction pathway is activated not only by endotoxin, but also by proinflammatory cytokines (e.g. TNF, IL-1), and environmental stress. The detection of p38 MAP kinase in the nucleus of stimulated cells suggests that p38 MAP kinase can mediate signaling to the nucleus [86]. The exposure of human neutrophils to, for example, endotoxin results in phosphorylation and activation of p38 MAP kinase in a concentration-dependent manner and with a maximum at 20–25 min [87]. Activation of the p38 MAP kinase by endotoxin occurs via LPS receptor CD14 and requires the presence of LBP [87]. A transient activation of p38 protein kinase by thrombin has been demonstrated (with maximal stimulation at 1 min) that might be involved in thrombin-mediated signaling events during platelet activation [88]. Similarly, the cytosolic phospholipase A2 activation by thrombin has been suggested to be mediated by the same protein kinase [89]. Beyaert et al. [64] reported that p38 MAP kinase is involved in TNF-induced gene expression and regulates, for example, IL-6 synthesis in response to TNF.

CSAIDs, such as pyridynil-imidazole compounds have been shown to inhibit TNFα and IL-1 production from human monocytes [90] by inhibiting a pair of closely related mitogen-activated protein kinase (MAP kinase) homologues, termed

CSBPs. Most recently, a specific inhibitor of p38 MAP kinase, SB203580, has been demonstrated to completely inhibit synthesis of IL-6 in TNF-stimulated cells without affecting TNF-induced cytotoxicity [64]. This inhibitor also suppressed the TNF-induced surface expression of endothelial adhesion molecule (VCAM-1) without affecting the VCAM-1 mRNA accumulation [91], indicating that the p38 MAP kinase signaling pathway regulates the endothelial expression of VCAM-1 at the post-transcriptional level. Thus, p38 MAP kinase might provide an interesting target for selective interference with TNF-induced gene activation.

Decrease in mRNA stability

Recent interest in thalidomide stems not from its properties as a sedative or anti-emetic [92], but from the observation of its efficacy as an immunomodulatory or immunosuppressive drug [93]. Many recent experiments have confirmed that thalidomide is indeed a powerful immunomodulant, and it has been used beneficially in settings such as vasculitis [94], a model of HIV [37], rheumatoid arthritis [95], sarcoidosis [96], chronic graft-versus-host disease [97], and prevention of rejection in transplantation [98]. Both *in vivo* and *in vitro* experiments have shown that a major effect of thalidomide is the selective down-regulation of TNF production by activated monocytes [99], but similar inhibitory effects have also been noted on IL-6 and, to a lesser extent, on IFNγ production. T cell proliferative responses seem relatively unaffected by thalidomide [100].

Only recently have the techniques become available to investigate the molecular mechanism(s) of action of thalidomide and its role in differential gene regulation. The experimental evidence to date points to thalidomide having selective effects on proinflammatory cytokines (mainly TNF) and suggests that its mechanism of action may be related to, or result in, alteration in the half-life of TNF mRNA [37]. There is only circumstantial evidence that this control is exerted in a cell-specific manner, and it appears likely that all cells capable of expressing TNF mRNA are equally affected, although, on a per cell basis, monocytes are the principal source of this cytokine. Glucocorticoids such as dexamethasone are known to downregulate nuclear factor κB (NFκB), a transcription factor common to many cytokine genes [101]. Various transcription factor families, including the NFATs (nuclear factors of activated T cells), are common to many T cell cytokines and some monokines [102]. Specific cytokine gene transcription is initiated by differential activation of various combinations of these and other transcription factors. This might explain the differences in expression of TNF (and other cytokines) when the effects of thalidomide are compared with steroids such as dexamethasone. Recent evidence has indicated that TNF is activated by a combination of transcription factors which include the ubiquitous NFκB and the more restricted NFATp and AFT-2/JUN [103], transcription factors not associated with most other cytokines. It therefore seems likely that a unique combination of transcription factor binding, part of which is thalidomide-sensitive, may account for the independent regulation of TNF mRNA activation and explain the steroid-sparing capacity of thalidomide [100].

Recently, structural modifications of thalidomide that produce analogues with enhanced TNF inhibitory activity have been examined [104, 105]. The researchers concerned have systematically examined a series of analogues and derivatives of thalidomide and have identified compounds which inhibit TNF production with IC50s at sub-molar levels (compared with thalidomide at 194 µM) and which are almost 500 times more potent than thalidomide [104]. These results indicate enormous potential for the development of effective TNF inhibitors, which should have clearly defined clinical applications, especially in the context of an overwhelming TNF production in the early stages of sepsis and septic shock. The highly effective TNF inhibitors described also appear to inhibit other cytokines and proliferative responses. To date, there are no published data on the toxicity of these compounds, and it is possible that they are considerably more cytotoxic than the parent molecule.

Reduction in translation

Corticosteroids are important anti-inflammatory endogenous mediators produced in response to inflammation, since it is well known that the hypothalamic-pituitary-adrenal axis is influenced by proinflammatory cytokines such as IL-1, IL-6, and TNF. Corticosteroids inhibit TNF formation at the translational level [36] and affect formation of IL-1 and IL-6 by interfering with the stability of specific mRNA [106] and via the glucocorticoid receptor by interference with various transcription factors [107]. There is also some indication that steroids reduce the secretion of IL-1. In human volunteers injected with corticosteroids just prior to an intravenous injection of endotoxin there are reduced levels of circulating IL-1β, TNF, and IL-6 [108, 109]. These reductions in IL-1β, TNF, and IL-6 take place without suppressing IL-1-Ra production [109]. Relevant to these experiments are studies showing that IL-6 and TNF induce endogenous corticosteroids [24], and that adrenalectomized mice have profoundly decreased resistance to IL-1- or TNF-mediated lethality [110]. Therefore, some studies suggest that IL-1- and TNF-induced endogenous corticosteroid production acts as an intrinsic anti-inflammatory negative feed-back mechanism.

However, several controlled clinical trials with high-dose corticosteroids in septic patients have failed to show an improvement in survival. A meta-analysis of these studies indicated no beneficial effects of high-dose corticoids in severe sepsis but gave evidence for an increased rate of opportunistic infections in patients recieving corticosteroids [111]. There is still controversy regarding the use of exogenous corticosteroids in sepsis and septic shock, since recent data suggest an increased need and a relative insufficiency of corticosteroids under septic conditions. Thus, low-dose hydrocortisone infusion may be beneficial [112].

Reduction in processing

It has been suggested that membrane-bound cytokines may be implicated in their paracrine activities in tissues, while systemic activities of cytokines may be associated with the secreted form [113].The release (shedding) of extracellular domains of many cell-surface proteins is mediated proteolytically and therefore can be altered by modification of the cell surface. Several studies suggest that the release of TNFα is mediated by serine proteinases [114]. Serine proteinase inhibitors were shown to suppress the secretion of TNFα without affecting TNFα mRNA levels [115]. Moreover, D-galactosamine-sensitized mice pretreated with serine proteinase inhibitor α-1-antitrypsin were not able to secrete TNFα in response to endotoxin, becoming fully protected against endotoxin-induced hepatitis [116]. Further reports suggest the implication of metalloproteinase in the processing of TNFα [117]. A series of hydroxamate inhibitors of matrix metalloproteinases have been shown to inhibit the release of TNFα without affecting cell-associated activity and to protect mice challenged with lethal doses of endotoxin [117–119]. Recently, peptide-hydroxamate metalloproteinease inhibitors have been reported to block the proteolytic processing (shedding/secretion) of transmembrane domain-containing cytokines and cytokine receptors TNFα, macrophage colony-stimulating factor (M-CSF), TGFα, stem cell factor (SCF), sTNFR-p55, sTNFR-p75, and IL-6 receptor [120]. Hydroxamate metalloproteinease either did not affect or augmented the shedding/secretion of cytokines lacking transmembrane-containing domain precursor (IL-1α, IL-1β, IL-6, IL-10) [120].

Conclusion

The host response to pathogens consists of a complex network that is still poorly understood. Based on the idea that an overproduction of secondary inflammatory mediators secreted into the bloodstream is harmful to the host, tremendous efforts have been made in the past decade to develop new drugs for the treatment of sepsis-related complications. Nonetheless, mortality rates of septic patients have not appreciably improved. Although overwhelming cytokine response may be detrimental, a complete blockade, e.g. by antibodies in peritonitis, also appears not to be beneficial. Thus, modulation of the cytokine response should be the goal. In this respect, in addition to the particular mode of functioning, synthetic drugs might be much cheaper than recombinant materials. For the development of new and more effective therapeutic strategies, however, our current knowledge of the basic pathophysiology of sepsis, the roles of the many inflammatory mediators, and their interaction with each other needs to be improved.

References

1 Pinsky MR, Vincent JL, Deviere J, Alegre M, Kahn RJ, Dupont E (1993) Serum cytokine levels in human septic shock. Relation to multiple-system organ failure and mortality. *Chest* 103: 565–575

2 Dinarello CA, Gelfand JA, Wolff SM (1993) Anticytokine strategies in the treatment of the systemic inflammatory response syndrome. *JAMA* 269: 1829–1835

3 Bone RC, Grodzin CJ, Balk RA (1997) Sepsis: a new hypothesis for pathogenesis of the disease process. *Chest* 112: 235–243

4 Moller DR, Wysocka M, Greenlee BM, Ma X, Wahl L, Trinchieri G, Karp CL (1997) Inhibition of human interleukin-12 production by pentoxifylline. *Immunology* 91: 197–203

5 Tracey KJ (1995) TNF and Mae West or: death from too much of a good thing [see comments]. *Lancet* 345: 75–76

6 Jansen PM, Boermeester MA, Fischer E, de Jong IW, Van der Poll T, Moldawer LL, Hack CE, Lowry SF (1995) Contribution of interleukin-1 to activation of coagulation and fibrinolysis, neutrophil degranulation, and the release of secretory-type phospholipase A2 in sepsis: studies in nonhuman primates after interleukin-1α administration and during lethal bacteremia. *Blood* 86: 1027–1034

7 Smith JW, 2d, Urba WJ, Curti BD, Elwood LJ, Steis RG, Janik JE, Sharfman WH, Miller LL, Fenton RG, Conlon KC et al (1992) The toxic and hematologic effects of interleukin-1α administered in a phase I trial to patients with advanced malignancies. *J Clin Oncol* 10: 1141–1152

8 Parrat JR, Sturgess RM (1975) *E. coli* endotoxin shock in the cat: treatment with indomethacin. *Brit J Pharmacol* 33: 485–488

9 Casey LC, Balk RA, Bone RC (1993) Plasma cytokine and endotoxin levels correlate with survival in patients with the sepsis syndrome [see comments]. *Ann Intern Med* 119: 771–778

10 Van der Poll T, Levi M, Hack CE, Ten Cate H, van Deventer SJ, Eerenberg AJ, de Groot ER, Jansen J, Gallati H, Buller HR et al (1994) Elimination of interleukin 6 attenuates coagulation activation in experimental endotoxemia in chimpanzees. *J Exp Med* 179: 1253–1259

11 Moore KW, O'Garra A, de Waal Malefyt R, Vieira P, Mosmann TR (1993) Interleukin-10. *Annu Rev Immunol* 11: 165–190

12 Chernoff AE, Granowitz EV, Shapiro L, Vannier E, Lonnemann G, Angel JB, Kennedy JS, Rabson AR, Wolff SM, Dinarello CA (1995) A randomized, controlled trial of IL-10 in humans. Inhibition of inflammatory cytokine production and immune responses. *J Immunol* 154: 5492–5499

13 Vannier E, Miller LC, Dinarello CA (1992) Coordinated antiinflammatory effects of interleukin 4: interleukin 4 suppresses interleukin 1 production but up-regulates gene expression and synthesis of interleukin 1 receptor antagonist. *Proc Natl Acad Sci USA* 89: 4076–4080

14   Chantry D, Turner M, Abney E, Feldmann M (1989) Modulation of cytokine production by transforming growth factor-beta. *J Immunol* 142: 4295–4300

15   Strieter RM, Remick DG, Ward PA, Spenger RN, Lynch JP, Larrick J, Kunkel SL (1988) Cellular and molecular regulation of tumor necrosis factor α production by pentoxifylline. *Biochem Biophys Res Commun* 155: 1230–1236

16   Semmler J, Gebert U, Eisenhut T, Moeller J, Schonharting MM, Allera A, Endres S (1993) Xanthine derivatives: comparison between suppression of tumour necrosis factor-alpha production and inhibition of cAMP phosphodiesterase activity. *Immunology* 78: 520–525

17   Giroir BP, Beutler B (1992) Effect of amrinone on tumor necrosis factor production in endotoxic shock. *Circ Shock* 36: 200–207

18   Endres S, Fülle HJ, Sinha B, Stoll D, Dinarello CA, Gerzer R, Weber PC (1991) Cyclic nucleotides differentially regulate the synthesis of tumour necrosis factor α and interleukin-1β by human mononuclear cells. *Immunobiology* 72: 56–60

19   Knudsen PJ, Dinarello CA, Strom TB (1986) Prostaglandins posttranscriptionally inhibit monocyte expression of interleukin 1 activity by increasing intracellular cyclic adenosine monophosphate. *J Immunol* 137: 3189–3193

20   Ghezzi P, Dinarello CA (1988) Interleukin-1 induces interleukin 1. III. Specific inhibition of interleukin-1 production by gamma interferon. *J Immunol* 140: 4238–4242

21   Scordamaglia A, Ciprandi G, Ruffoni S, Caria M, Paolieri F, Venuti D, Canonica GW (1988) Theophylline and the immune response: *in vitro* and *in vivo* effects. *Clin Immunol Immunopathol* 48: 238–245

22   Brandwein SR (1986) Regulation of interleukin-1 production by mouse peritoneal macrophages. Effects of arachidonic acid metabolites, cyclic nucleotides, and interferons. *J Biol Chem* 261: 8624–8630

23   Tannenbaum CS, Hamilton TA (1989) Lipopolysaccharide-induced gene expression in murine peritoneal macrophages is selectively suppressed by agents that elevate intracellular cAMP. *J Immunol* 142: 1274–1280

24   Zabel P, Wolter DT, Schonharting MM, Schade UF (1989) Oxpentifylline in endotoxaemia. *Lancet* 2: 1474–1477

25   Waage A, Sorensen M, Stordal B (1990) Differential effect of oxpentifylline on tumour necrosis factor and interleukin-6 production [letter; comment]. *Lancet* 335: 543

26   Ward A, Clissold SP (1987) Pentoxifylline: A review of its pharmacodynamic and pharmacokinetic properties and its therapeutic efficacy. *Drugs* 34: 50–97

27   Rieneck K, Diamant M, Haahr PM, Schonharting M, Bendtzen K (1993) *In vitro* immunomodulatory effects of pentoxifylline. *Immunol Lett* 37: 131–138

28   Zabel P, Schade UF (1993) Pentoxifylline as an anti-tumor necrosis factor alpha agent. *Immunol Infect Dis* 3: 175–180

29   Funk JO, Ernst M, Schönharting MM, Zabel P (1995) Pentoxifylline exerts synergistic immunomodulatory effects with dexamethasone or cyclosporine. *Int J Immunopharmacol* 17: 1007–1016

30   Thanhauser A, Reiling N, Bohle A, Toellner KM, Duchrow M, Scheel D, Schluter C,

Ernst M, Flad HD, Ulmer AJ (1993) Pentoxifylline: a potent inhibitor of IL-2 and IFNγ biosynthesis and BCG-induced cytotoxicity. *Immunology* 80: 151–156

31 Rott O, Cash E, Fleischer B (1993) Phosphodiesterase inhibitor pentoxifylline, a selective suppressor of T helper type 1- but not type 2-associated lymphokine production, prevents induction of experimental autoimmune encephalomyelitis in Lewis rats. *Eur J Immunol* 23: 1745–1751

32 Hussein A, Meyrick B, Graber S, Berry Lj, Brigham KL (1988) Attenuation of endotoxin-induced cytotoxicity and prostacyclin production in cultured bovine pulmonary artery endothelial cells by phosphodiesterase inhibition. *Exp Lung Res* 14: 637–654

33 Eigler A, Sinha B, Hartmann G, Endres S (1997) Taming TNF: strategies to restrain this proinflammatory cytokine. *Immunol Today* 18: 487–492

34 Schade UF (1989) The role of prostacyclin in the protective effects of pentoxifylline and other xanthine derivatives in endotoxin action in mice. *Eicosanoids* 2: 183–188

35 Rall TW (1982) Evolution of the mechanism of action of methylxanthines: from calcium mobilizers to antagonists of adenosine receptors. *Pharmacologist* 24: 277–282

36 Han J, Thompson P, Beutler B (1990) Dexamethasone and pentoxifylline inhibit endotoxin-induced cachectin/tumor necrosis factor synthesis at separate points in the signaling pathway. *J Exp Med* 172: 391–394

37 Moreira AL, Sampaio EP, Zmuidzinas A, Frindt P, Smith KA, Kaplan G (1993) Thalidomide exerts its inhibitory action on tumor necrosis factor α by enhancing mRNA degradation. *J Exp Med* 177: 1675–1680

38 Schade UF (1990) Pentoxifylline increases survival in murine endotoxin shock and decreases formation of tumor necrosis factor. *Circ Shock* 31: 171–181

39 Hadjiminas DJ, McMasters KM, Robertson SE, Cheadle WG (1994) Enhanced survival from cecal ligation and puncture with pentoxifylline is associated with altered neutrophil trafficking and reduced interleukin-1β expression but not inhibition of tumor necrosis factor synthesis. *Surgery* 116: 348–355

40 Zabel P, Leimenstoll G, Schröder P, Elfeldt R, Schlaak M, Niedermayer W (1991) Pentoxifylline suppresses OKT3-induced tumor necrosis factor α formation in renal transplant recipients. *Z Tx Med* 3: 62–65

41 Dezube BJ, Pardee AB, Chapman B, Beckett LA, Korvick JA, Novick WJ, Chiurco J, Kasdan P, Ahlers CM, Ecto LT et al (1993) Pentoxifylline decreases tumor necrosis factor expression and serum triglycerides in people with AIDS. NIAID AIDS Clinical Trials Group [see comments]. *J Acquir Immune Defic Syndr* 6: 787–794

42 Dezube BJ, Sherman ML, Fridovich Keil JL, Allen Ryan J, Pardee AB (1993) Down-regulation of tumor necrosis factor expression by pentoxifylline in cancer patients: a pilot study. *Cancer Immunol Immunother* 36: 57–60

43 Zabel P, Entzian P, Dalhoff K, Schlaak M (1997) Pentoxifylline in treatment of sarcoidosis. *Am J Respi. Crit Care Med* 155: 1665–1669

44 Zeni F, Pain P, Vindimian M, Gay JP, Gery P, Bertrand M, Page Y, Page D, Vermesch R, Bertrand JC (1996) Effects of pentoxifylline on circulating cytokine concentrations and hemodynamics in patients with septic shock: results from a double-blind, randomized, placebo-controlled study. *Crit Care Med* 24: 207–214

45 Staubach KH, Schröder J, Stüber F, Gehrke K, Traumann E, Zabel P (1998) Effect of pentoxifylline in sepsis – results of a double-blind, randomized, placebo-controlled study. *Arch Surg* 133: 94–100

46 Hoffmann H, Markewitz A, Kreuzer E, Reichert K, Jochum M, Faist E (1998) Pentoxifylline decreases the incidence of multiple organ failure after major cardio-thoracic surgery. *Shock* 9: 235–240

47 Zabel P, Schade FU, Schlaak M (1993) Inhibition of endogenous TNF formation by pentoxifylline. *Immunobiology* 187: 447–463

48 Gebert U, Okyayuz-Baklouti I, Thorwart W (1987) Tertiary hydroxyalkylxantines, procedure for their preparation, drugs containing them, and their use. *Chem Abstr* 106: 213–218

49 Hatherill JR, Yonemaru M, Zheng H, Hoffmann H, Fujishima S, Ishizaka A, Raffin TA (1989) Attenuation of acute lung injury in septic guinea-pigs by a new xanthine derivative (HWA-138). *Pharmatherapeutica* 5: 407–415

50 Hoffmann H, Weiss M, Frank G, Birg A, Schönharting MM, Jochum M (1995) Amelioration of endotoxin-induced acute lung injury in pigs by HWA 138 and A 80 2715: new analogs of pentoxifylline. *Shock* 4: 166–170

51 Bahrami S, Redl H, Buurman WA, Schlag G (1992) Influence of the xanthine derivate HWA138 on endotoxin-related coagulation disturbances: effect in non-sensitized vs D-galactosamine sensitized rats. *Thromb Haemost* 68: 418–423

52 Bengtsson A, Redl H, Schlag G, Mollnes TE, Hogasen K (1996) Effect on complement activation and cytokine (TNFα and IL-8) release of infusion of anti-TNF-antibodies or a xanthine derivate (HWS 138) in septic baboons. *Acta Anaesth Scand* 40: 244–249

53 Bahrami S, Yu Y-H, Redl H, Schlag G (1995) Acute lung injury by endotoxin-.induced mediators: prevention by HWA138, a new xanthine derivative. *J Lab Clin Med* 125: 487–492

54 Boogaerts MA, Meeus P, Scheers W, Declercq M, Vande Broeck J, Verhoef G. (1990) Pentoxifylline and analogues: effects on normal and diseased granulocyte function *in vitro*. In: Hakim J, Mandell GL, Novick WJ (eds): *Proceedings of the Workshop on Pentoxifylline and Analogues: Effects on leucocyte function*. Sait Paul de Vece, France, 9–16

55 Bahrami S, Redl H, Schlag G, Leichtfried G, Ceska M, Strieter RM (1991) Comparison of the efficacy of different xanthine derivates to reduce endotoxin-induced mortality and/or cytokine production: *in vivo* and *in vitro* studies. *Circ Shock* 34: 140

56 Bahrami S, Yao Y-M, Shiga H, Leichtfried G, Redl H, Schlag G (1996) Comparison of the efficacy of pentoxifylline and albifyllin (HWA 138) on endotoxin-induced cytokine production, coagulation disturbances, and mortality. *Shock* 5: 424–428

57 Netea MG, Blok WL, Kullberg B-J, Bemelmans M, Vogels MTE, Buurman WA, van der Meer JWM (1995) Pharmacologic inhibitors of tumor necrosis factor production exert differential effects in lethal endotoxemia and in infection with live microorganisms in mice. *J Infect Dis* 171: 393–399

58 Pahan K, Namboodiri AM, Sheikh FG, Smith BT, Singh I (1997) Increasing cAMP attenuates induction of inducible nitric-oxide synthase in rat primary astrocytes. *J Biol Chem* 272: 7786–7791

59 Szabo C, Hasko G, Zingarelli B, Nemeth ZH, Salzman AL, Kvetan V, Pastores SM, Vizi ES (1997) Isoproterenol regulates tumour necrosis factor, interleukin-10, interleukin-6 and nitric oxide production and protects against the development of vascular hyporeactivitiy in endotoxaemia. *Immunology* 90: 95–100

60 Yoshimura T, Kurita C, Nagao T, Usami E, Nakao T, Watanabe S, Kobayashi J, Yamazaki F, Tanaka H, Inagaki N et al (1997) Inhibition of tumor necrosis factor-alpha and interleukin-1-beta production by β-adrenoceptor agonists from lipopolysaccharide-stimulated human peripheral blood mononuclear cells. *Pharmacology* 54: 144–152

61 Fortenberry JD, Huber AR, Owens ML (1997) Inotropes inhibit endothelial cell surface adhesion molecules induced by interleukin-1β. *Crit Care Med* 25: 303–308

62 Van der Poll T, Calvano SE, Kumar A, Coyle SM, Lowry SF (1997) Epinephrine attenuates down-regulation of monocyte tumor necrosis factor receptors during human endotoxemia. *J Leukoc Biol* 61: 156–160

63 Spinas GA, Bloesch D, Keller U, Zimmerli W, Cammisuli S (1991) Pretreatment with ibuprofen augments circulating tumor necrosis factor-alpha, interleukin-6, and elastase during acute endotoxinemia. *J Infect Dis* 163: 89–95

64 Beyaert R, Cuenda A, Vanden-Berghe W, Plaisance S, Lee JC, Haegeman G, Cohen P, Fiers W (1996) The p38/RK mitogen-activated protein kinase pathway regulates interleukin-6 synthesis response to tumor necrosis factor. *EMBO J* 15: 1914–1923

65 Granowitz EV, Clark BD, Vannier E, Callahan MV, Dinarello CA (1992) Effect of interleukin-1 (IL-1) blockade on cytokine synthesis: I. IL-1 receptor antagonist inhibits IL-1-induced cytokine synthesis and blocks the binding of IL-1 to its type II receptor on human monocytes. *Blood* 79: 2356–2363

66 Dinarello CA. (1996) Cytokines as mediators in the pathogenesis of septic shock. In: Rietschel ET Wagner H (eds): *Pathology in septic shock*. Springer-Verlag, Berlin, Heidelberg, 133–165

67 Jorres A, Dinter H, Topley N, Gahl GM, Frei U, Scholz P (1997) Inhibition of tumour necrosis factor production in endotoxin-stimulated human mononuclear leukocytes by the prostacyclin analogue iloprost: cellular mechanisms. *Cytokine* 9: 119–125

68 Fletcher JR, Ramwell PW (1980) Indomethacin improves survival after endotoxin in baboons. *Adv Prostaglandin Thromboxan Leukot Res* 7: 821–828

69 Haupt MT, Jastremski MS, Clemmer TP, Metz CA, Goris GB (1991) Effect of ibuprofen in patients with severe sepsis: a randomized, double-blind, multicenter study. The Ibuprofen Study Group [see comments]. *Crit Care Med* 19: 1339–1347

70 Bernard GR, Wheeler AP, Russell JA, Schein R, Summer WR, Steinberg KP, Fulkerson WJ, Wright PE, Christman BW, Dupont WD et al (1997) The effects of ibuprofen on the physiology and survival of patients with sepsis. The Ibuprofen in Sepsis Study Group [see comments]. *N Engl J Med* 336: 912–918

71 Schade UF, Burmeister I, Engel R (1987) Increased 13-hydroxyoctadecadienoic acid content in lipopolysaccharide stimulated macrophages. *Biochem Biophys Res Commun* 147: 695–700

72 Sirko SP, Schindler R, Doyle MJ, Weisman SM, Dinarello CA (1991) Transcription,

translation and secretion of interleukin 1 and tumor necrosis factor: effects of tebufelone, a dual cyclooxygenase/5-lipoxygenase inhibitor. Eur. *J Immunol* 21: 243–250

73 Meydani SN, Dinarello CA (1993) Influence of dietary fatty acids on cytokine production and its clinical implications. *Nutr Clin Pract* 8: 65–72

74 Zon G (1995) Antisense phosphorothioate oligodeoxynucleotides: introductory concepts and possible molecular mechanisms of toxicity. *Toxicol Lett* 82–83: 419–424

75 Lefebvre dHellencourt C, Diaw L, Guenounou M (1995) Immunomodulation by cytokine antisense oligonucleotides. *Eur Cytokine Netw* 6: 7–19

76 Webber S, Zheng R, Kamal A, Withnall M, Karlsson JA (1997) IFNγ production from human Th1 cells in controlled by Raf kinase. *Int Arch Allergy Immunol* 113: 275–278

77 Ding M, Zhang M, Wong JL, Voskuhl RR, Ellison GW (1996) Antisense blockade of inducible nitric oxide synthase in glial cells derived from adult SJL mice. *Neurosci Lett* 220: 89–92

78 Marzo AL, Fitzpatrick DR, Robinson BW, Scott B (1997) Antisense oligonucleotides specific for transforming growth factor β2 inhibit the growth of malignant mesothelioma both *in vitro* and *in vivo*. *Cancer Res* 57: 3200–3207

79 Ojwang JO, Mustain SD, Marshall HB, Rao TS, Chaudhary N, Walker DA, Hogan ME, Akiyama T, Revankar GR, Peyman A et al (1997) Modified antisense oligonucleotides directed against tumor necrosis factor receptor type I inhibit tumor necrosis factor α-mediated functions. *Biochemistry* 36: 6033–6045

80 Stein CA, Cheng Y-C (1993) Antisense oligonucleotides as therapeutic agents – is the bullet really magical? *Science* 261: 1004–1012

81 Wagner RW (1994) Gene inhibition using antisense oligodeoxynucleotides. *Nature* 372: 333–335

82 Gibson I (1996) Antisense approaches to the gene therapy of cancer – 'Recnac'. *Cancer Metastasis Rev* 15: 287–299

83 Knee R, Murphy RP (1997) Regulation of gene expression by natural antisense RNA transcripts. *Neurochem Int* 31: 379–392

84 Weiss B, Davidkova G, Zhang SP (1997) Antisense strategies in neurobiology. *Neurochem Int* 31: 321–348

85 Han J, Lee J-D, Bibbs L, Ulevitch RJ (1994) A MAP kinase targeted by endotoxin and hyperosmolarity in mammalian cells. *Science* 265: 808–811

86 Raingeaud J, Whitmarsh AJ, Barrett T, Derijard B, Davis RJ (1996) MKK3- and MKK6-regulated gene expression is mediated by the p38 mitogen-activated protein kinase signal transduction pathway. *Mol Cell Biol* 16: 1247–1255

87 Nick JA, Avdi NJ, Gerwins P, Johnson GL, Worthen GS (1996) Activation of a p38 mitogen-activated protein kinase in human neutrophils by lipopolysaccharide. *J Immunol* 156: 4867–4875

88 Kramer RM, Roberts EF, Strifler BA, Johnstone EM (1995) Thrombin induces activation of p38 MAP kinase in human platelets. *J Biol Chem* 270: 27395–27398

89 Kramer RM, Roberts EF, Hyslop PA, Utterback BG, Hui KY (1995) Differential activa-

tion of cytosolic phospholipase A2 (cPLA2) by thrombin and thrombin receptor agonist peptide in human platelets. Evidence for activation of cPLA2 independent of the mitogen-activated protein kinases ERK1/2. *J Biol Chem* 270: 14816–14823

90 Lee JC, Laydon JT, McDonnell PC, Galagher TF, Kumar S, Green D, McNulty D, Blumenthal MJ, Heys JR, Landvatter SW et al (1994) A protein kinase involved in the regulation of inflammatory cytokine biosynthesis. *Nature* 372: 739–746

91 Pietersma A, Tilly BC, Gaestel M, de Jong N, Lee JC, Koster JF, Sluiter W (1997) p38 mitogen activated protein kinase regulates endothelial VCAM-1 expression at the post-transcriptional level. *Biochem Biophys Res Commun* 230: 44–48

92 Hennies HH, Günzler WA, Flohe L (1984) Influence of supimide on brain neurotransmitter systems of rats and mice. *Arzneimittelforschung* 34: 1471–1480

93 Powell RJ (1996) New roles for thalidomide [editorial]. *BMJ* 313: 377–378

94 Postema PT, den Haan P, van Hagen PM, van Blankenstein M (1996) Treatment of colitis in Behcet's disease with thalidomide. *Eur J Gastroenterol Hepatol* 8: 929–931

95 Gutierrez Rodriguez O, Starusta Bacal P, Gutierrez Montes O (1989) Treatment of refractory rheumatoid arthritis—the thalidomide experience. *J Rheumatol* 16: 158–163

96 Carlesimo M, Giustini S, Rossi A, Bonaccorsi P, Calvieri S (1995) Treatment of cutaneous and pulmonary sarcoidosis with thalidomide. J Am Acad Dermatol 32: 866–869

97 Vogelsang GB, Farmer ER, Hess AD, Altamonte V, Beschorner WE, Jabs DA, Corio RL, Levin LS, Colvin OM, Wingard JR et al (1992) Thalidomide for the treatment of chronic graft-versus-host disease [see comments]. *N Engl J Med* 326: 1055–1058

98 Vogelsang GB, Hess AD, Gordon G, Brundrette R, Santos GW (1987) Thalidomide induction of bone marrow transplantation tolerance. *Transplant Proc* 19: 2658–2661

99 Sampaio EP, Sarno EN, Galilly R, Cohn ZA, Kaplan G (1991) Thalidomide selectively inhibits tumor necrosis factor α production by stimulated human monocytes. *J Exp Med* 173: 699–703

100 McHugh SM, Rowland TL (1997) Thalidomide and derivatives: immunological investigations of tumor necrosis factor alpha (TNF) inhibition suggest drugs capable of selective gene regulation. *Clin Exp Immunol* 110: 151–154

101 Beauparlant P, Hiscott J (1996) Biological and biochemical inhibition of the NF-kappa B/Rel proteins and cytokine synthesis. *Cytokine Growth Factor Rev* 7: 175–190

102 Rao A (1994) NF-ATp: a transcription factor required for the co-ordinate induction of several cytokine genes. *Immunol Today* 15: 274–281

103 Tsai EY, Jain J, Pesavento PA, Rao A, Goldfeld AE (1996) Tumor necrosis factor α gene regulation in activated T cells involves ATF-2/Jun and NFATp. *Mol Cell Biol* 16: 459–467

104 Muller GW, Corral LG, Shire MG, Wang H, Moreira A, Kaplan G, Stirling DI (1996) Structural modifications of thalidomide produce analogs with enhanced tumor necrosis factor inhibitory activity. *J Med Chem* 39: 3238–3240

105 Corral LG, Muller GW, Moreira AL et al (1996) Selection of noval analogs of thalidomide with enhanced tumor necrosis factor α inhibitory activity. *Mol Med* 2: 506–515

106 Amano Y, Lee SW, Allison AC (1993) Inhibition by glucocorticoids of the formation of

interleukin-1α, interleukin-1β, and interleukin-6: mediation by decreased mRNA stability. *Mol Pharmacol* 43: 176–182

107 Beato M (1989) Gene regulation by steroid hormones. *Cell* 56: 335–344

108 Rock CS, Coyle SM, Keogh CV, Lazarus DD, Hawes AS, Leskiw M, Moldawer LL, Stein TP, Lowry SF (1992) Influence of hypercortisolemia on the acute-phase protein response to endotoxin in humans. *Surgery* 112: 467–474

109 Santos AA, Scheltinga MR, Lynch E, Brown EF, Lawton P, Chambers E, Browning J, Dinarello CA, Wolff SM, Wilmore DW (1993) Elaboration of interleukin 1-receptor antagonist is not attenuated by glucocorticoids after endotoxemia. *Arch Surg* 128: 138–143

110 Fantuzzi G, Ghezzi P (1993) Glucocorticoids as cytokine inhibitors: role in neuroendocrine therapy of inflammatory diseases. Mediator Inflamm 2: 263–270

111 Lefering R, Neugebauer EA (1995) Steroid controversy in sepsis and septic shock: a meta-analysis [see comments]. *Crit Care Med* 23: 1294–1303

112 Briegel J, Kellermann W, Forst H, Haller M, Bittl M, Hoffmann GE, Buchler M, Uhl W, Peter K (1994) Low-dose hydrocortisone infusion attenuates the systemic inflammatory response syndrome. The Phospholipase A2 Study Group. *Clin Investig* 72: 782–787

113 Kriegler M, Perez C, DeFay K, Albert I, Lu SD (1988) A novel form of TNF/cachectin is a cell surface cytotoxic transmembrane protein: ramifications for the complex physiology of TNF. *Cell* 53: 45–53

114 Robache-Gallea S, Morand V, Bruneau JM, Schoot B, Tagat E, Realo E, Chouaib S, Roman-Roman S (1995) *In vitro* processing of human tumor necrosis factor α. *J Biol Chem* 270: 23688–23692

115 Scuderi P (1989) Suppression of human leukocyte tumor necrosis factor secretion by the serine protease inhibitor p-toluenesulfonyl-L-arginine methyl ester (TAME). *J Immunol* 143: 168–173

116 Niehorster M, Tiegs G, Schade UF, Wendel A (1990) *In vivo* evidence for protease-catalysed mechanism providing bioactive tumor necrosis factor alpha. *Biochem Pharmacol* 40: 1601–1603

117 Mohler KM, Sleath PR, Fitzner JN, Cerretti DP, Alderson M, Kerwar SS, Torrance DS, Otten-Evans C, Greenstreet T, Weerawarna K et al (1994) Protection against a lethal dose of endotoxin by an inhibitor of tumor necrosis factor processing. *Nature* 370: 218–220

118 McGeehan GM, Becherer JD, Bast RC, Boyer CM, Champion B, Connolly KM, Conway JG, Furdon P, Karp S, Kidao S et al (1994) Regulation of tumour necrosis factor α processing by a metalloproteinase inhibitor. *Nature* 370: 558–561

119 Gearing AJH, Beckett P, Christodoulou M, Churchill M, Clements J, Davidson AH, Drummond AH, Galloway WA, Gilbert R, Gordon JL et al (1994) Processing of tumour necrosis factor α precursor by metalloproteinases. *Nature* 370: 555–557

120 Gallea-Robache S, Morand V, Millet S, Bruneau JM, Bhatnagar N, Chouaib S, Roman-Roman S (1997) A metalloproteinase inhibitor blocks the shedding of soluble cytokine receptors and processing of transmembrane cytokine precursors in human monocyte cells. *Cytokine* 9: 340–346

Neutralizing antibodies and receptor constructs

Edward Abraham

Division of Pulmonary Sciences and Critical Care Medicine, Box C272, University of Colorado Health Sciences Center, 4200 E. Ninth Avenue, Denver, CO 80262, USA

Proinflammatory cytokines, including interleukin 1 (IL-1) and tumor necrosis factor (TNF), appear to play an important role in contributing to organ system dysfunction and mortality in septic patients [1]. Clinical trials investigating the endogenously produced anti-IL-1 agent, interleukin 1 receptor antagonist (IL-1ra), yielded disappointing results [2]. Several large studies have examined anti-TNF therapies in patients with sepsis, and the results of these studies, although generally negative, still suggest that there may be benefit from anti-TNF therapies in sharply defined groups of critically ill patients with overwhelming infections [3].

The two major approaches taken to neutralizing TNF have involved either monoclonal anti-TNF antibodies or fusion protein constructs in which the extramembrane portion of the p55 (Type I) or p75 (Type II) TNF receptor is joined to the Fc fragment of a human IgG1 antibody (Fig. 1). There are several differences in TNF binding kinetics and efficiency between these two methodologies which may be significant in the clinical utility of each approach.

The monoclonal anti-TNF antibodies used in clinical trials have either been entirely murine in origin or humanized. As would be expected, almost all patients receiving the murine monoclonal antibodies develop HAMAs (human anti-mouse antibodies) [4]. The level of antibody response in patients given humanized anti-TNF antibodies or TNF receptor fusion protein complexes is minimal, allowing repeated administration for chronic diseases, such as rheumatoid arthritis. However, in the setting of severe sepsis or septic shock, where a single dose of the anti-TNF antibodies is given, the incidence of clinically significant serum sickness in patients who received murine monoclonal antibodies is less than 1% and the clinical significance of HAMA development appears to be minimal [4].

The binding affinity of TNF receptor fusion proteins for TNFα appears to be more than 50 times greater than that of monoclonal anti-TNF antibodies, allowing significantly lower doses to be administered [5, 6, 7]. Additionally, a single TNF receptor fusion protein molecule can bind to two TNFα components of the circulating TNFα trimer, effectively preventing TNF receptor clustering on the cell surface, and thereby diminishing TNF receptor induced intracellular signaling. In con-

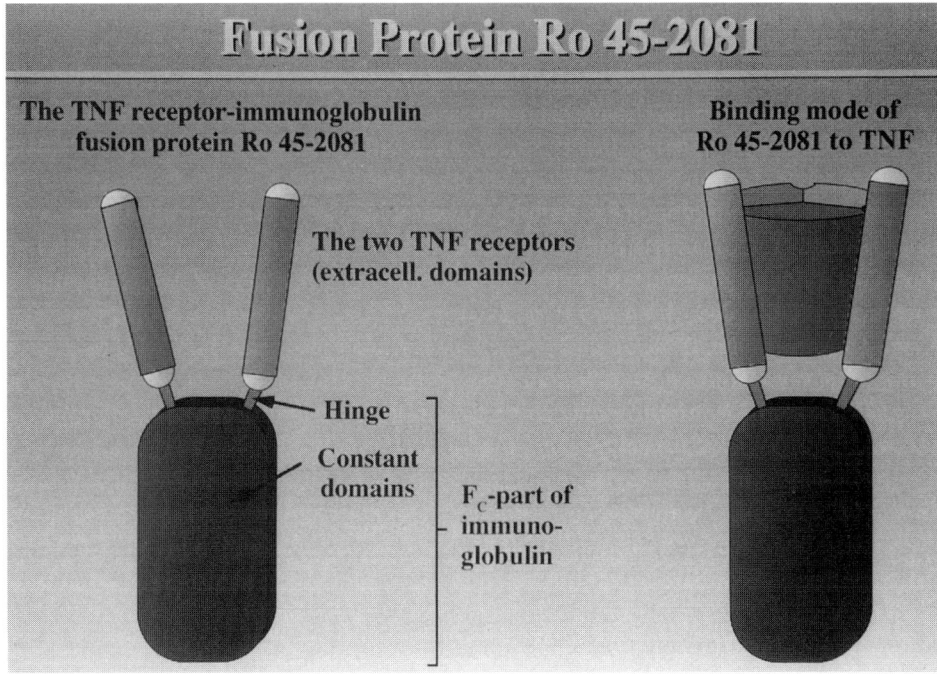

Figure 1
Structure of the p55 (type I) tumor necrosis factor receptor (TNFR)-IgG1 immunoglobulin Fc
fusion protein (Ro 45-2081). The extramembrane sequence of two p55 receptors are joined
to the Fc sequence of an IgG1 immunoglobulin molecule. The p75 (type II) tumor necrosis
factor receptor fusion protein is similar except that the extramembrane portion of the p75
TNFR is substituted for the fragment of the p55 TNFR. The resulting fusion protein is able to
bind to two of the three components of the circulating TNF trimer, thereby preventing TNF
receptor clustering on the cell surface and resultant intracellular signaling.

trast, several anti-TNF antibodies must bind to the circulating TNF trimer in order to prevent interactions between two or more TNF receptors on the cell surface. TNF receptor fusion proteins bind both TNFα and TNFβ whereas the monoclonal anti-TNF antibodies only bind TNFα. Although there is some evidence in animal models that TNFβ may contribute to physiological instability in sepsis [8], the role of TNFβ in humans with severe infections remains undetermined at present, and the potential utility of blocking TNFβ induced toxicity in septic patients is unknown.

Anti-TNF antibodies

Pretreatment of endotoxemic or bacteremic animals with anti-TNFα antibodies results in a clear improvement in survival and amelioration of organ system dysfunction [9, 10]. In some models of Gram-negative or Gram-positive bacteremia, administration of anti-TNFα antibodies at the time of initiation of the bacteremic insult or even shortly thereafter (i.e. within the first hour) is still associated with a significant survival benefit [11, 12]. However, the use of such antibodies at later timepoints in endotoxemia or bacteremia models does not appear to be associated with any clear benefits.

Because of the substantial differences between preclinical models, where large doses of endotoxin or bacteria are used in otherwise normal animals, and the clinical setting, where infection most commonly develops slowly in patients with underlying medical problems, it has been difficult to extrapolate the beneficial results using anti-TNFα antibodies in endotoxemia or bacteremia models to critically ill patients with life-threatening infections. Although there are still several ongoing trials examining anti-TNFα antibodies, the results with almost 5000 patients already included in such studies suggest that the benefit of such therapies, if it exists at all, will be limited to relatively small subgroups of patients.

Although several small studies [13, 14] suggested that anti-TNFα antibody therapy could improve physiological parameters, such as cardiac output in septic patients, the initial study which indicated that such therapy could improve survival was the NORASEPT I trial, which examined a murine IgG1 monoclonal antibody in the treatment of severe sepsis and septic shock [4]. Entry criteria for this study in patients with the clinical diagnosis of infection included the presence of at least one organ system dysfunction (i.e. decreased urine output, hypoxemia, lactic/metabolic acidosis, altered mental status, or disseminated intravascular coagulation (DIC)) for less than 12 h prior to enrollment. Separate randomization lists were used for patients with or without shock at the time of study entry. A total of 994 patients were entered in NORASEPT I, of which approximately half were in shock at the time of randomization. Overall, there was no statistically significant benefit associated with anti-TNF therapy. However, in the prospectively defined subgroup of patients with septic shock, a statistically significant reduction in mortality was present during the first two weeks following therapy with either 7.5 mg/kg or 15 mg/kg monoclonal anti-TNFα antibody compared to placebo. At day 28 after anti-TNFα therapy, the reduction in mortality among septic shock patients was 17% compared to those receiving placebo. In contrast, no benefit was found with anti-TNF- therapy in patients who were not in shock at study entry.

In the NORASEPT I shock patients, the beneficial effect of anti-TNFα antibodies on survival appeared within the first 24 h after enrollment, with the greatest separation between the survival curves for placebo and anti-TNF antibody treated patients occurring within this time window. Approximately 60% of the placebo

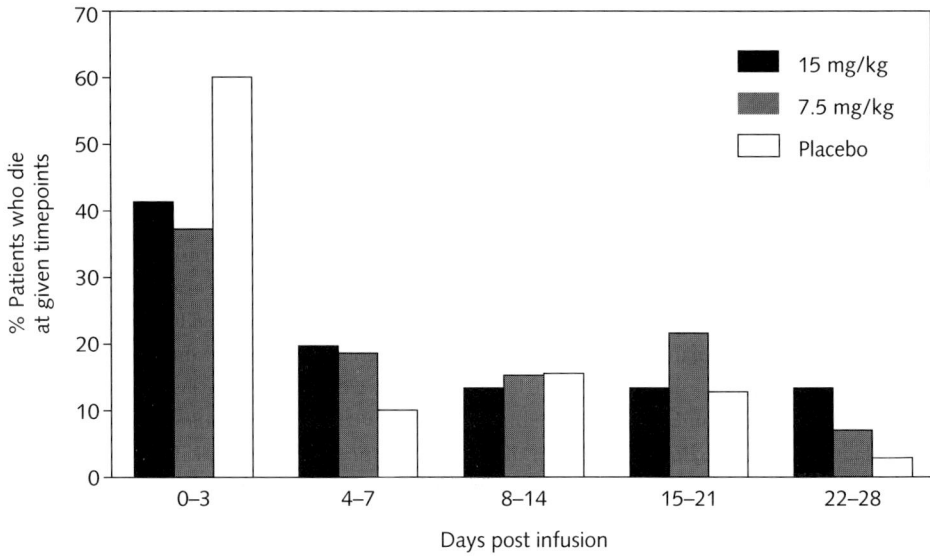

Figure 2
Percentage of septic shock patients treated with monoclonal anti-tumor necrosis factor-α antibodies compared to placebo who died during the indicated postinfusion time points in the NORASEPT I trial [4]. Note that almost 60% of the total number of deaths in placebo-treated patients occurred within the first three days after study enrollment.

deaths occurred within the first three days of the study (Fig. 2). Treatment with 7.5 mg/kg monoclonal anti-TNFα antibodies was associated with a 49% reduction in mortality versus placebo at day three after study enrollment.

A second study (INTERSEPT) with the same murine monoclonal anti-TNFα antibody used in the NORASEPT I study was undertaken in 14 countries, primarily in Europe [15]. Although the INTERSEPT study initially enrolled septic patients with and without shock, after the results of NORASEPT I were available, only shock patients were entered into INTERSEPT. A total of 564 patients, of which 420 were in septic shock, were enrolled in the INTERSEPT study. Day 28 mortality was reduced by 14.5% in patients who received 3 mg/kg monoclonal anti-TNFα antibody, with no reduction in mortality found in the patients given 15 mg/kg. There was no evidence in the INTERSEPT trial of early survival benefit (i.e. within the first three days after anti-TNF antibody infusion) similar to what had been seen in NORASEPT I. Additionally, whereas 60% of the placebo deaths among patients in shock occurred within the first three study days in the NORASEPT I trial, less than 45% of placebo deaths occurred within this period in the INTERSEPT study.

A recently completed study (NORASEPT II) enrolled 1900 patients with septic shock and examined the potential utility of 7.5 mg/kg of the murine monoclonal anti-TNFα antibody [16]. No improvement in survival was found in septic shock patients treated with the monoclonal anti-TNFα antibody compared to those who received placebo. All-cause mortality at day 28 was 40.3% in monoclonal anti-TNFα antibody treated patients compared to 42.8% in placebo-treated patients. Even though the APACHE II scores, day 28 mortality rates, sex ratio, and percentage of patients with one or more organ failures present at baseline were similar in NORASEPT I and NORASEPT II, there did appear to be substantial differences in patient survival patterns. Whereas more than 60% of the deaths in the placebo arm of NORASEPT I occurred in the first three days after study entry, the mean time to death in the placebo group of NORASEPT II was more delayed, averaging 6.8 days. These differences in survival may reflect improvement between the two studies in the supportive care provided to patients with septic shock resulting in better survival from the initial hypotensive episode and associated immediate complications, a period where proinflammatory cytokine release, including that for TNFα, may be greatest. If advances in management have permitted critically ill septic patients to better survive the initial state of accelerated cytokine expression, then this would diminish the efficacy of therapies, such as anti-TNFα antibodies, aimed at modulating the early proinflammatory response.

An additional concern in interpreting the NORASEPT II data revolves around the efficacy of the anti-TNF antibody used in inhibiting TNFα. Even though only a minority of patients had detectable circulating TNFα at baseline and post-treatment time points, therapy with the monoclonal anti-TNF antibody used in this study did not completely eliminate the presence of plasma TNFα levels. Therefore, there remains a question as to the ability of the anti-TNF antibody in the doses used in NORASEPT I, INTERSEPT, and NORASEPT II to actually block TNF activity.

The utility of the F(ab')$_2$ fragments of a murine IgG3 monoclonal antibody to TNFα has been examined in patients with severe sepsis or septic shock [17]. There were 122 patients entered in the clinical trial, and no increase in survival from sepsis for the patients receiving anti-TNF treatment was present in the overall study population. However, a retrospective stratification of patients by interleukin-6 (IL-6) concentration suggested beneficial effects for the drug in patients (n = 37) with baseline circulating IL-6 concentrations greater than 1000 pg/ml, with mortality decreasing from 80% in the placebo group to 35% in patients who received the highest dose (1 mg/kg) of the anti-TNFα therapy. However, a larger subsequent study was unable to substantiate the hypothesis that a beneficial response to anti-TNFα therapy could be predicted by IL-6 levels at the time of enrollment. There is, however, another ongoing study in Canada and the U.S. which is examining the predictive value of IL-6 levels in defining patients who may respond to anti-TNF therapy.

Soluble TNF receptor fusion protein complexes

In preclinical studies, soluble TNF receptor fusion protein complexes using either the human p55 or the p75 TNF receptor joined with the Fc portion of a human IgG1 molecule were effective in improving survival when administered before endotoxin infusion [6, 18]. In at least one model of Gram-negative bacteremia with *E. coli*, however, minimal improvement in survival was found when the p75 TNF receptor fusion protein was used whereas the p55 receptor fusion protein reduced mortality [18]. In human volunteers given endotoxin, administration of p75 TNF receptor fusion protein blocked plasma TNF bioactivity and decreased circulating levels of IL-1β, IL-8, IL-1 receptor antagonist (IL-1ra), and granulocyte-colony stimulating factor (G-CSF) [19]. However, increases in cardiac index, heart rate, and decreases in systemic vascular resistance index were not affected by p75 TNF receptor fusion protein. Interestingly, a high dose of p75 TNF receptor fusion protein (60 mg/m^2) was less effective than a lower dose (10 mg/m^2) in decreasing circulating levels of cytokines, epinephrine, or cortisol.

Two clinical studies have reported results using soluble TNF receptor constructs as anti-TNF agents. In the first of these studies, the molecule used consisted of the extramembrane components of the human type II (p75) receptor joined to the Fc portion of a human IgG1 antibody molecule [20]. Patients (n = 141) with septic shock, with or without associated organ system dysfunction, were entered into the study. A statistically significant (p = 0.014) dose dependent increase in mortality was found in patients treated with this p75 soluble TNF receptor construct, with mortality rising from 30% in the placebo group to 53% in the patients treated with the highest dose (1.5 mg/kg) of the anti-TNF compound.

A 498 patient study examined the role of a p55 TNF receptor fusion protein construct in which separate randomization lists were used for patients with severe sepsis with or without early shock and also for those with refractory septic shock [21]. The doses of the p55 TNF receptor complex used in this study (0.008 mg/kg, 0.042 mg/kg, and 0.08 mg/kg) were substantially lower than those administered in the p75 TNF receptor complex clinical trial. In this study, refractory septic shock was defined as hypotension that was unresponsive to fluid for at least two hours prior to enrollment associated with at least one organ dysfunction (i.e. hypoxemia, metabolic acidosis, decreased urine output, or DIC). The severe sepsis group consisted of patients having at least two organ dysfunctions, with or without fluid unresponsive hypotension for less than two hours prior to enrollment. The drug under study had to be administered within four hours of patient enrollment, meaning that the maximal duration of fluid unresponsive hypotension in severe sepsis patients was six hours.

Therapy with 0.08 mg/kg of the p55 TNF receptor fusion protein complex, but not other doses, was associated with a 36% reduction (p = 0.07) in day 28 mortality in the prospectively defined patient group with severe sepsis with or without early septic shock. In contrast, no apparent beneficial effects were seen with any dose of the p55 receptor complex in patients with refractory septic shock.

There are several possible explanations for the marked differences in the outcomes of septic patients treated with the p55 or p75 TNF receptor fusion protein constructs. Clearly, the most important reason for the improvement in outcome with the p55 TNF receptor complex may be the relatively more restrictive entry criteria for the study investigating this molecule. In particular, hypotensive patients also had to have evidence of sepsis-induced organ system dysfunction, whereas only hypotension was required in the study examining the p75 TNF receptor fusion protein complex. Additionally, hypotension could not be present for more than six hours in the p55 TNF receptor fusion protein study, while patients could still be enrolled in the p75 TNF receptor protein study with periods of hypotension as long as 24 hours.

The enhanced mortality associated with treatment with the p75 TNF receptor molecule may be related to the extremely high doses used in the study. Although potency estimates are difficult to quantitate, soluble TNF receptor fusion proteins appear to inactivate TNFα more than fifty times as well as the monoclonal antibodies [7], so that therapy with a dose of 1.5 mg/kg of the p75 TNF receptor fusion protein would be expected to completely neutralize TNFα for a prolonged period, especially given the long half life of the compound (> 60 hours). TNFα is an essential component of normal inflammatory responses, and prolonged neutralization of its activity may have potent immunosuppressive effects leading to increased mortality.

An additional possible reason for the seemingly opposite effects of the p75 and the p55 TNF receptor fusion proteins in septic patients relates to the differing kinetic affinities of the two molecules. Although both molecules rapidly bind TNFα, TNFα is released much more quickly from the p75 receptor complex than from the p55 fusion protein [18]. These differences in kinetic affinity may have *in vivo* significance. In a series of experiments in mice given intravenous infusions of *E. coli*, therapy with the p75 TNF receptor complex decreased the magnitude of the initial rise in circulating TNFα which occurred in untreated mice after the administration of *E. coli* [18]. However, whereas TNFα rapidly disappeared from the circulation in untreated mice, administration of the p75 TNF receptor complex was associated with prolonged increases in circulating levels of TNFα. In contrast, in bacteremic mice treated with the p55 TNF receptor complex molecule, no TNFα was present in the circulation at any time after the *E. coli* infusion.

Approximately 5000 patients have been included in studies investigating anti-TNF therapies. Four of the Phase II studies, compromising over 2000 patients, showed survival benefits in patients treated with the anti-TNF agent. However, subsequent Phase III studies have been unable to confirm such a benefit. Taken together, the results from the anti-TNF clinical trials do not provide strong support for this therapeutic approach in broad groups of critically ill patients with sepsis. However, there remains reason to believe that some critically ill patient populations may benefit from anti-TNF therapies. In particular, the results with the Phase II study investigating the p55 TNF receptor complex molecule suggest that patients with severe sepsis causing the failure of at least two organ systems, with or without the presence of shock of less than six hours duration, may benefit from such therapy. This hypothesis is presently being investigated in a 1340 patient Phase III study.

References

1   Abraham E (1997) Emerging therapies for sepsis and septic shock. *West J Med* 166: 195–200

2   Opal SM, Fisher CJ, Pribble JP, Dhainaut J-F, Vincent J-L, Brase R, Lowry SF, Sadoff JC, Slotman GJ, Levy H et al (1997) The confirmatory interleukin-1 receptor antagonist trial in severe sepsis: a phase III randomized, double-blind, placebo-controlled, multicenter trial. *Crit Care Med* 25: 1115–1124

3   Grau GE, Maennel DN (1997) TNF inhibition and sepsis – sounding a cautionary note. *Nature Med* 3: 1193–1195

4   Abraham E, Wunderink R, Silverman H, Perl T, Nasraway S, Levy H, Bone R, Wenzel R, Balk R, Allred R, Pennington J, Wherry J (1995) Monoclonal antibody to human tumor necrosis factor alpha (TNF MAb): Efficacy and safety in patients with the sepsis syndrome. *JAMA* 273: 934–941

5   Ashkenazi A, Marsters SA, Capon DJ, Chamow SM, Figari IS, Pennica D, Goeddel DV, Palladino MA, Smith DH (1991) Protection against endotoxic shock by a tumor necrosis factor receptor immunoadhesin. *Proc Natl Acad Sci USA* 88: 10535–10539

6   Van Zee KJ, Moldawer LL, Oldenburg HAS, Thompson WZ, Stackpole SA, Montegut WJ, Rogy MA, Meschter C, Gallati H, Schiller CD et al (1996) Protection against lethal *Escherichia coli* bacteremia in baboons (Papio anubis) by pretreatment with a 55-kDa TNF receptor (CD120a)-Ig fusion protein, Ro 45-2081. *J Immunol* 156: 2221–2230

7   Haak-Frendscho M, Marsters SA, Mordenti J, Brady S, Gillett NA, Chen SA, Ashkenazi A (1994) Inhibition of TNF by a TNF receptor immunoadhesin. *J Immunol* 152: 1347–1353

8   Sriskandan S, Moyes D, Lemm G, Cohen J (1996) Lymphotoxin-α (TNF-α) during sepsis. *Cytokine* 8: 933–937

9   Tracey KJ, Fong Y, Hesse DG, Manogue KR, Lee AT, Kuo GC et al (1987) Anticachectin/TNF monoclonal antibodies prevent septic shock during lethal bacteremia. *Nature* 330: 662–664.

10 Fong Y, Tracey KJ, Moldawer LL et al (1989) Antibodies to cachectin/TNF reduce interleukin-1 and interleukin-6 appearance during lethal bacteremia. *J Exp Med* 170: 1627–1633.

11 Hinshaw LB, Tekamp-Olson P, Chang AC et al (1990) Survival of primates in LD 100 septic shock following therapy with antibody to tumor necrosis factor (TNF). *Circ Shock* 30: 279–292.

12 Hinshaw LB, Emerson TE Jr., Taylor FB Jr., Chang ACK, Duerr M, Peer GT, Flournoy DJ, White GL, Kosanake SD, Murray CK, Xu R, Passey RB, Fournel MA (1992) Lethal *S. aureus* shock in primates: prevention of death with anti-TNF antibody. *J Trauma* 33: 568–573.

13 Fisher CJ, Opal SM, Dhainaut J-F, Stephens S, Zimmerman JL, Nightingale P, Harris SJ, Schein RMH, Panacek EA, Vincent J-L et al (1993) Influence of an anti-tumor necrosis factor monoclonal antibody on cytokine levels in patients with sepsis. *Crit Care Med* 21: 318–327

14 Dhainaut J-F A, Vincent J-L, Richard C, Lejeune P, Martin C, Fierobe L, Stephens S, Ney UM, Sopwith M (1995) CDP571, a humanized antibody to human tumor necrosis factor-α: Safety, pharmacokinetics, immune response, and influence of the antibody on cytokine concentrations in patients with septic shock Crit Care Med 23: 1461–1469

15 Cohen J, Carlet J, for the INTERSEPT Study Group (1996) INTERSEPT: An international, multicenter, placebo-controlled trial of monoclonal antibody to human tumor necrosis factor-α in patients with sepsis. *Crit Care Med* 24: 1431–1440

16 Abraham E, and the NORASEPT II Study Group (1997) Effect of murine monoclonal antibodies to human tumor necrosis factor (BAY x 1351) in patients with septic shock. *Chest* 112: 47S

17 Reinhart K, Wiegand-Lohnert C, Grimminger F, Kaul M, Withington S, Treacher D, Eckart J, Willatts S, Bouza C, Krausch D et al (1996) Assessment of the safety and efficacy of the monoclonal anti-tumor necrosis factor antibody-fragment, MAK 195F, in patients with sepsis and septic shock: A multicenter, randomized, placebo-controlled, dose-ranging study. *Crit Care Med* 24: 733–742

18 Evans TJ, Moyes D, Carpenter A, Martin R, Loetscher H, Lesslauer W, Cohen J (1994) Protective effect of 55- but not 75-kD soluble tumor necrosis factor receptor-immunoglobulin G fusion proteins in an animal model of gram-negative sepsis. *J Exp Med* 180: 2173–2179

19 Suffredini AF, Reda D, Banks SM, Tropea M, Agosti JM, Miller R (1995) Effects of recombinant dimeric TNF receptor on human inflammatory responses following intravenous endotoxin administration. *J Immunol* 155: 5038–5045

20   Fisher CJ, Agosti JM, Opal SM, Lowry SF, Balk RA, Sadoff JC, Abraham E, Schein RMH, Benjamin E, and the Soluble TNF Receptor Sepsis Study Group (1996) Treatment of patients with septic shock with tumor necrosis factor receptor Fc fusion protein. *N Engl J Med* 334: 1697–1702

21 Abraham E, Glauser MP, Butler T, Lew D, Gelmont D, Laterre PF, Kudsk K, Bruining HA, Otto C, Tobin E, Zwingelstein C, Lesslauer W, Leighton A (1997) p55 tumor necrosis factor receptor fusion protein in the treatment of patients with severe sepsis and septic shock: A placebo controlled, randomized, double-blind, multi-center clinical trial. *JAMA* 277: 1531–1538

Immunomodulation following shock and sepsis

René Zellweger[1,2]*, Alfred Ayala[1,2], Ping Wang[1,2] and Irshad H. Chaudry[1,2,3]

[1]Center for Surgical Research and [2]Departments of Surgery, [3]Molecular Pharmacology, Physiology and Biotechnology, Brown University School of Medicine and Rhode Island Hospital, Middle House II, 593 Eddy Street, Providence, RI 02903, USA; *Present address: Department of Trauma Surgery, University of Zurich, 8091 Zurich, Switzerland

General introduction

Despite the introduction of broad-spectrum antibiotics, sepsis is one of the most important causes of multiple organ failure (MOF) which accounts for 70,000 deaths in the USA each year [1]. Infection is also an important cause of mortality in the severely traumatized patient and is responsible for 50–70% of all burn-related deaths [2–3].

The immune system produces cytokines and other humoral factors to protect the host when threatened by inflammatory agents, microbial invasion, or injury. In some cases this complex defense network successfully restores normal homeostasis, but in other instances the overproduction of immunoregulatory mediators may actually prove deleterious to the host. All biological processes require a balance of activity that can be hazardous to the host in excess and alternatively imperil the patient/animal to opportunistic infectious agents if decreased or eliminated. This process of appropriate balance is essential whether it is with respect to blood pressure, heart rate, respiration, gut function, tumor necrosis factor (TNF), interleukin-1 (IL-1), nitric oxide (NO), prostacyclin, and thromboxane, or the endothelial-leukocyte adhesion molecules (ELAMs) and their mRNA's [4–7]. There is no doubt about the ability of various mediators of inflammation to produce toxic or deleterious effects when administered in human volunteers or animals. Despite the rapid development of antibiotics and vasopressor medications, septic shock remains a major cause of mortality in intensive care units [8]. In this regard, studies suggest that the majority of the deleterious effects of septic shock are due to the stimulation of the host's own immune response by bacterial toxins [8].

The exciting research being carried out on receptors, mediators, inhibitors and stimulators, blocking agents, and antibodies, has led to speculation about breakthroughs and magic bullets for various human diseases. Many new and established pharmaceutical companies have helped develop many agents which could have great impact on human diseases. Animal trials so far have been impressive.

A large number of agents have been used to improve cell and organ function following thermal injury, blunt and penetrating trauma, hemorrhagic shock, peritonitis, severe sepsis and septic shock. These agents include ATP-MgCl$_2$, non-anti-coagulant heparin, pentoxyfylline, interferon-γ, chloroquine, platelet activating factor (PAF) antagonists, calcium channel blockers, cyclooxygenasee inhibitors, phospholipase A$_2$ inhibitors, antibodies to cytokines, growth hormone and insulin-like growth factor 1, erythropoeitin, nutritional immunomodulation, NO inhibitors, sex hormones and/or antagonists. This chapter will not attempt to describe all the immunomodulators which have been used following various adverse circulatory conditions, but rather the focus will be limited to describing some of the effects of the recently used immunomodulators following hemorrhagic shock, sepsis, and septic shock and their potential mechanism of action under those conditions.

Adenosine triphosphate-magnesium chloride (ATP-MgCl$_2$)

It is known that decreased high-energy phosphates contribute to organ dysfunction following shock and studies by Chaudry et al. [9–10] have shown that ATP-MgCl2 treatment after hemorrhagic shock improves tissue ATP levels and organ function. Hirasawa et al. [11] have given ATP-MgCl$_2$ to anuric MOF patients with some beneficial effects. It is important to note that this agent can be used safely in trauma patients, but should be given after fluid resuscitation since it reduces afterload [12]. Recently, Meldrum et al. [13] showed that prolonged sepsis in the mouse, produced by cecal ligation and puncture (CLP), caused a significant decrease in lymphocyte ATP levels which were correlated with decreased proliferative capacity in response to mitogenic stimulation. Treatment with ATP-MgCl$_2$ at the onset of sepsis significantly increased lymphocyte ATP levels and proliferative response. Improved lymphocyte function correlated with a significant increase in overall survival at day three (20% CLP vs. 70% CLP/ATP-MgCl$_2$; P < 0.05). The authors concluded that decreased lymphcyte ATP levels may be the cause of defective lypmhocyte proliferative capacity in late sepsis, since adjuvant treatment with ATP-MgCl$_2$ improved both lymphocyte ATP levels and lymphocyte proliferative capacity [13]. Moreover, intraperitoneal ATP-MgCl$_2$ administration decreased lethality from sepsis [13].

Although studies have demonstrated that ATP-MgCl$_2$ produces beneficial effects following various adverse circulatory conditions [14], until recently little was known as to whether this agent had any salutary effect on the depressed vascular endothelial cell function (i.e. the decreased release of endothelium-derived NO) during sepsis. To study this, Wang et al. [15] administered ATP-MgCl$_2$ (50 µmol/kg body wt) or an equivalent volume of normal saline over 90 min intravenously at 1 h after CLP in male Sprague Dawley rats. At 5 and 10 h after CLP (i.e. hyperdynamic stages of polymicrobial sepsis [16]), the thoracic aorta was isolated for measurement of vascular relaxation. Administration of ATP-MgCl$_2$ at 1 h after the onset of sepsis maintained acetylcholine-induced vascular relaxation at both time points of hyperdynamic sepsis without altering endothelium-independent vascular relaxation [15]. Whether the salutary effect of ATP-MgCl$_2$ on endothelial cell function extends into the late stage of sepsis or whether delayed administration of ATP-MgCl$_2$ after the onset of sepsis also produces salutary effects on endothelial cell function remains to be determined.

Nonanticoagulant heparin

From previous studies [17, 18] we know that a novel non-anticoagulant heparin (i.e. GM 1892) produces various beneficial effects such as improved splenocyte and peritoneal macrophage immune functions as well as cardiovascular and hepatocellular function after hemorrhage and resuscitation. Furthermore, GM 1892 decreased susceptibility to sepsis [17] and a recent study by Morrison et al. [19] indicated that the novel non-anticoagulant heparin prevented vascular endothelial cell dysfunction during hyperdynamic sepsis in rats.

Calcium channel blockers

A number of investigators [20–22] have shown that calcium channel blockers have beneficial effects on cell and organ function after ischemia or endotoxic shock. The beneficial effects of calcium channel blockers has been postulated to be due to inhibition of the massive influx of extracellular calcium into cells after injury or shock [20–22].

Meldrum et al. [23] examined the effects of diltiazem administration at a dose of 400 or 800 µg/kg body weight following hemorrhage. Their results indicated that hemorrhaged-induced depression in lymphocyte IL-2, IL-3, IL-6, as well as interferon-γ productive capacity was restored by diltiazem treatment [23]. In additional studies, animals were subjected to sepsis three days following hemorrhage and resuscitation. The results demonstrated that diltiazem also improved the survival of animals following hemorrhage and subsequent sepsis to rates comparable to those seen in non-hemorrhage control animals subjected to sepsis [23]. These data suggest that there is an association between low-dose diltiazem treatment, restoration of lymphokine synthesis, macrophage antigen presentation function and decreased susceptibility to sepsis following hemorrhage. Thus, the adjuvant use of diltiazem, or potentially other calcium channel blockers might offer a new therapeutic modality in the treatment of immunosuppression and for decreasing susceptibility to sepsis following low-flow conditions.

Chloroquine

Chloroquine is used not only as an antimalarial agent [24], but also for the treatment of rheumatoid arthritis [25]. It has been suggested that chloroquine exerts its therapeutic effect in the treatment of arthritis by inhibiting the inflammatory events underlying this disease process [25]. *In vitro* studies have shown that chloroquine inhibits tritiated thymidine incorporation into lymphocytes in a dose-dependant manner by interfering with the accessory functions of monocytes. Moreover, studies by Authi and Tragnor [26] showed that chloroquine inhibited phospolipase A_2 activity leading to decreased production of prostanoids. *In vitro* studies of Ertel et al. [27] showed that chloroquine selectively inhibits TNF and IL-6 release by peritoneal macrophages. Furthermore, chloroquine treatment also decreased the mortality of septic mice after hemorrhage to levels comparable to those of sham-operated mice [28]. Studies by Zhu et al. [29] indicated that chloroquine downregulated LPS-induced TNFα gene expression. Based on these results, it can be suggested that chloroquine's ability to reduce the release of TNF from macrophages is due, at least in part, to the disruption of TNF gene transcription. Thus, because of its unique ability to selectively inhibit the release of inflammatory cytokines and prostaglandins, chloroquine may be a useful adjunct in the clinical setting for the treatment of shock-induced immunodepression and for decreasing the susceptibility to sepsis following hemorrhage.

Cyclooxygenase inhibitors

Several experimental and clinical studies have suggested that after mechanical trauma [30] or burn injury [31], prostaglandin E_2 (PGE_2) may play a detrimental role in inducing a defective immune response [32, 33]. Ertel et al. [34] determined whether the systemic administration of the cyclooxygenase inhibitor ibuprofen following hemorrhage and resuscitation had any beneficial effects on the susceptibility to sepsis. For such studies, mice were subjected to CLP three days following hemorrhage and resuscitation. The results indicated that all animals in the vehicle-treated group died within three days following the onset of sepsis, while the mortality rate of the sham-operated animals subjected to sepsis was 50% through day six. Ibuprofen treatment after hemorrhage significantly prolonged survival time and increased overall survival rate of animals following CLP when compared to the vehicle-treated group. Furthermore, there was no significant difference in survival between ibuprofen-treated hemorrhage animals and the sham operated group [34]. Thus, blockade of cyclooxygenase with ibuprofen significantly decreased the susceptibility to sepsis following hemorrhage and resuscitation. Moreover, Faist et al. [35] have made considerable progress in immunomodulation to decrease the likelihood of infection by blocking the post-traumatic increase in PGE_2 with indomethacin and immune stimulation with thymopentin.

Phospholipase A_2

Vadas et al. [36] found a relation between increased levels of non-pancreatic phospholipase A_2 (PLA_2) and hypotension in sepsis and adult respiratory distress syndrome (ARDS). The gut mucosa contains a high concentration of PLA_2 [37, 38], which can be excessively activated in the presence of splanchinic hypoperfusion and may generate proinflammatory lipid mediators such as lysophospholipids (precursors of PAF) and arachidonic acid (the primary substrate for eicosanoids [39]. Furthermore, PLA_2 is released during sepsis [36, 40] and is partly under the control of TNF [40]. In view of this, inhibitors of PLA_2 should also be considered for preventing the release of proinflammatory mediators.

Platelet activating factor (PAF)

Bioactive phospholipids, derived from the activation and release of PLA_2, may also play a role in the host systemic inflammatory response to sepsis. Among these phospholipids, PAF, produced by a variety of cells (endothelial cells, platelets, leucocytes, monocytes, and lymphocytes), is an important trigger of cell-to-cell interaction, leading to the release of important inflammatory mediators. Platelet-activating factor is expressed rapidly by endothelial cells during shock in response to various stimuli (e.g. thrombin, histamine, leukotrienes) [41] and may be responsible for the earliest adherence of polymorphonuclear leukocytes (PMNs) to endothelial cells (in addition to P-selectin) via the PAF receptors. Cytokines such as IL-1, IL-6 and TNF can synthesize PAF in endothelial cells [42]. Increased PAF release has been reported in septic patients [43, 44] and high amounts of platelet-associated PAF have also been observed in patients with sepsis [44]. Since increased PAF levels are characteristic of sepsis and shock, PAF is considered to be an important toxic mediator which is partially responsible for producing the increased membrane permeability [41] under those conditions.

A number of specific PAF receptor antagonists, both naturally occurring or chemically synthesized, have been identified. PAF-receptor antagonists inhibit the specific binding of PAF to platelets, PAF-induced platelet aggregation, PAF-induced hypotension, and LPS-induced hypotension. PAF inhibitors also appear to attenuate endotoxin-induced pulmonary vascular abnormalities and prevent extravascular fluid accumulation in the lungs. Most significantly, PAF inhibitors appear to prolong survival in endotoxemic animals [45] Recent studies have shown that PAF antagonist (Ro 24-4736, a thienodiazepine) administration after hemorrhage and resuscitation prevented splenocyte immunodepression in mice [46]. In another study, Redl et al. [47] evaluated the effect of the PAF antagonist BN 52021 in ovine endotoxin shock and showed that the pulmonary vasculature and lung fluid balance disruption produced by LPS was markedly reduced by treatment with the PAF antagonist. In a clinical trial including 120 patients with Gram-negative sepsis, BN-52021 administration was associated with a 42% decrease in mortality compared with placebo [48].

Inflammatory cytokines

Characterization of the mechanisms regulating the production and action of inflammatory cytokines, especially those of T cell origin, could eventually lead to effective prophylaxis or therapy for septic shock. T cell activation is a complex process and requires the participation of many proteins, of which the interaction and function have yet to be completely clarified. An important understanding from such studies is that, without proper costimulation, ligation of the T cell receptor (TCR) alone not only leads to an inability to proliferate and to produce cytokines but also results in an unresponsiveness to further stimulation, a phenomenon referred to as anergy [49]. Ligation of the membrane associated costimulatory molecules and the TCR is a prerequisite for optimal immunological function of the T cell. Among many costimulatory molecules identified to date, CD28 is by far the most potent. CD28, a member of the Ig superfamily and forms a disulfide-linked homodimer of a 44-kDa glycoprotein expressed on the T cell surface. CD28 and CTLA-4, a closely related molecule, have been shown to modulate the mitogenic stimulation of T cells [50–53] by interacting with B7.1 (BB1; CD80) and B7.2 (CD86) on the surface of antigen presenting cells (APCs) [54]. This function of CD28 has been attributed to its ability to enhance the transcription of cytokine genes, to stabilize their messages, to inhibit anergy, and to prevent programmed cell death [55–57]. Wang et al. [58] found that both the septic shock syndrome and death could be prevented by administration of anti-CD28 Abs. The protection induced by anti-CD28 Ab was associated with a decrease in TNFα levels in the circulation. In addition, serum from anti-CD28 Ab-treated mice was capable of inhibiting the production of TNFα by bone marrow-derived macrophages following treatment with LPS, indicating that anti-CD28 Ab induced production of soluble factors that subsequently inhibited the production of TNFα. Wang et al. [58] confirmed that one of the factors present in the serum was IL-10 since anti-CD28 Ab treatment stimulated the expression of IL-10 both in splenocytes and in T cell lines. Furthermore, injection of anti-IL-10 Abs could abolish the protective effect of anti-CD28 Ab in septic shock. Anti-IL-10 Ab could also suppress the anti-CD28 Ab-induced inhibition of TNFα production, either *in vivo* or *in vitro*. They concluded that ligation of CD28 induces expression of IL-10, which in turn suppresses TNFα production and prevents septic shock [58].

Interferon-γ (IFNγ)

Studies by Livinston et al. [59] demonstrated that the capacity of rats to ward off infection after fixed-pressure hemorrhagic shock (35 mmHg for 1 h duration followed by resuscitation) is enhanced by combined IFNγ and antibiotic therapy. In additional studies, Malangoni et al. [60] showed that IFNγ combined with cefoxitin reduced the development of polymicrobial soft-tissue infections. Hershman et al. [61] found that IFNγ treatment enhanced survival after *Klebsiella pneumonia* infection in mice. Thus, it could be suggested that IFNγ alone or in combination with antibiotics can reduce the spread of infection. Ertel et al. [62] administered 4 x 10^4 units/kg body weight recombinant murine IFNγ following hemorrhage and resuscitation in mice and demonstrated that administration of this agent restored the depressed macrophage antigen presentation capacity of peritoneal macrophages, as well as Ia expression, on these macrophages. The depressed release of IL-1 and TNF was also increased by IFNγ treatment and the depressed splenocyte proliferation was restored. Furthermore, IFNγ decreased the lethality from sepsis following hemorrhage [62]. These data therefore indicate that IFNγ is a potent agent for the treatment of hemorrhagic shock-induced immunosuppression and for increasing the ability of the host to combat bacterial infections following hemorrhage.

Growth hormone and insulin-like growth factor-1

Growth hormone (GH) belongs to the somatolactogen family of hormones [63] and is an anabolic hormone that improves protein metabolism in critical illness [64, 65]. Growth hormone is also the major regulator stimulating the synthesis and secretion of insulin-like growth factor I (IGF-I) from various tissues. Moreover, the anabolic effects of GH on protein metabolism are mediated mainly by IGF-I [66]. Inoue et al. [66] recently showed in a murine sepsis model that exogenous GH and IGF-1 increased peritoneal exudative cell numbers, reduced viable bacterial counts in the peritoneal lavage fluid and the liver, and consequently prolonged survival in mice with sepsis. Furthermore, these hormones exerted modulatory effects on local and systemic cytokine production (TNF, IL-1, IL-6). These authors [66] therefore concluded that administration of GH and IGF-1 effectively improves host defense via immunomodulation.

Erythropoietin

Patients with chronic infections and inflammatory diseases often exhibit low serum erythropoietin (Epo) levels in relation to the blood hemoglobin concentration [67]. *In vitro* studies utilizing Epo-producing human hepatoma cells and isolated perfused rat kidneys have shown that proinflammatory cytokines such as IL-1 and TNFα inhibit Epo gene expression [68–70]. Sepsis is perhaps the most severe example of a systemic inflammatory reaction. The clinical characteristics of the sepsis syndrome include fever, hypotension, hypoglycemia, disseminated intravascular coagulation and increased vascular permeability [5, 71]. IL-1, IL-6 and TNFα play an important role in the development of these host responses to infection. Approximately 50% of the patients die because of refractory hypotension or progressive failure of multiple organ systems [71]. Anemia due to hemorrhage and hemolysis in association with suppressed erythropoiesis worsens the clinical course. In contrast to the prognostic value of elevated plasma TNFα levels in patients with sepsis, measurements of IL-1β are thought to be of little significance for monitoring [5, 72]. Very high IL-6 levels were earlier detected by bioassay of plasma from septic patients and studies indicate that the level of immunoreactive IL-6 correlates with mortality rates in patients with sepsis [72–75]. However, although associated with the patients' outcome as a whole, the plasma concentration of IL-6 alone is not considered to be a clinically useful prognostic predictor for the individual patient [75]. TNFα, IL-1α and IL-1β have been shown to suppress the *in vitro* synthesis of Epo in human hepatoma cell cultures [68–70] and isolated perfused rat kidneys [69]. Therefore, these proinflammatory cytokines are thought to play an important role in the defective production of Epo in distinct acute and chronic inflammatory renal and nonrenal diseases, including nephritis, renal allograft rejection, autoimmune diseases and malignancies [67, 76]. There has been one earlier report showing low Epo bioactivity detected *in vitro* in the plasma of infants with sepsis [77]. Studies done by Abel et al. [78] in critically ill patients with documented sepsis indicate that Epo production is not generally lowered in septic patients, despite the increased levels of proinflammatory cytokines. However, they propose that increasingly high Epo levels is a negative prognostic indicator in septic patients since it increases IL-6 levels and APACHE II scores. The mechanisms responsible for the final increase in circulation Epo are still unclear. Septic shock is associated with decreased tissue perfusion and hypoxia [71] which may induce Epo gene expression. Alternatively, specific cytokines may stimulate Epo production. IL-6, which is produced excessively in septic shock, has been shown to stimulate Epo gene expression in the human hepatic cell line Hep3B [69]. Since IL-6 has been shown to inhibit Epo production in isolated perfused rat kidneys [69, 79], the effects of IL-6 on hepatic Epo synthesis deserve further consideration.

Dietary manipulation

Current nutritional formulations contain *n*-6 polyunsaturated acids (PUFA's) as a primary fat source. However, a great deal of attention has recently been focused on the potential use of *n*-3 PUFAs (i.e. ω-3 fatty acids) which are found in high concentration in fish oil. Studies have shown that these ω-3 fatty acids, which include eicosapentaenoic acid and decosahexaenoic acid, are rapidly and preferentially incorporated into membrane phospholipids and thus reduce the production of arachidonic acid metabolites. It is this effect which is thought to be responsible for some of the anti-inflammatory and immunostimulatory effects associated with diets high in ω-3 fatty acids. Experimental studies indicate that the severity of arthritis [80], systemic lupus erythematosus [81] and amyloidosis [82] are markedly reduced if diets high in ω-3 fatty acids are given. Studies in humans have demonstrated that the synthesis of the inflammatory cytokines TNF and IL-1 could be decreased by dietary supplementation with ω-3 fatty acids [83]. Animal studies showed that diets high in ω-3 fatty acids led to a significant decrease in the synthesis and release of PGE_2 by endotoxin-stimulated macrophages [84, 85]. In addition, mortality was significantly reduced by using diets supplemented with ω-3 fatty acids in a chronic model of sepsis [86]. These results are in line with data of two clinical trials in which fish oil was shown to have a restorative effect on the depressed cellular immunity of patients in intensive care units [87] and in patients after major surgery [88, 89]. However, a significant decrease of infectious complications or mortality in such patients could not be demonstrated. Nonetheless, a prospective clinical study in burn patients, however, has shown that the use of a diet containing fish oil significantly reduced wound infection, shortened hospital stays, and reduced deaths when compared to other standard enteral formulations [90]. Collectively, these studies would suggest that a diet containing fish oil given to malnourished, immunocompromised patients awaiting elective surgery with a high postoperative risk of sepsis should be useful in preventing postoperative infectious complications.

Sex hormones

Several clinical and epidemiological studies indicate gender differences in the susceptibility to and morbidity from sepsis [91–95]. Immune functions in normal males and females has been reported to be influenced by sex steroids [96, 97]. In this regard, it appears that better maintained immune functions in females are not only due to physiological levels of female sex-steroids, but also at least in part because of the markedly lower level of immunosuppressive androgenic hormones [98]. Studies from our laboratory showed that hemorrhage in mice markedly decreased the ability of peritoneal and splenic macrophages to release IL-1 and IL-6 two hours after hemorrhaged [99]. This was associated with increased mRNA expression for IL-1 and IL-6 and increased serum corticosterone levels. Administration of prolactin following hemorrhage attenuates the increased mRNA expression for IL-1β and IL-6 in peritoneal macrophage (pMØ) and splenic macrophages (sMØ) [99]. Furthermore, the cytokine release capacity and blood corticosterone levels were comparable to the values in sham animals [99]. Prolactin also significantly improved the survival of animals subjected to sepsis after hemorrhage [99]. Previous studies from our laboratory indicate a profound suppression of TNFα, IL-1β and IL-6 release capacity by pMØ and sMØ during late sepsis (24 h after CLP), which is associated with severe host immunosuppression [100, 101]. However, prolactin as well as metoclopramide (a dopamine antagonist, which has been reported to increase prolactin secretion and circulating plasma levels [102]) treatment after the onset of sepsis resulted in significant upregulation of constitutive and inducible cytokine gene expression in both MØ polulation, when compared to septic-untreated and sham-operated mice [103]. Thus, prolactin and metoclopramide enhance the depressed MØ gene expression and may be useful in improving cell-mediated immunity during sepsis. In line with this is a recent experimental study [94] which determined in a prospective and randomized manner whether the cell-mediated immune response during sepsis differs in females vs. males, and whether the survival rate in females is different than in males after a septic insult. After anesthesia, male and proestrus (a stage at which the female sexual hormones are highest) female mice underwent cecal ligation and puncture (CLP) to induce sepsis. The mice were killed at 24 h after the onset of sepsis. Splenocyte proliferative capacity and splenocyte IL-2 and IL-3 release were markedly decreased in male, but not in female, septic mice. Furthermore, the survival rate of septic female proestrus mice was significantly higher than in comparable male mice. These results support the concept that the immune response of females differs from males, and that females in proestrus state are immunologically better positioned to meet the challenge of sepsis [94]. Alternatively, to the extent that androgens contribute to the marked immune depression seen following hemorrhage, it is worth noting that recent studies indicate that testosterone receptor-blockade in males following hemorrhage restored the depressed immune functions and improved survival following hemorrhage and the induction of subsequent sepsis [104, 105].

Potential limitations in the application of experimental therapeutic agents at the bedside

The success in the use of immunomodulatory agents following hemorrhage and sepsis in rodent models appears to be promising in the development of new therapeutic concepts for the treatment of immunosuppression and for decreasing the mortality from sepsis in humans. However, careful evaluation of both the benefits and potential adverse effects of therapy is needed before widespread clinical use can be envisioned. As discussed in the other chapters in this book, studies in rodent models of endotoxemia and bacteremia indicated that neutralization of endotoxin, as well as TNFα biological activity, markedly decreased the morbidity and mortality in these animals. However, clinical trials in humans following septic shock have thus far not yielded remarkable results, which might suggest that factors other than endotoxin or

TNFα may be important for producing the pathophysiological problems in patients. The reason for the lack of benefits in patients receiving anti-TNFα or anti-endotoxin antibodies is most likely due to the polymicrobial nature of sepsis which involves gram negative bacteria, gram positive bacteria, and fungus. Therefore, animal models which only involve endotoxin or gram negative bacteria may not accurately mimic the clinical condition of sepsis and thus the unremarkable outcome of clinical trials with anti-TNFα or anti-endotoxin treatment is not surprising.

The accurate modeling of human trauma patients in animals is extremely complex and difficult since a number of important differences exist between animal models of shock/sepsis and patients in shock/sepsis. Human patients, following trauma, receive multiple interventions which include blood transfusions, colloid, inotropic agents, anti-inflammatories, antibiotics, analgesics and anesthetics. Some of these agents have been shown to have immunosuppressive properties. Furthermore, it is unclear if these agents act in a synergistic manner in suppressing immune function. In impending animal studies of trauma, the effect of these agents on immune function will need to be evaluated in order to more accurately replicate the human patient. Other factors that are clearly important to patient outcome following trauma include gender, age, nutritional status, socioeconomic background, and preexisting disease or infection which may also profoundly influence the immune response. These factors will also need to be accurately examined in future experimental studies. The importance of identifying multiple agents that can restore immune function following trauma and sepsis is that these immunomodulators may have different degrees of efficacy, or the efficacy may be counteracted by the additional interventions the patient receives such as epinephrine etc., during intensive care stays.

Summary and conclusion

Sepsis produces severe immunosuppression and is associated with high morbidity and mortality [106, 107]. Treatment strategies for sepsis include the use of antibiotics, debridement of infected or necrotic tissues, and intensive life-support procedures such as dialysis, mechanical ventilation, and vasoactive drug administration [108]. However, the incidence of sepsis and the mortality associated with sepsis remain high [107]. Therefore, new strategies for the prevention of severe sepsis are required. A large number of experimental studies indicate beneficial effects of agents such as ATP-MgCl$_2$, pentoxifylline, non-anticoagulant heparin, calcium channel blockers, chloroquine, cyclooxygenase inhibitors, PAF antagonists, anti-endotoxin Abs, TNF Abs, IL-1ra, soluble TNF receptors etc., following trauma and sepsis (using primarily models of endotoxemia or bacteremia).

As mentioned in this and other chapters, a number of agents such as anti endotoxin Abs, TNF Abs, IL-1ra, soluble TNF receptors or binding proteins etc., have been and are being examined in the clinical arena. However, if the efficacy of these agents is to be established and maximized, it will be extremely important to not only clearly define the pathobiology of shock/sepsis state but also the patient population who will benefit from these new modalities. It should also be noted that indisputable modeling of human trauma patients in animals is arduous since a number of important differences exist between animal models of shock and sepsis and patients in shock or sepsis. An example of this is that human patients, following trauma, receive multiple modalities which include blood transfusions, colloid, inotropic agents, anti- inflammatory agents, antibiotics, analgesics and anesthetics. Some of the above-mentioned agents have been shown to have immonusuppressive properties. Moreover, it is unclear if these agents act in a synergistic and/or additive manner in suppressing immune function. Experimental animal models, on the other hand, have usually been designed to keep the model as "simple" as possible and thus they do not undergo the same magnitude/diversity of trauma nor are they subjected to multiple interventions including the concurrent use of pressor agents. In future animal studies of trauma/sepsis, the effects of inotropic agents, antibiotics, analgesics, etc. on immune function will need to be evaluated in order to more accurately replicate the human patient. Additional factors that follow trauma and sepsis such as age, gender, nutritional status, socioeconomic background, and pre-existing disease(s) also influence the immune responses and are important components in patient outcome following trauma and sepsis. These factors should also be thoroughly considered and examined in future experimental studies. Identifying multiple agents that can restore immune function following trauma/sepsis is important since some of those immunomodulators may have different degrees of efficacy. Moreover, the efficacy of some of these agents may be counteracted by accessory interventions such as epinephrine etc., which the patient receives during their stay in the intensive care unit.

Acknowledgment
This work was supported by USPHS grant RO1 GM 37127.

References

1   Fry DE, Pearlstein L, Fulton RL, Polk HC Jr. (1980) Multiple system organ failure. The role of uncontrolled infection. *Arch Surg* 115: 136–140

2   Polk HC Jr (1979) Consensus summary on infection. *J Trauma* 19: 894–896

3   Curreri PW, Luterman A, Braun DW, Shires GT (1980) Burn injury. Analysis of survival and hospitalization time for 937 patients. *Ann Surg* 192: 472–478

4   Redl H, Nikolai A, Kneidinger R, Schlag G (1993) Endothelial and leukocyte activation in experimental polytrauma and sepsis. *Behring Inst Mitt* 92: 218–228

5   Molloy RG, Mannick JA, Rodrick ML (1993) Cytokines, sepsis and immunomodulation. *Br J Surg* 80 289–297

6   Cerami A (1992) Inflammatory Cytokines. *Clin Immunol Immunopathol* 62: S3–S10

7   Baue AE (1994) Multiple organ failure, multiple organ dysfunction syndrome, and the systemic inflammatory response syndrome – where do we stand? *Shock* 2: 385–397

8   Baron RL (1993) Pathophysiology of septic shock and implications for therapy. *Clin Pharm* 12: 829–845

9   Chaudry IH (1983) Cellular mechanisms in shock and ischemia and their correction. *Am J Physiol* 245: R117–R134

10 Harkema JM, Chaudry IH (1992) Magnesium-adenosine triphosphate in the treatment of shock, ischemia, and sepsis. *Crit Care Med* 20: 263–275

11 Hirasawa H, Sugai T, Ohtake Y et al (1990) Energy metabolism and nutritional support in anuric multiple organ failure patients. In: Tanaka T, Okada A (eds): *Nutritional support in organ failure*. Elsevier, Amsterdam, 439–446

12 Liebscher G, Shapiro MJ, Barner H, Daake C, Moskoff M, Durham RM, Baue AE: ATP-MgCl$_2$ as and afterload reducing agent. *Crit Care Med* 1992; 21: S200 (abstract)

13 Meldrum DR, Ayala A, Chaudry IH (1994) Energetics of lymphocyte "burnout" in late sepsis: Adjuvant treatment with ATP-MgCl$_2$ improves energetics and decreases lethality. *J Surg Res* 56: 537–542

14 Harkema JM, Singh G, Wang P, Chaudry IH (1992) Pharmacologic agents in the treatment of ischemia, hemorrhagic shock, and sepsis. *J Crit Care* 7: 189–216

15 Wang P, Wood TH, Ba ZF, Chaudry IH (1996) Depressed vascular endothelial cell function during hyperdynamic sepsis: restoration with ATP-MgCl$_2$ administration. *Surg Forum* 47: 48–50

16 Wang P, Chaudry IH (1996) Editorial review: Mechanism of hepatocellular dysfunction during hyperdynamic sepsis. *Am J Physiol* 270: R927–R938

17 Wang P, Ba ZF, Reich SS, Zhou M, Holme KR, Chaudry IH (1996) Effects of nonanticoagulant heparin on cardiovascular and hepatocellular function after hemorrhagic shock. *Am J Physiol* 270: H1294–H1302

18 Zellweger R, Ayala A, Zhu XL, Holme KR, DeMaso CM, Chaudry IH (1995) A novel non-anticoagulant heparin improves splenocyte and peritoneal macrophage immune function after trauma-hemorrhage and resuscitation. *J Surg Res* 59: 211–218

19 Morrison AM, Wang P, Chaudry IH (1996) A novel nonanticoagulant heparin prevents vascular endothelial cell dysfunction during hyperdynamic sepsis. *Shock* 6: 46–51

20 Maitra SR, Sayeed MM (1987) Effect of diltiazem on intracellular Ca^{2+} mobilization in hepatocytes during endotoxic shock. *Am J Physiol* 253: R545–R548

21 Hess ML, Warner MF, Smith JM, Manson NH, Greenfield LJ (1983) Improved myocardial hemodynamic and cellular function with calcium channel blockade (verapamil) during canine hemorrhagic shock. *Circ Shock* 10: 119–130

22 Westfall MV, Sayeed MM (1989) Effect of diltiazem on skeletal muscle 3-0-methylglucose transport in bacteremic rats. *Am J Physiol* 256: R716–R721

23 Meldrum DR, Ayala A, Perrin MM, Ertel W, Chaudry IH (1991) Diltiazem restores IL-

2, IL-3, IL-6 and IFN-gamma synthesis and decreases susceptibility to sepsis following hemorrhage. *J Surg Res* 51: 158–164

22 Rollo IM (1980) Drugs used in the chemotherapy of malaria. In: Goodman LS, Gilman AG (eds): *Pharmacological basis of therapeutics*. MacMillan Publishing, New York, 1038–1060

25 Freedman A (1956) Chloroquine and rheumatoid arthritis: short term controlled trial. *Ann Rheum Dis* 15: 251–257

26 Authi KS, Tragnor JR (1979) Effects of anti-malarial drugs on phospholipase A_2. *Br J Pharmacol* 66: 496–501

27 Ertel W, Morrison MH, Ayala A, Chaudry IH (1991) Chloroquine attenuates hemorrhagic shock-induced suppression of Kupffer cell antigen presentation and major histocompatibility complex class II antigen expression through blockade of tumor necrosis factor and prostaglandin release. *Blood* 7: 1781–1788

28 Ertel W, Morrison MH, Ayala A, Chaudry IH (1992) Chloroquine attenuates hemorrhagic shock induced immunosuppression and decreases susceptibility to sepsis. *Arch Surg* 127: 70–76

29 Zhu X, Ertel W, Ayala A, Morrison MH, Perrin MM, Chaudry IH (1993) Chloroquine inhibits macrophage tumor necrosis factor-α mRNA transcription. *Immunology* 80: 122–126

30 Faist E, Mewes A, Bader CC, Strasser T, Alkan SS, Rieber P, Heberer G (1987) Prostaglandin E_2 dependent suppression of interleukin-2 production in patients with major trauma. *J Trauma* 27: 837–848

31 Miller-Graziano CL, Fink M, Wu JY, Szabo G, Kodys K (1988) Mechanisms of altered monocyte prostaglandin E_2 production in severely injured patients. *Arch Surg* 123: 293–299

32 Walker C, Kristensen F, Bettens F, DeWeck AL (1983) Lymphokine regulation of activated (G_1) lymphocytes: prostaglandin E_2-induced inhibition of interleukin 2 production. *J Immunol* 130: 1770–1773

33 Knapp W, Baumgartner G (1978) Monocyte-mediated suppression of human B lymphocyte differentiation *in vitro*. *J Immunol* 121: 1177–1183

34 Ertel W, Morrison MH, Meldrum DR, Ayah A, Chaudry IH (1992) Ibuprofen restores cellular immunity and decreases susceptibility to sepsis following hemorrhage. *J Surg Res* 53: 55–61

35 Faist E, Markewith A, Endres S, Fuchs D, Hültner L, Lang (1993) Progress in anti-infective perioperative immunomodulatory therapy with simultaneous administration of blocking and enhancing agent. In: Faist E, Meakins J, Schildberg FW (eds): Host defense dysfunction in trauma, shock and sepsis. Springer-Verlag, Berlin, Heidelberg, 1109–1129

36 Vadas P, Przanski W, Stefanski E (1988)Pathogenesis of hypotension in septic shock: correlation of circulating phospholipase A_2 levels with circulatory collapse. *Crit Care Med* 16: 1–7

37   Dennis EA, Rhee SG, Billah MM, Hannun A (1991) Role of phospholipase in generating lipid second messengers in signal transduction. *Faseb J* 5: 2068 (abstract)

38   Mansbach CM (1990) Phospholipases: old enzymes with new meaning. *Gastroenterology* 98: 1369–1382

39   Koike K, Moore EE, Moore FA, Carl VS, Pitman JM, Banerjee A (1992) Phospholipase A$_2$ inhibition decouples lung injury from gut ischemia reperfusion. *Surgery* 112: 173–178

40   Redl H, Schlag G, Schiesser A, Davies J (1993) Tumor necrosis factor is a mediator of phospholipase release during bacteremia in baboons. *Am J Physiol* 264: H2119

41   Schlag G, Redl H (1996) Mediators of Injury and Inflammation. *World J Surg* 20: 406–410

42   Hosford D, Koltai M, Braquet P (1993) Platelet-activating factor in shock, sepsis, and organ failure. In: Schlag G, Redl H (eds.): *Pathophysiology of shock, sepsis, and organ failure*. Springer-Verlag, Berlin, Heidelberg, 502–517

43   Bussolino, F, Procellini MG, Varese L, Bosia A (1987) Intravascular release of platelet-activating factor in children with sepsis. *Thromb Res* 48: 619–620

44   Lopez-Diez F, Nieto ML, Femandez-Gallardo S, Gijon MA, Sanchez-Crespo M (1989) Occupancy of platelet receptors for platelet activating factor in patients with septicemia. *J Clin Invest* 83: 1733–1740

45   Verhoef J, Hustinx WMN, Frasa H, Hoepelman AIM (1996) Issues in the adjunct therapy of severe Sepsis Antimicrobiol Chemotherapy 38: 167–182

46   Zellweger R, Ayala A, Schmand JF, Morrison MH, Chaudry IH (1995) Platelet activating factor antagonist administration after hemorrhage-resuscitation prevents splenocyte immunodepression. *J Sur Res* 59: 366–370

47   Redl H, Vogl C, Schiesser A, Paul E, Thurnher M, Bahrami S, Schlag G (1990) Effect of the PAF antagonist BN 52021 in ovine endotoxin shock. *J Lipid Mediat* 2 Suppl: S195–S201

48   Dhainaut JFA, Tenaillon A, Le Tulzo Y, Schlemmer B, Solet JP, Wolff M, Holzappel L, Zeni F, Dreyfuss D, Mira JP, deVathaire F, Guinot P (1994) Platelet activating factor receptor antagonist BN 52021 in the treatment of severe sepsis: a randomized, double-blind, placebo-controlled, multicenter clinical trial. *Crit Care Med* 22: 1720–1728

49   Zanders ED, Lamb JR, Feldman M, Green N, Beverlt PCL (1983) Tolerance of T cells is associated with membrane antigen changes. *Nature* 303: 625–627

50   Hara T, Fu SM, Hansen JA (1985) Human T cell activation, IL: a new T cell activation pathway used by a major T cell population via a disulfide bonded dimer of a 44-kilodalton peptide (9.3 antigen). *J Exp Med* 161: 1513–1524

51   Ledbetter JA, Martin PJ, Spooner CE, Wofsy D, Tsu TT, Beatty PG, Gladstone P (1985) Antibodies to Tp67 and Tp44 augment and sustain proliferative responses of activated T cells. *J Immunol* 135: 2331–2336

52   Linsley PS, Ledbetter JA (1993) The role of the CD28 receptor during T cell responses to antigen. *Annu Rev Immunol* 11: 191–212

53 Gross JA, Calla E, Allison FP (1992) Identification and distribution of the costimulatory receptorCD28 in the mouse. *J Immunol* 149: 380–388

54 Linsley PS, Greene JL, Brady W, Bajorath J, Ledbetter JA, Peach R (1994) Human B7-1 (CD80) and B7-2 (CD86)bind with similar avidities but distinct kinetics to CD28 and CTLA-4 receptors. *Immunity* 1: 793–801

55 Green JM, Thompson CB (1994) Modulation of T cell proliferative response by accessory cell interactions. *Immunol Res* 13: 234–243

56 Shi Y, Radvanyi LG, Shaw P, Green DR, Miller R, Mills GB (1995) CD28-mediated signaling *in vivo* prevents activation-induced apoptosis in the thymus and alters peripheral lymphocytes homeostasis. *J Immunol* 155: 1829–1837

57 Boise LH, Minn AJ, Noel PJ, June CH, Accavitti MA, Lindsten T, Thompson CB (1995) CD28 costimulation can promote T cell survival by enhancing the expression of Bcl-XL. *Immunity* 3: 87–98

58 Wang R, Fang Q, Zhang L, Randvany L, Sharma A, Noben-Trauth N, Mills GB, Shi Y (1997) CD 28 ligation prevents bacterial toxin-induced septic shock in mice by inducing IL-10 expression. *J Immunol* 158: 2856–2861

59 Livingston DH, Malangoni M (1988) Interferon-gamma restores immune competence after hemorrhagic shock. *J Surg Res* 45: 37–43

60 Malangoni MA, Livingston DH, Sonnenfeld G, Polk HC (1990) Interferon gamma and tumor necrosis factor alpha. *Arch Surg* 125: 444–446

61 Hersham MJ, Pietsch JD, Trachtenberg L, Mooney THR, Shields RE, Sonnenfeld G (1989) Protective effects of recombinant human tumor necrosis factor alpha and interferon against surgically simulated wound infection in mice. *Br J Surg* 76: 1282–1286

62 Ertel W, Morrison MH, Ayala A, Dean RE, Chaudry IH (1992) Interferon-gamma attenuates hemorrhage induced suppression of macrophage and splenocyte functions and decreases susceptibility to sepsis. *Surgery* 111: 177–187

63 Arkins S, Dantzer R, Kellew KW (1993) Somatolactogens, somatomedins, and immunity. *J Dair Sc* 76: 2437–2450

64 Chwals WJ, Bistrian BR (1991) Role of exogenous growth hormone and insulin-like growth factor I in malnutrition and acute metabolic stress: a hypothesis. *Crit Care Med.* 19: 1317–1322

65 Voerman HJ, Strack van SchijndelRJM, de Boer H, van der Veen EA, Thijs LG (1992) Growth hormone: secretion and administration in catabolic adult patients, with emphasis on the critically ill patient. *Neth J Med* 41: 229–244

66 Inoue T, Saito H, Fukushima R, Inaba T, Lin MT, Fukatsu K, Muto T (1995) Growth Hormone and insulin-like growth factor I enhance host defense in a murine sepsis model. *Arch Surg* 130: 1115–1122

67 Means RT, Krantz SB (1992) Progress in understanding the pathogenesis of the anemia of chronic disease. *Blood* 80: 1639–1647

68 Faquin WC, Schneider TJ, Goldberg MA (1992) Effect of inflammatory cytokines on hypoxia-induced erythropoietin production. *Blood* 79: 1987–1994

69 Jelkmann W, Pagel H, Wolff M, Fandrey J (1992) Monokines inhibiting erythropoietin

production in human hepatoma cultures and in isolated perfused rat kidneys. *Life Sci* 50: 301–308

70   Fandrey, Huwiler A, Frede S, Pfeilschifter J, Jelkmann W (1994) Distinct signaling pathways mediate phorbol-ester-induced and cytokine-induced inhibition of erythropoietin gene expression. *Eur J Biochem* 226: 335–340

71   Parrillo J (1993) Pathogenetic mechanisms of septic shock. *N Engl J Med* 328: 1471–1477

72   Waage A, Brandtzag P, Halstensen A, Kierulf P, Espevik T (1989) The complex pattern of cytokines in serum from patients with menigococcal septic shock. *J Exp Med* 169: 333–338

73   Endo S, Inada K, Inoue Y, Kuwata Y, Suzuki M, Yamashita H, Hoshi S, Yosshida M (1992) Two types of septic shock classified by the plasma levels of cytokines and endotoxin. *Circ Shock* 38: 264–274

74   Damas P, Lesoux D, Nys M, Vrindts Y, DeGroote D, Franchimont P (1992) Cytokines serum level during severe sepsis in human Il-6 as a marker of severity. *Ann Surg* 215: 356–362

75   Calandra T, Gerain J, Heumann D, Baumgartner Jd, Glauser MP (1991) High circulating levels of interleukin-6 in patients with septic shock: evolution during sepsis, prognostic value, and interplay with other cytokines. *Am J Med* 91: 23–29

76   Jelkmann W (1992) Erythropoietin: structure, control of production, and function. *Physiol Rev* 72: 449–489

77   Soboleva MK, Manakova TE (1993) Plasma erythropoietin activity in infants with sepsis. *Bull Exp Biol Med* 115: 545–548

78   Abel J, Spannbrucker N, Fandrey J, Jelkmann W (1996) Serum erythropoietin levels with sepsis and septic shock. *Eur J Haemato* 57: 359–363

79   Jelkmann W, Fandrey J, Frede S, Pagel H (1994) Inhibition of erythropoietin production by cytokines. Implications for the anemia involved in inflammatory states. *Ann NY Acad Sci* 718: 300–309

80   Kremer JM, Bigauoette J, Michaled AV, Timchalk MA, Lininger L, Rynes RI, Huyck C, Zieminsk J, Bartholomew LE (1985): Effects of manipulation of dietary fatty acids on clinical manifestations of rheumatoid arthritis. *Lancet* i: 184–187

81   Robinson DR, Prickett JD, Polisson R, Steinberg AD, Levine L (1985) The protective effect of dietary fish oil on murine lupus. *Prostaglandins* 30:51–75

82   Cathcart ES, Leslie CA, Meydani SN, Hayes KC (1987) A fish oil diet retards experimental amyloidosis, modulates lymphocyte function and decreases macrophages arachidonate metabolism in mice. *J Immunol* 139: 1850–1854

83   Endres S, Ghorbani R, Kellew VE, Georgilis K, Lonnemann G, Van deer Meer JW, Cannon JG, Rogers TS, Klempner MS, Weber PC, Schaefer EJ, Wolff SM, Dinarello CA (1989) The effect of dietary supplementation with n-3 polyunsaturated fatty acids on the synthesis of interleukin-1 and tumor necrosis factor by mononuclear cells. *N Engl J Med* 320: 265–271

84   Biliar TR, Bankey PE, Swingen BA, Curran RD, West MA, Holman RT, Simmons RL,

Cerra FB (1988) Fatty acid intake and Kupffer cell function: fish oil alters eicosanoid and monokine production to endotoxin stimulation. *Surgery* 104: 343–349

85 Lokesh BR, Sayers TJ, Kinsella JE (1990) Interleukin-1 and tumor necrosis factor synthesis by mouse peritoneal macrophages is enhanced by dietary n-3 polyunsaturated fatty acids. *Immunol Letters* 23: 281–286

86 Barton RG, Wells CL, Carlson A, Singh R, Sullivan JJ, Cerra FB (1991) Dietary omega-3 fatty acids decrease mortality and Kupffer cell prostaglandin E2 production in a rat model of chronic sepsis. *J Trauma* 31: 768–774

87 Cerra FB, Lehman S, Konstantinides N, Shronts EP, Holman R (1990) Effect of enteral nutrient on *in vitro* test of immune function in ICU patient: a preliminary report. *Nutrition* 6: 84–87

88 Leberman MD, Shou J, Torres AS, Weintraub F, Goldfine J, Sigal R, Daly JM (1990) Effects of nutrient substrates on immune function. *Nutrition* 6: 88–91

89 Cerra FB, Lehmann S, Konstantinides N, Dzik J, Fish J, Konstantinides F, LiCari JJ, Holman RT (1991) Improvements in immune function in ICU patients by enteral nutrition supplemented with arginine, RNA and Menhaden Oil is independent of nitrogen balance. *Nutrition* 7: 193–199

90 Alexander JW, Gottschlich MM (1990) Nutritional immunomodulation in burn patients. *Crit Care Med* 18: S149–S153

91 Bone RC (1992) Toward an epidemiology and natural history of SIRS (systemic inflammatory response syndrome). *JAMA* 268: 3452–3455

92 Center for Disease Control: Mortality Patterns – United States, 1989.(1992) *Morbidity Mortality Wkly Rpt* 41: 121–125

93 McGowan JE, Barnes MW, Finland N (1975) Bacteremia at Boston City Hospital: occurrence and mortality during 12 selected years (1935–1972) with special reference to hospital-acquired cases. *J Infect Dis* 132: 316–335

94 Zellweger R, Wichmann MW, Ayala A, Stein S, DeMaso CM, Chaudry IH (1997) Females in proestrus state maintain splenic immune functions and tolerate sepsis better than males. *Crit Care Med* 25: 106–110

95 Wichmann M, Zellweger R, DeMaso C, Ayala A, Chaudry IH.(1996) Enchanced immune responses in females, as oppose to decreased responses in males following haemorrhagic shock and resuscitation. *Cytokine* 8: 853–863

96 Homo-Delarche F, Fitzpatrick F, Christeff N, Nunez EA, Bach JF, Dardenne M (1991) Sex steroids, glucocorticoids, stress and autoimmunity. *J Steroid Biochem Molec Biol* 40: 619–637

97 Wichmann, Ayala A, Chaudry IH (1997) Male sex steriods are responsible for depressing macrophage immune function after trauma-hemorrhage. *Am J Physiol* 273: C1335–C1340

98 Luster MI, Pfeifer RW, Tucker AN (1985) Influence of sex hormones on immunoregulation with specific reference to natural and environmental estrogens. In: Thomas JA, Korach KS, McLachlan JA (eds): *Endocrine toxicology.* Raven Press, New York, 67–83

99 Zellweger R, Zhu XH, Wichmann MW, Ayala A, DeMaso CM, Chaudry IH (1996) Pro-

lactin administration following hemorrhagic shock improves macrophage cytokine release capacity and decreases mortality form subsequent sepsis. *J Immunol* 157: 5748–5754

100 Ayala A, Kisala JM, Felt JA, Perrin MM, Chaudry IH (1992) Does endotoxin tolerance prevent the release of inflammatory monokines (IL-1, IL-6, or TNF) during sepsis? *Arch Surg* 127: 191–197

101 Ayala A, Chaudry IH. (1996) Immune dysfunction in murine polymicrobial sepsis: mediators, macrophages, lymphocytes and apoptosis. *Shock* 6: S27–S38

102 Ehrenkranz RA, Ackermann BA (1986) Metoclopramide effect on faltering milk production by mothers of premature infants. *Pediatrics* 78: 614–620

103 Zhu ZH, Zellweger R, Wichmann MW, Ayala A, Chaudry IH (1997) Effects of prolactin and metoclopramide on macrophage cytokine gene expression in late sepsis. *Cytokine* 6 437–446

104 Wichmann MW, Angele MK, Ayala A, Cioffi WG, Chaudry IH (1997) Flutamide:A novel agent for restoring the depressed cell-mediated immunity following soft-tissue trauma and hemorrhagic shock. *Shock* 8: 242–248

105 Angele MK, Wichmann MW, Ayala A, Cioffi WG, Chaudry IH (1997) Testosterone receptor blockade after hemorrhage in males: restoration of the depressed immune functions and improved survival following subsequent sepsis. *Arch Surg* 132: 1207–124

106 Mainous MR, Deitch EA (1994) Nutrition and infection. *Surg Clin North Am.* 74: 659–676

107 Dunn D (1994) Gram-negative bacterial sepsis and sepsis syndrome. *Surg Clin North Am* 74: 621–635

108 Natanson C, Hoffman WD, Suffredini AF, Eichacker PQ, Danner RL (1994) Selected treatment strategies for septic shock based on proposed mechanisms of pathogenesis. *Ann Intern Med* 120: 771–783

Gene therapy – an alternative approach for anti-cytokine therapies

Michael A. Rogy

University of Vienna, AKH Wien, Department of Surgery, Währingergürtel 18–20, A-1090 Wien, Austria

Background

Over the past ten years, anticytokine therapies for the treatment of septic shock, adult respiratory distress syndrome (ARDS) and systemic inflammatory response syndrome (SIRS) have progressed from the laboratory to the clinic. It is now generally accepted that overproduction of several classes of proteins produced by inflammatory cells, termed pro-inflammatory cytokines, contribute to the pathological consequences of septic shock [1, 2]. Neutralizing an exaggerated endogenous tumor necrosis factor α (TNFα) response with anti-TNFα antibodies [3, 4], soluble TNF receptor immunadhesins [5, 6], or downregulating TNFα production with interleukin-10 (IL-10) pretreatment [7, 8] confers survival to otherwise lethal endotoxemia. Presently, clinical trials are underway with monoclonal antibodies and immunadhesins directed against TNFα in patients with sepsis syndrome [9]. Similarly, efforts to block an exaggerated interleukin-1 (IL-1) production, primarily with the use of IL-1 receptor antagonist (IL-1ra), have shown variable results in preclinical studies [10, 11] and early clinical trials [12].

However, current therapeutic approaches, although conceptually sound, are inherently inefficient. Firstly, these natural antagonists or inhibitors of pro-inflammatory cytokines have short biological half-lives, ranging from minutes to hours [5, 10, 13]. Secondly, pro-inflammatory cytokine levels are often several times higher in the inflamed tissue compartment than they are in the plasma [14, 15] and thus, inhibitors that are given parenterally must be done so in large quantities to reach and saturate all tissue pools. In fact, some inhibitors are sequestered almost entirely in the plasma compartment [16] and may not reach interstitial pools. Finally, exaggerated cytokine production may contribute to pathology in one body compartment while, simultaneously, production in another compartment may actually have beneficial effects. Thus, systemic administration of cytokine inhibitors at levels sufficient to neutralize exaggerated cytokine production in one organ may also block the presumably beneficial aspects of cytokine production in another.

Cytokines in Severe Sepsis and Septic Shock, edited by H. Redl and G. Schlag†
© 1999 Birkhäuser Verlag Basel/Switzerland

To develop an alternative approach for anticytokine therapies in acute inflammation, gene transfer of cytokine inhibitors or the use of catalytic ribozymes directed against pro-inflammatory cytokine mRNA are being considered as a novel drug delivery system. Although gene transfer and transfection studies are being actively pursued for patients with somatic gene disorders, and for modulating the genetic basis of cancer, diabetes, and other chronic diseases (for reviews see [17–19]), gene transfer as an acute therapeutic modality for sepsis, surgical injury, and acute inflammation is clinically not being as actively pursued [20]. However, the capability to deliver cytokine inhibitors or antagonists directly to the local site of inflammation, where exaggerated pro-inflammatory cytokine production is occurring, makes non-stable gene transfer a powerful alternative to systemic administration.

Efforts to accentuate beneficial components of the acute phase or inflammatory response by targeting such organs as the liver with low dose human TNFα, IL-6 or IL-1 (α or β) may present an alternative means to improve outcome to infection/ injury, particularly in models of immune suppression and organ injury. In this manner the utility of gene transfer in clinically relevant models of infection and sepsis is explored. In particular, the advantages of gene transfer as a novel drug delivery system for the treatment of septic shock, multisystem organ failure (MSOF) and inflammatory response syndromes is determined for possible future clinical trials.

Role of pro-inflammatory cytokines in the pathogenesis of sepsis/MSOF

The reported mortality to septic shock varies between 25–50%. Although controversy exists over the frequency and morbidity associated with sepsis and septic shock, there is agreement that the incidence of septic shock is increasing and mortality rates are remaining relatively constant despite marked improvements in antimicrobial therapies and pulmonary and vascular support. Even with constant improvements in supportive care, increases in immuno-compromised diseases like AIDS, as well as the ageing of the population, have resulted in an increased preposition to sepsis and septic shock.

In 1986/87, Beutler et al. demonstrated that overproduction of the pro-inflammatory cytokine, TNFα, was antecedent to shock and death [21–24]. Initial studies demonstrated that the panoply of host responses seen in lethal endotoxemia or Gram-negative bacteremia could be reproduced in healthy animals simply by administering recombinant TNFα. In subsequent studies in mice and *Papio* (baboon), the authors demonstrated that an exaggerated endogenous TNFα response was inhibitable with polyclonal and monoclonal antibodies, and contributed to the mortality associated with endotoxemia and Gram-negative bacteremia [4]. Since 1987, when the studies were first reported, there have been at least 15 studies confirming the central role that TNFα plays in acute Gram-negative bacteremia and endotoxemia (for review see [25]).

Similarly, in 1988, Waage and colleagues [26] and Schreiber et al. [27] each reported that TNFα toxicity could be potentiated by coadministration of either IL-1 or lipopolysaccharide. As early as 1989, Fong et al. [28] reported that blocking an endogenous TNFα response in Gram-negative septic shock with monoclonal antibodies led to an attenuated IL-1 and IL-6 response. In 1991, Ohlssen et al. [11] and subsequently Dinarello et al. [29], Norton et al. [30] and Fisher et al. [10] reported that blocking an endogenous IL-1 response with IL-1 receptor antagonist (IL-1ra) also improved survival and reduced tissue damage associated with lethal Gram-negative bacteremia.

Since then a considerable body of knowledge has developed to explain the mechanism and pathways by which the pro-inflammatory cytokines initiate and propagate shock, tissue damage, and the sepsis syndrome. Investigators have implicated additional pro-inflammatory cytokines in the pathogenesis of overwhelming Gram-negative infections or endotoxemia, including interferon-γ, IL-6, LiF/Factor D and IL-12 [30–32]. Although the role that each of these specific cytokines play in the pathogenesis of septic shock is still being resolved, there is general agreement that endogenous production of TNFα and IL-1 are central to initiating and sustaining the pro-inflammatory cytokine cascade. These two mediators, in particular TNFα, appear very early in the inflammatory response, and their synthesis and release begins within minutes of macrophage activation [33, 34]. The early release to TNFα initiates a subsequent cascade of other cytokines and mediators. When TNFα or IL-1 are inhibited with either antibodies or receptor antagonists, the major components of the inflammatory response are suppressed [24, 34].

It has only been recently recognized that the integrated cytokine response to infection and injury is complex and that ultimately the host response to infection depends not only upon the absolute concentrations of IL-1 and TNFα, but also upon the presence of cytokine inhibitors and anti-inflammatory cytokines. It is now generally accepted that the catastrophic host responses to overwhelming bacterial infections represent an aberrant relationship between pro-inflammatory cytokines, TNFα and IL-1, and their naturally occurring inhibitors. In lethal bacteremia and endotoxemia the concentrations of TNFα and IL-1β in the plasma are far greater than can be neutralized by the corresponding levels of shed TNF receptors (TNFR) (p55 & p75) or IL-1ra [5, 35]ß. Similarly, in ongoing inflammatory processes, such as those which occur in hospitalized patients with systemic inflammatory response syndrome (SIRS) or sepsis syndrome, the mechanisms which ultimately down-regulate pro-inflammatory cytokine release are ineffective. This is due in part to the continued external stimuli which ongoing infectious or inflammatory processes invoke. In such cases repeated or persistent pro-inflammatory cytokine synthesis (TNFα, IL-1) contributes to the hemodynamic instability, coagulopathy, and multi-organ dysfunction that occurs. In both septic shock and SIRS the beneficial aspects of pro-inflammatory cytokine production (including stimulation of non-specific host immunity, increased antigen specific T cell proliferation, macrophage and NK-cell bactericidal capacity) are offset by the adverse consequences of continued exposure to elevated TNFα and IL-1 concentrations.

Successful anticytokine approaches to the treatment of septic shock or sepsis syndrome associated with bacteremia or endotoxemia have been directed at either suppressing the pro-inflammatory cytokine (TNFα or IL-1) response, such as with IL-10 or transforming growth factor β (TGFβ), or blocking TNFα and IL-1 activity with antibodies, or by increasing pharmacologically the levels of cytokine inhibitors with recombinant IL-1ra and soluble TNF receptors. The preclinical rodent and subsequent primate studies which demonstrated efficacy with either antibodies (anti-TNFα mAb) or cytokine inhibitors (IL-1ra or soluble TNF receptors TNFR) in lethal endotoxemia and Gram-negative bacteremia prompted the initiation of clinical trials in patients with sepsis syndrome and shock. The initial promising Phase II report of improved outcome in patients with sepsis syndrome treated with IL-1ra [12] could only be confirmed in the Phase III trials with a subgroup of critically ill patients with predicted mortalities of greater than 24% by APACHE III scores [35]. In fact, clinical trials with IL-1ra have been discontinued, and IL-1ra is no longer under clinical investigation. Beneficial results from the anti-TNFα monoclonal antibody studies have also been conditional. For example, Fisher reported an improvement in outcome only in those patients with detectable plasma TNFα9.

In light of the observation that these clinical studies can only confirm the utility of anticytokine therapies for the treatment of shock and sepsis syndrome in very selected patient populations, interest has focused primarily on identifying prospective patients that may benefit from such therapies. In fact, retrospective analysis of Phase II and III clinical trials with TNFα antibodies and IL-1 inhibitors revealed that only some patient subpopulations benefited from anticytokine therapies, whereas there was a trend towards increased mortality in other patient populations [9, 12, 35]. In particular, anti-IL-1 and anti-TNFα therapies appeared to be most helpful in patients who had organ failure or were already in shock, whereas they were least beneficial (and potentially harzadous) in patients at risk of developing septic shock but not as critically ill.

The inability of these several clinical trials to unequivocally demonstrate efficacy of this novel approach does not indicate a failure of the underlying concept, but rather a failure in its implementation. Such results are not surprising given the fact that cytokines have both concurrent beneficial and pathological roles. In fact, Echtenacher and others demonstrated that blocking an endogenous TNFα response made a non-lethal peritonitis model lethal [36–38]. Similarly, van der Meer and Czyprinski demonstrated that administration of IL-1 improved outcome to a variety of Gram-negative bacterial infections and blocking an endogenous IL-1 response inhibited antimicrobial processes [39–45]. Such results suggest that an endogenous pro-inflammatory cytokine response can have beneficial effects, and efforts to block an endogenous TNFα or IL-1 response may have untoward negative effects.

We believe that identifying the optimal patient population who can benefit from such therapies will only partially address the problems associated with the current approaches for delivering anticytokine therapies. A major difficulty with the current strategy of infusing systemically either inhibitors of IL-1 (IL-1ra) or TNFα (monoclonal antibodies or soluble receptors), or infusing anti-inflammatory mediators (such as glucocorticoids, IL-4, TGFβ, IL-10 or IL-13) is that systemic administration is an imprecise means of directing an anticytokine therapy to individual body compartments where exaggerated production is occurring. Similarly, because such therapies are inherently aimed at blocking cytokines primarily in the vasculature, but also in all organs of the body, they can be potentially hazardous to some patient populations where an organ-specific cytokine production may have beneficial antimicrobial functions.

Systemic administration of cytokine inhibitors may in fact be an inappropriate means to block the paracrine actions of a cytokine. Only recently has a greater appreciation for the paracrine nature of TNFα and IL-1 been recognized. Both IL-1 and TNFα are known to exist in cell-associated forms and retain some biological activity [43, 44]. Ginsberg et al. reported in mice suffering adeno-virus induced hemorrhagic pneumonia, local, but not systemic, production of TNFα and IL-1 [14]. TNFα and IL-1 levels in the lung were often in excess of 10 ng/ml whereas plasma concentrations were less than 50 pg/ml and could not be detected by either immuno-or bioassays. Similarly, in rats expiring from a thermal injury and *Pseudomonas* infection, local, but not systemic, TNFα production was reported [46, 47]. Ulich has reported lung TNFα levels exceeding 10 ng/ml in mice following intratracheal instillation of lipopolysaccharide (LPS) whereas levels in the plasma were less than 100 pg/ml [48, 49]. Similar findings have been seen with patients with ARDS [15, 50]. In such patients, TNFα was recovered from the lungs of patients with ARDS at levels as high as 15 ng/ml, whereas concentrations in the plasma were only 100 pg/ml. Thus, systemic administration of cytokine inhibitors must be given at levels sufficient to block the elevated concentrations in the tissues but not in the plasma compartment. This is exceedingly problematic since anti-TNFα monoclonal antibodies, soluble receptor fusion proteins, and even IL-1ra, are primarily sequestered in the plasma compartment [5, 10, 16, 17].

Systemic administration of cytokine inhibitors is also problematic since the natural antagonists or inhibitors of TNFα and IL-1 often have short biological halflives, ranging from minutes to hours [5, 10]. For example, Fisher et al. reported that in the septic primate, IL-1ra has a biological half-life (beta phase) of approximately 21 minutes [10]. To sustain therapeutic plasma concentrations of 10–15 µg/ml, IL-1ra and soluble TNF receptors have to be given at concentrations of 1.5–2 mg/kg

BW/hr, or approximately 2.5 g/day, for as long as the patient is septic. Such an approach may not be cost-effective. To some extent, these problems have been obviated by the use of antibodies or TNF receptors that are joined to the FC and hinge region of human IgG. These 'Chimeric fusion' proteins have a biological half life of between 20–60 hours [6, 16, 17].

Finally, exaggerated pro-inflammatory cytokine production may contribute to the pathology in one body compartment while, simultaneously, production in another compartment may actually have beneficial effects. There has been little examination into the differential organ response to a variety of lethal and non-lethal infections or inflammation. The implications of these findings are considerable. Systemic administration of cytokine inhibitors at levels sufficient to exit the plasma pool in quantities sufficient to neutralize exaggerated TNFα production in one tissue compartment may also block the presumably beneficial aspects of cytokine production in other tissue compartments. This latter point may explain some of the experimental observations where TNFα inhibition is associated with adverse outcome.

In 1986, Beutler and Cerami characterized TNFα's actions as being two sides of the same coin [51]. Even at that time it was understood that the biological actions of pro-inflammatory cytokines were in general beneficial to the host. Since then, considerable experimental data has arisen to suggest that an endogenous TNFα or IL-1 response is critical to a normal, non-specific host response that serves to reduce the amount of tissue damage and the likelyhood of a secondary bacterial infection. It has been well recognized that endogenous TNFα and IL-1 production contributes to the antimicrobial responses against several intracellular pathogens, such as listeria and pneumocystis [52]. An endogenous TNFα and IL-1 response, particularly in the liver and spleen, are essential to the anti-listerial response. In addition, there is also increasing appreciation of a beneficial role for TNF and IL-1 in the host response to Gram-negative bacterial infections [38, 53]. Dinarello reported that some IL-1 production was critical in newborn rodents [53]. He demonstrated that exaggerated IL-1 production could be lethal as well as an inadequate IL-1 production in a murine model of Gram-negative infection. In two day old rats infected with *Klebsiella*, mortality normally approached 100% and high levels of IL-1 could be documented. When excess quantities of IL-1 were inhibited with low dose IL-1ra, mortality declined to under 20%. However, when rats were treated with sufficient IL-1ra to completely block all of IL-1's actions, mortality increased to nearly 100%. Thus, the findings confirm that some IL-1 production is essential for eliciting an antimicrobial response, but either too much or too little is disadvantageous.

For the reasons described above, we propose that gene transfer of anti-inflammatory cytokines or cytokine inhibitors represents a more efficient means to block pro-inflammatory cytokine action in tissue compartments than does the systemic administration of these same agents.

Use of gene transfer to deliver anticytokine therapies directly to organs and tissues

In the past three years, significant progress has been made in the development of gene therapy. There have been several excellent reviews of the various technologies available for human gene therapy [17–19]. These reviews in general have focused on currently available methods to deliver human genes to distant organs. Invariably, the emphasis of these studies has been to correct germ line abnormalities, such as those associated with the cystic fibrosis transmembrane conductance regulator, ornithine-transcarbamylase, adenosine desaminase, Duchenne type muscular dystrophy, and LDL receptor, among others [18, 19]. Such approaches in general are aimed at either supplanting defective genes, or altering immune cell phenotype. We propose to employ gene transfer as a novel drug delivery system to transiently mitigate the inflammatory response in individual tissues and organs. We believe that coupling gene transfer technologies with surgical intervention and manipulation ultimately offers a unique means to modify the post-surgical and inflammatory response, by either down-regulating inflammatory processes in tissues where exaggerated pro-duction occurs, or in cases where upregulating the inflammatory response may stim-ulate antimicrobial processes. Thus, gene transfer technologies will be an integral component of the surgeon's armament, aimed at modulating wound healing, tissue regeneration, and decreasing inflammatory cell-mediated injury.

The specific goals of gene therapy for sepsis and acute inflammation therefore differ in some important regards from efforts to correct germ-line disorders. Where-as the treatment of such germ-line disorders as adenosine deaminase (ADA) defi-ciency-induced severe combined immune deficiency (SCID) or cystic fibrosis seeks a stable integration of the foreign gene into the target tissue genome [54–60], the goal of gene transfer in sepsis or acute inflammation is a transient, non-stable transfor-mation that results in maximal gene expression lasting days and at most weeks. In the case of downregulating an inflammatory response, stable integration of the gene for an anti-inflammatory cytokine or cytokine inhibitor with a viral promotor-enhancer into the target cell genome could have adverse long lasting effects, includ-ing immune suppression and oncogenesis. Such stable transfections are therefore not desirable. In addition to non-stable transfection, gene therapy approaches in sepsis are aimed at targeting several cell populations simultaneously in a single organ or tissue, such as pulmonary macrophages, or epithelial and endothelial cells in the lung. Under ideal conditions, the target cell population in sepsis is one in which excessive production of the pro-inflammatory cytokines IL-1 and TNFα occurs.

We have considered non-viral methods of gene transfer

Cationic liposomes have often been historically dismissed as an inefficient means of gene transfer *in vivo* [61]. This has been due historically to the relatively low transfection efficiencies that are observed *in vitro* when compared to viral transfection systems [62]. In addition, due to the lack of quality control in liposome preparation and their rapid peroxidation, results have often been unreproducible and, in some cases, liposomes have been directly toxic to some cell populations [62]. The *in vivo* use of liposomes for gene transfer, however, began in earnest after the report of Felgner's group at Syntex in 1987 that liposome-mediated DNA transfection can be simple, inexpensive, reproducible, and more efficient than other commonly employed non-viral techniques [61]. In general, cationic liposome technology has progressed markedly since 1987 when Lipofectin Reagent® [*N*-[1-(2,3,-dioleyloxy) propyl]-*N,N,N*-trimethylammonium chloride] (DOTMA) was first developed [63]. Lipofectin® was cytotoxic to some cell lines and expensive to manufacture. Second generation liposomes were created using mixtures of the cationic lipid (DOTMA) and neutral lipids (usually a variant of dioleyl-L-a-phosphatidyl-ethanolamine DOPE) [64]. With these newer formulations, transfection efficiencies increased to almost 75%, values approaching those seen with viral transfection schemes [64]. Ramila Philip and Robert Debs have also shown that some degree of tissue specific transgene expression can be achieved by varying the composition of the cationic lipid [66–68]. In general, these cationic lipids spontaneously form multilamellar vesicles that can either be used to capture intact DNA, or can be sonicated to form small unilamellar vesicles. DNA interacts spontaneously with solutions of both these vesicles to form lipid:DNA complexes. It is presumed that the ionic interactions occur between the positively charged lipid and the negatively charged phosphate group of the DNA [64].

The positively charged lipid from the liposome interacts not only with the negatively charged DNA but also with negatively charged cell membranes. These liposomes also undergo membrane fusion or transient membrane destabilization with the plasmalemma or endosome in order to achieve delivery of DNA into the cytoplasm while avoiding degradation in the lysosomal compartment. This process is independent of cellular receptors and should be present in most cell types. Once inside the cell, the DNA migrates to the nucleus where, depending upon the presence of *cis* acting sequence elements such as the long terminal repeats (LTR's) of retrovirus, the DNA is either integrated into genomic DNA or is transcribed in an episomal fashion [18]. This migration of transgenic material to the nucleus can be enhanced by coating the DNA with HMG-1, histones that permit more rapid transit through nuclear membrane pores [69].

Conceptually, it is the same whether entry of the DNA is facilitated by viral packaging and binding to specific cellular receptors, as occurs with viral transfection schemes, or endocytosis and plasma membrane interactions, as occurs with liposomes. Once the foreign DNA is incorporated into the cell, transgene expression is driven by additional *cis*-acting regulatory sequences which include transcriptional promoters and enhancers as well as the host cell's RNA polymerase and transcriptional initiation factors. Mammalian transcriptional promoters are required for transcription of sequences within mammalian cells. The choice of transcriptional promoter also determines which RNA polymerase will transcribe the foreign DNA.

Commonly, *in vivo* studies with cationic liposomes have utilised mammalian expression vectors containing the cytomegalovirus (CMV) immediate-early transcriptional promoter and enhancer [65–69]. The CMV promoter is transcribed by RNA polymerase II and has the advantage of directing high levels of expression in a variety of tissues, including lung, kidney and vascular endothelium in most mammalian species [70].

Cationic liposomes and plasmids containing the CMV early promoter and enhancer for transfer of foreign DNA have been reported by Debs, Philip, Felgner and others [65–68]. In studies described by Debs and Philip, cationic liposomes and CMV promoter vectors, which contained reporter genes such as chloramphenicol acetyl transferase (CAT), were administered intravenously, intraperitoneally, and by inhalation to healthy animals. Debs has extensively analyzed the tissues transfected following intravenous administration of liposomes and CMV promoter and enhancer-driven CAT (CMV-CAT) expression vectors. Evidence of CAT expression was documented for up to 63 days following intravenous injection, and CAT activity was present in the lung, spleen, liver, heart, kidney, and lymph nodes, as well as in the thymus, uterus, ovary, skeletal muscle, intestine and colon of transfected mice [65]. The highest CAT expression was observed in lung and spleen when expressed as per mg protein. Immunohistochemistry studies revealed that there were three different cellular patterns of CAT expression following intravenous injection. CAT expression was generalized throughout the lung affecting both endothelial and epithelial cells. However, in the spleen, liver, lymph nodes and bone marrow, CAT expression was limited to extravascular parenchymal cells. Thus, in these tissues, circulating liposome:DNA complexes appeared to readily extravasate across the vascular endothelium. In the heart and kidney, however, CAT expression was limited to mostly endothelial cells with little expression by parenchymal cells. Therefore liposome-directed gene transfer for sepsis will not be limited by the inability to reach target cell populations. In practice, the difficulty will be to direct gene transfer to those cell populations that are responsible for exaggerated proinflammatory cytokine production.

Debs and colleagues also examined CAT expression following inhalation of liposome:CMV-CAT DNA [68]. Inhalation of liposomes complexed to CMV-CAT vectors resulted in high levels of CAT expression in the lungs of the animals for periods up to 21 days. No CAT expression was observed in any other tissue suggesting that uptake of the liposome:DNA mixture was limited to the lung. Using a polyclonal antisera directed against CAT, immunohistochemical analysis of lung sections showed a pattern of diffuse staining for CAT activity that involved both bronchiolar and alveolar components. Bronchiolar epithelium had the highest CAT immunoactivity, but CAT immunoactivity was also recovered from alveolar lining cells.

Table 1 - Survival and peak TNFα concentrations in LPS-D-galN mice pretreated with lipo-somes containing pCMV/p55 or pcD-SR-a/IL-10

Experiment #	pCMV/p55 survived/total	pcD/SR-a/hIL-10 survived/total	relevant DNA/liposomes survived/total
1	4/6	6/6	1/6
2	3/6	4/6	0/6
3	3/6	6/6	1/6
totals	10/18	16/18	2/18
TNFα, pg/ml	2080 ± 810	190 ± 60	2690± 660

Table 2 - Lung TNF and myeloperoxidase levels in mice after intratracheal LPS administration and gene transfer

	pCMV/p55	pcD/SR-a/hIL-1	liposomes	control
TNF/a, pg/g	500 ± 43	146 ± 58	382 ± 66	<100
MPO, U/g	53.2 ± 1.3	26.4 ± 5	58.7 ± 6.2	1.7 ± 1.7

Targeting gene transfer to the kidney has also been accomplished. Isaka and colleagues infused liposomes and coding sequences for human TGFβ into the renal artery of mice with genetic susceptibility to lupus and recovered immune reactive human TGFβ from the kidney [71]. TGFβ activity was not recovered from the contralateral kidney or any other tissue suggesting that targeted expression is feasible by regional iv. administration. Furthermore, with the increasing understanding of the immunological and genetic basis of carcinogenesis, gene transfer is also becoming a valid option for cancer therapy [72].

We conducted over the past years several gene therapy studies in murine models with septic shock and acute inflammation. To evaluate whether gene therapy aimed at inhibiting an endogenous TNF response could improve outcome in a model of more direct TNF dependence, gene therapy was employed prior to lethal LPS D-galactosamine [73]. 48 h after gene transfer, mice were injected intraperitoneally with 250 ng LPS and 18 mg D-GalN. Lethality in this LPS-D-GalN model has been previously shown to be more dependent on an exaggerated TNFα response, since treatment of mice with TNF receptor immunoadhesins or the use of TNF receptor (p55)-deficient mice results in reduced mortality. Our results from three separate experiments demonstrated that gene transfer with either IL-10 or p55 improves sur-

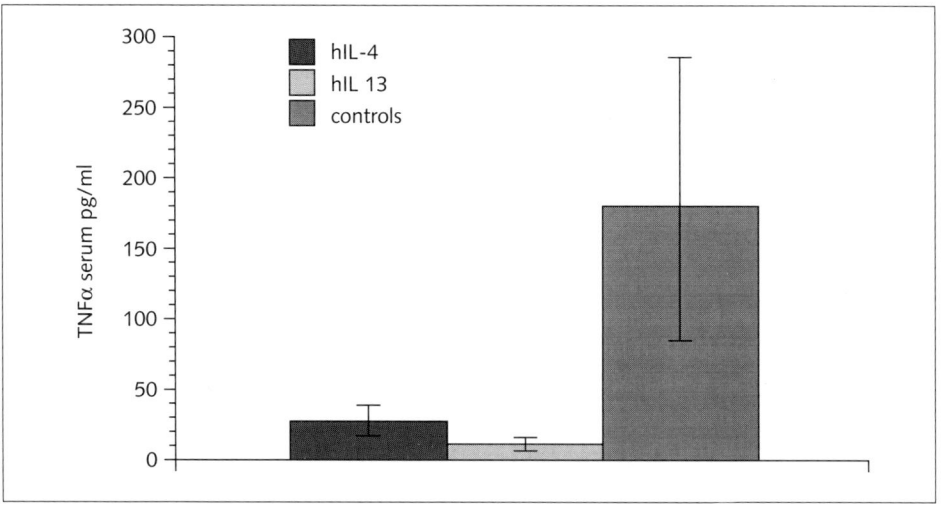

Figure 1

TNFα immunoactivity in the serum (pg/ml) from mice 90 min after challenge with a lethal experimental septic shock. 2 days prior to induction of septic shock, the mice were transfected intraperitoneally with 200 μg pcD hIL-4, 200 μg pJFE14 hIL-13 or 200 μg pMP6 complexed to 100 nmol DDAB:DOPE cationic liposomes. The results represent the average of three different experiments with six mice per group in each experiment. Mice pretreated with hIL-4 or hIL-13 display a down regulation of TNFα response to a lethal LPS-D-GalN challenge, p < 0.05.

vival (Tab. 1). In additional studies, intratracheal administration of IL-10 DNA-liposome complexes 48 h before an intratracheal LPS challenge reduced pulmonary TNFα levels by 62% and decreased neutrophil infiltration in the lung by 55% as measured by myeloperoxidase activity (both p < 0.05). This effect was not seen with the p55 gene transfer (Tab. 2). In retrospect, it is not surprising that gene transfer with p55 was less effective than IL-10 after i.p. and intratracheal LPS challenge, given the magnitude of TNFα response. In contrast to transfection with the modified p55, the increased effectiveness of IL-10 gene transfer highlights a therapeutic advantage associated with cytokines that directly inhibit pro-inflammatory cytokine production rather than competing for ligand binding.

These results encouraged us to consequently perform another study with other anti-inflammatory cytokines, namely IL-4 and IL-13 [74]. Gene transfer with hIL-4 reduced the serum TNFα production in response to endotoxin/D-GalN by 80% from 113.1 pg/ml in mock-transfected animals to 22.2 pg/ml (p < 0.05), whereas human IL-13 gene transfer reduced serum TNFα levels by 90% (113.1 pg/ml to 11.6 pg/ml; p < 0.05) (Fig. 1). Survival was improved from 20% to over 83% in

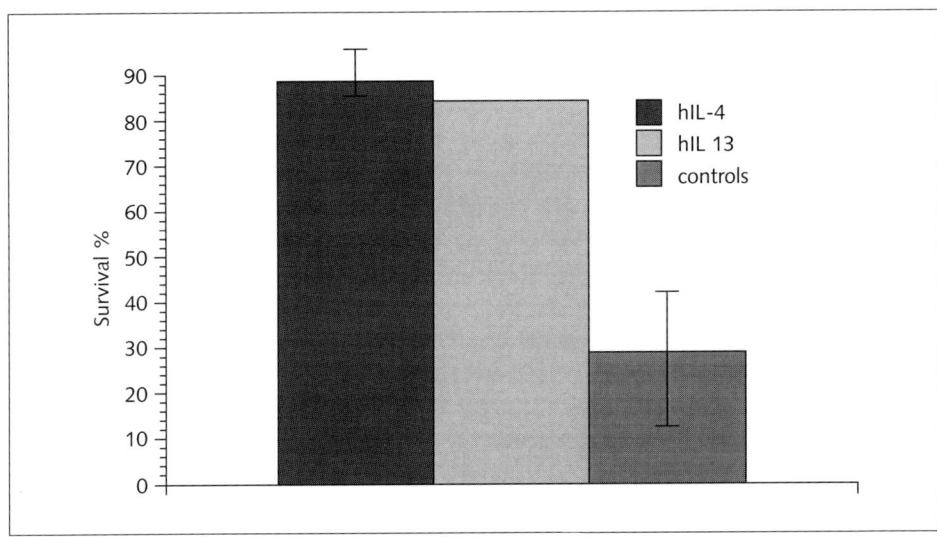

Figure 2
48 h survival of mice challenged with a lethal experimental septic shock. 2 days prior to induction of septic shock, the mice were transfected interperitoneally with 200 μg pcD hIL-4, 200 μg pJFE14 hIL-13 or 200 μg pMP6 complexed to 100 nmol DDAB:DOPE cationic liposomes. The results represent the average of three different experiments with six mice per group in each experiment. Mice pretreated with hIL-4 or hIL-13 demonstrated a significant improve in survival, p < 0.001.

both treatment groups (p < 0.001) (Fig. 2). Our data demonstrate a potent *in vivo* anti-inflammatory action of both IL-4 and IL-13. In addition the immune functions of peritoneal macrophages are significantly ameliorated in both treatment groups, herein IL-13 demonstrates a better macrophage immune modulation than IL-4 (p < 0.05) (Fig. 3).

Our results underscore several advantages for the use of gene transfer as a treatment option for septic shock or other acute inflammatory episodes. First, the specificity of targeting inhibitors to specific organs is greatly increased. Second, the gene transfer scheme permits a continued expression of these inhibitors for several days, allowing for prolonged delivery of a short lived antagonist. However, since the gene transfer is ultimately transient and the plasmid DNA remains episomal, expression efficiencies decline after 48 hours [66]. Therefore, the risk of a stable transfection and incorporation of a gene for a potentially immunosuppressive agent under a constitutive promoter is remote. Finally, local cytokine inhibitors or antagonists can be directed away from organs where the putative beneficial effects of pro-inflammatory cytokines are occurring.

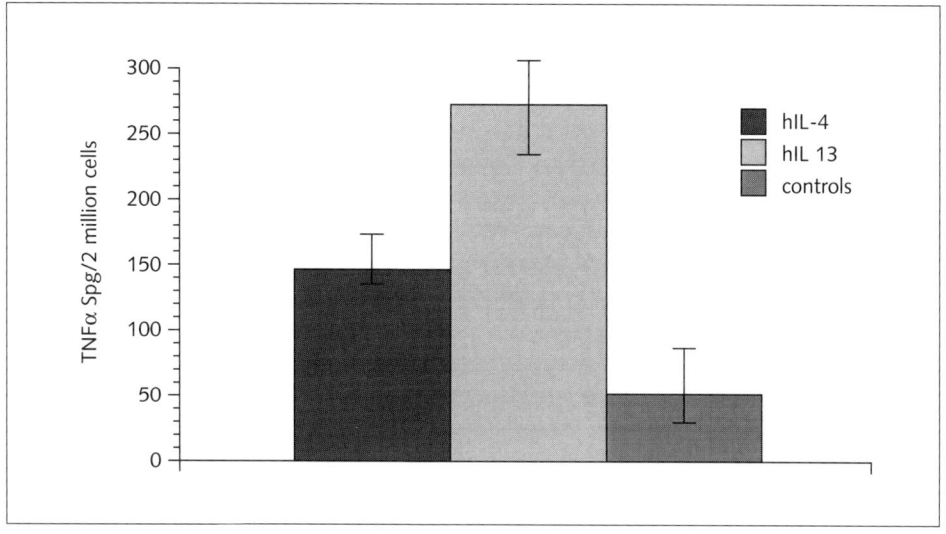

Figure 3
TNFα secretion by primary cultures of peritoneal macrophages from mice 48 h after challenge with a lethal experimental septic shock. 2 days prior to induction of septic shock, the mice were transfected intraperitoneally with 200 μg pcD hIL-4, 200 μg pJFE14 hIL-13 or 200 μg pMP6 complexed to 100 nmol DDAB:DOPE cationic liposomes. 48 h after challenge with septic shock, peritoneal macrophages were isolated from sunivors. 2×10^6 macrophages in 1 ml complete medium were plated into 6 well microtiter plates at 37° C in 5% CO_2. 90 min later, the cells were washed and adherent cells were cultured further in 1 ml complete medium containing 1 μg LPS. 18 h later the supernatants were aspired and analyzed for TNFα immunoactivity by ELISA. Surviving mice pretreated with hIL-4 or hIL-13 respond more potent than controls, $p < 0.01$.

References

1   Bone RC (1991) The pathogenesis of sepsis. *Ann Intern Med* 115: 457–469
2   Fong Y, Moldawer LL, Shires GT, Lowry SF (1990) The biologic characteristics of cytokines and their implication in surgical injury. *Surg Gynecol Obstet* 170: 363–378
3   Hinshaw LB, Tekamp Olson P, Chang AC, Lee PA, Taylor FB Jr, Murray CK, Peer GT, Emerson TE Jr, Passey RB, Kuo GC (1990) Survival of primates in LD100 septic shock following therapy with antibody to tumor necrosis factor (TNF alpha). *Circ Shock* 30: 279–292
4   Tracey KJ, Fong Y, Hesse DG, Manogue KR, Lee AT, Kuo GC, Lowry SF, Cerami A (1987) Anti-cachectin/TNF monoclonal antibodies prevent septic shock during lethal bacteraemia. *Nature* 330: 662–664

5   Van Zee KJ, Kohno T, Fischer E, Rock CS, Moldawer LL, Lowry SF (1992) Tumor necrosis factor soluble receptors circulate during experimental and clinical inflammation and can protect against excessive tumor necrosis factor alpha *in vitro* and *in vivo*. *Proc Natl Acad Sci USA* 89: 4845–4849

6   Lesslauer W, Tabuchi H, Gentz R, Brockhaus M, Schlaeger EJ, Grau G, Piguet PF, Pointaire P, Vassalli P, Loetscher H (1991) Recombinant soluble tumor necrosis factor receptor proteins protect mice from lipopolysaccharide-induced lethality. *Eur J Immunol* 21: 2883–2886

7   Howard M, Muchamuel T, Andrade S, Menon S (1993) Interleukin 10 protects mice from lethal endotoxemia. *J Exp Med* 177: 1205–1208

8   Gerard C, Bruyns C, Marchant A, Abramowicz D, Vandenabeele P, Delvaux A, Fiers W, Goldman M, Velu T (1993) Interleukin 10 reduces the release of tumor necrosis factor and prevents lethality in experimental endotoxemia. *J Exp Med* 177: 547–550

9   Fisher CJ Jr, Opal SM, Dhainaut JF, Stephens S, Zimmerman JL, Nightingale P, Harris SJ, Schein RM, Panacek EA, Vincent JL et al (1993) Influence of an anti-tumor necrosis factor monoclonal antibody on cytokine levels in patients with sepsis The CB0006 Sepsis Syndrome Study Group [see comments]. *Crit Care Med* 21: 318–327

10   Fischer E, Marano MA, Van Zee KJ, Rock CS, Hawes AS, Thompson WA, DeForge L, Kenney JS, Remick DG, Bloedow DC et al (1992) Interleukin-1 receptor blockade improves survival and hemodynamic performance in *Escherichia coli* septic shock but fails to alter host responses to sublethal endotoxemia. *J Clin Invest* 89: 1551–1557

11   Ohlsson K, Bjork P, Bergenfeldt M, Hageman R, Thompson RC (1990) Interleukin-1 receptor antagonist reduces mortality from endotoxin shock. *Nature* 348: 550–552

12   Fisher CJ Jr, Slotman GJ, Opal SM, Pribble JP, Bone RC, Emmanuel G, Ng D, Bloedow DC, Catalano MC et al (1994) IL-1ra Sepsis Syndrome Study Group Initial evaluation of human recombinant interleukin-1 receptor antagonist in the treatment of sepsis syndrome A rnadomized open-label, placebo-controlled multicenter trial. *Crit Care Med* 22: 12–21

13   Fischer E, Marano MA, Barber AE, Hudson A, Lee K, Rock CS, Hawes AS, Anderson TD, Benjamin WR, Lowry SF, Moldawer LL (1991) Comparison between effects of interleukin-1alpha administration and sublethal endotoxemia in primates. *Am J Physiol* 261: R442–R452

14   Ginsberg HS, Moldawer LL, Sehgal PB, Redington M, Kilian PL, Chanock RM, Prince GA (1991) A mouse model for investigating the molecular pathogenesis of adenovirus pneumonia. *Proc Natl Acad Sci USA* 88: 1651–1655

15   Suter PM, Suter S, Girardin E, Roux Lombard P, Grau GE, Dayer JM (1992) High bronchoalveolar levels of tumor necrosis factor and its inhibitors interleukin-1 interferon and elastase, in patients with adult respiratory distress syndrome after trauma, shock, or sepsis. *Am Rev Respir Dis* 145: 1016–1022

16   Ashkenazi A, Marsters SA, Capon DJ, Chamow SM, Figari IS, Pennica D, Goeddel DV, Palladino MA, Smith DH (1991) Protection against endotoxic shock by a tumor necrosis factor receptor immunoadhesin. *Proc Natl Acad Sci USA* 88: 10535–10539

17   Anderson WF(1992) Human gene therapy. *Science* 256: 808–813

18   Mulligan RC (1993) The basic science of gene therapy. *Science* 260: 926–932

19   Morsy MA, Mitani K, Clemens P, Caskey T (1993) Progress toward human gene therapy. *JAMA* 270, No 19: 2338–2345

20   Rogy MA, Lutge B, Espat NJ Copeland, EM Moldawer, LL (1994) Human TNF receptor and Interleukin-10 gene transfer in the mouse reduces mortality to lethal endotoxemia. *Surgical Forum* XLV: 21–23

21   Tracey KJ, Wei H, Manogue KR, Fong Y, Hesse DG, Nguyen HT, Kuo GC, Beutler B, Cotran RS, Cerami A et al (1988) Cachectin/tumor necrosis factor induces cachexia, anemia and inflammation. *J Exp Med* 167: 1211–1227

22   Tracey KJ, Lowry SF, Fahey TJ, Albert JD, Fong Y, Hesse D, Beutler B, Manogue KR, Calvano S, Wei H et al (1987) Cachectin/tumor necrosis factor induces lethal shock and stress hormone responses in the dog. *Surg Gynecol Obstet* 164: 415–422

23   Beutler B, Krochin N, Milsark IW, Luedke C, Cerami A Control of cachectin (tumor necrosis factor) synthesis: mechanisms of endotoxin resistance. *Science* 232: 977–980 1986

24   Cerami A (1993) Tumor necrosis factor as a mediator of shock, cachexia and inflammation. *Blood Purif* 11: 108–117

25   Bone RC (1993) Monoclonal antibodies to tumor necrosis factor in sepsis: help or harm? [editorial; comment]. *Crit Care Med* 21: 311–312

26   Waage A, Espevik T (1988) Interleukin 1 potentiates the lethal effect of tumor necrosis factor alpha/cachectin in mice. *J Exp Med* 167: 1987–1992

27   Rothstein JL, Schreiber H (1988) Synergy between tumor necrosis factor and bacterial products causes hemorrhagic necrosis and lethal shock in normal mice. *Proc Natl Acad Sci USA* 85: 607–611

28   Fong Y, Tracey KJ, Moldawer LL, Hesse DG, Manogue KB, Kenney JS, Lee AT, Kuo GC, Allison AC, Lowry SF et al (1989) Antibodies to cachectin/tumor necrosis factor reduce interleukin 1 beta and interleukin 6 appearance during lethal bacteremia. *J Exp Med* 170: 1627–1633

29   Wakabayashi G, Gelfand JA, Burke JF, Thompson RC, Dinarello CA (1991) A specific receptor antagonist for interleukin 1 prevents *Escherichia coli*-induced shock in rabbits. *FASEB J* 5: 338–343

30   Alexander HR, Doherty GM, Venzon DJ, Merino MJ, Fraker DL, Norton JA (1992) Recombinant interleukin-1 receptor antagonist (IL-1ra): effective therapy against gram-negative sepsis in rats. *Surgery* 112: 188–193

31   Block MI, Berg M, McNamara MJ, Norton JA, Fraker DL, Alexander HR (1993) Passive immunization of mice against D factor blocks lethality and cytokine release during endotoxemia. *J Exp Med* 178: 1085–1090

32   Beutler BA, Milsark IW, Cerami A (1985) Cachectin/tumor necrosis factor: production, distribution and metabolic fate *in vivo*. *J Immunol* 135: 3972–3977

33   Granowitz EV, Vannier E, Poutsiaka DD, Dinarello CA (1992) Effect of interleukin-1

(IL-1) blockade on cytokine synthesis: II IL-1 receptor antagonist inhibits lipopolysaccharide-induced cytokine synthesis by human monocytes. *Blood* 79: 2364–2369

34   Fischer E, Van Zee KJ, Marano MA, Rock CS, Kenney JS, Poutsiaka DD, Dinarello CA, Lowry SF, Moldawer LL (1992) Interleukin-1 receptor antagonist circulates in experimental inflammation and in human disease. *Blood* 79: 2196–2200

35   Fisher CJ Jr, Dhainaut J-FA, Opal SM, Pribble JP, Balk RA, Slotman GJ, Iberti TJ, Rackow EC, Shapiro MJ, Greenman RL, Reines HD, Shelly MP, Thompson BW, LaBrecque JF, Catalano MA, Knaus WA, Sadoff JC (1994) Recombinant human interleukin 1 receptor antagonist in the treatment of patients with sepsis syndrome: Results from a randomized, double-blind, placebo-controlled trial. *JAMA* 271: 1836–1843

36   Echtenacher B, Falk W, Mannel DN, Krammer PH (1990) Requirement of endogenous tumor necrosis factor/cachectin for recovery from experimental peritonitis. *J Immunol* 145: 3762–3766

37   Kenefick KB, Adams JL, Steinberg H, Czuprynski CJ (1994) *In vivo* administration of a monoclonal antibody against the type I IL-1 receptor inhibits the ability of mice to eliminate Mycobacterium paratuberculosis. *J Leukocyte Biol* 55: 719–722

38   Haak Frendscho M, Kurtz RS, Czuprynski CJ (1991) rIL-1 alpha enhances adoptive transfer of resistance to Listeria monocytogenes infection. *Microb Pathog* 10: 385–392

39   Czuprynski CJ, Haak Frendscho M, Maroushek N, Brown JF (1992) Effects of recombinant human interleukin-6 alone and in combination with recombinant interleukin-1 alpha and tumor necrosis factor alpha on antibacterial resistance in mice. *Antimicrob Agents Chemother* 36: 68–70

40   Roll JT, Young KM, Kurtz RS, Czuprynski CJ (1990) Human rTNF alpha augments anti-bacterial resistance in mice: potentiation of its effects by recombinant human rIL-1 alpha. *Immunology* 69: 316–322

41   van der Meer JW, Vogels M, Curfs JH, Eling WM (1993) Interleukin-1 as a possible agent for treatment of infection. *Eur J Clin Microbiol Infect Dis* 12 Suppl 1: S73–S77

42   van der Meer JW, Helle M, Aarden L (1989) Comparison of the effects of recombinant interleukin 6 and recombinant interleukin 1 on nonspecific resistance to infection. *Eur J Immunol* 19: 413–416

43   Perez C, Albert I, DeFay K, Zachariades N, Gooding L, Kriegler M (1990) A nonsecretable cell surface mutant of tumor necrosis factor (TNF) kills by cell-to-cell contact. *Cell* 63: 251–258

44   Kriegler M, Perez C, DeFay K, Albert I, Lu SD (1988) A novel form of TNF/cachectin is a cell surface cytotoxic transmembrane protein: ramifications for the complex physiology of TNF. *Cell* 53: 45–53

45   Mathison JC, Wolfson E, Ulevitch RJ (1988) Participation of tumor necrosis factor in the mediation of gram negative bacterial lipopolysaccharide-induced injury in rabbits. *J Clin Invest* 81: 1925–1937

46   Marano MA, Moldawer LL, Fong Y, Wei H, Minei J, Yurt R, Cerami A, Lowry SF (1988) Cachectin/TNF production in experimental burns and Pseudomonas infection. *Arch Surg* 123: 1383–1388

47   Keogh C, Fong Y, Marano MA, Seniuk S, He W, Barber A, Minei JP, Felsen D, Lowry SF, Moldawer LL (1990) Identification of a novel tumor necrosis factor alpha/cachectin from the livers of burned and infected rats. *Arch Surg* 125: 79–84

48   Ulich TR, Guo K, del Castillo J (1989) Endotoxin-induced cytokine gene expression *in vivo*. I Expression of tumor necrosis factor mRNA in visceral organs under physiologic conditions and during endotoxemia. *Am J Pathol* 134: 11–14

49   Ernsberger U, Sendtner M, Rohrer H (1989) Proliferation and differentiation of embryonic chick sympathetic neurons: effects of ciliary neurotrophic factor. *Neuron* 2: 1275–1284

50   Hyers TM, Tricomi SM, Dettenmeier PA, Fowler AA (1991) Tumor necrosis factor levels in serum and bronchoalveolar lavage fluid of patients with the adult respiratory distress syndrome. *Am Rev Respir Dis* 144: 268–271

51   Beutler B, Cerami A (1986) Cachectin and tumour necrosis factor as two sides of the same biological coin. *Nature* 320: 584–588

52   Rothe J, Lesslauer W, Lotscher H, Lang Y, Koebel P, Kontgen F, Althage A, Zinkernagel R, Steinmetz M, Bluethmann H (1993) Mice lacking the tumour necrosis factor receptor 1 are resistant to TNF-mediated toxicity but highly susceptible to infection by Listeria monocytogenes. *Nature* 364: 798–802

53   Mancilla J, Garcia P, Dinarello CA (1993) The interleukin-1 receptor antagonist can either reduce or enhance the lethality of Klebsiella pneumoniae sepsis in newborn rats. *Infect Immun* 61: 926–932

54   Cournoyer D, Caskey CT (1993) Gene therapy of the immune system. *Annu Rev Immunol* 11: 297–329

55   Salmons B, Gunzburg WH (1993) Targeting of retroviral vectors for gene therapy. *Hum Gene Ther* 4: 129–141

56   Roe T, Reynolds TC, Yu G, Brown PO (1993) Integration of murine leukemia virus DNA depends on mitosis. *EMBO J* 12: 2099–2108

57   Ellison V, Abrams H, Roe T, Lifson J, Brown P (1990) Human immunodeficiency virus integration in a cell-free system. *J Virol* 64: 2711–2715

58   Donahue RE, Kessler SW, Bodine D, McDonagh K, Dunbar C, Goodman S, Agricola B, Byrne E, Raffeld M, Moen R et al (1992) Helper virus induced T cell lymphoma in non-human primates after retroviral mediated gene transfer. *J Exp Med* 176: 1125–1135

59   Kotin RM, Siniscalco M, Samulski RJ, Zhu XD, Hunter L, Laughlin CA, McLaughlin S, Muzyczka N, Rocchi M, Berns KI (1990) Site-specific integration by adeno-associated virus. *Proc Natl Acad Sci USA* 87: 2211–2215

60   Rosenfeld MA, Siegfried W, Yoshimura K, Yoneyama K, Fukayama M, Stier LE, Paakko PK, Gilardi P, Stratford-Perricaudet LD, Perricaudet M, Jallat S, Pavirani A, Lecocq JP, Crystal RG (1991) Adenovirus-Mediated Transfer of a Recombinant 1-Antitrypsin Gene to the Lung Epithelium in Vivo. *Science* 252: 431–434

61   Felgner PL, Gadek TR, Holm M, Roman R, Chan HW, Wenz M, Northrop JP, Ringold GM, Danielson M (1987) Lipofection: A highly efficient, lipid-mediated DNA-transfection procedure. *Proc Natl Acad Sci USA* 84: 7413–7417

62 Felgner PL, Ringold GM (1989) Cationic liposome-mediated transfection. *Nature* 337: 387–388

63 Felgner PL, Rhodes G (1991) Gene therapeutics. *Nature* 349: 351–352

64 Felgner JH, Kumar R, Sridhar CN, Wheeler CJ, Tsai YJ, Border R, Ramsey P, Martin M, Felgner PL (1994) Enhanced gene delivery and mechanism studies with a novel series of cationic lipid formulations. *J Biol Chem* 269: 2550–2561

65 Zhu N, Liggitt D, Liu Y, Debs R (1993) Systemic gene expression after intravenous DNA delivery into adult mice. *Science* 261: 209–211

66 Philip R, Liggitt D, Philip M, Dazin P, Debs R (1993) *In vivo* gene delivery Efficient transfection of T lymphocytes in adult mice. *J Biol Chem* 268: 16087–16090

67 Debs R, Pian M, Gaensler K, Clements J, Friend DS, Dobbs L (1992) Prolonged transgene expression in rodent lung cells. *Am J Respir Cell Mol Biol* 7: 406–413

68 Stribling R, Brunette E, Liggitt D, Gaensler K, Debs R (1992) Aerosol gene delivery *in vivo*. *Proc Natl Acad Sci USA* 89: 11277–11281

69 Kaneda Y, Kunimitsu I, Uchida T (1989) Increased Expression of DNA Cointroduced with Nuclear Protein in Adult Rat Liver. *Science* 243: 375–378

70 Schmidt E, Christoph G, Zeller R, Leder P (1990) Cytomegalovirus enhancer: a pan-active control element in transgenic mice. *Mol Cell Biol* 10: 4406–4411

71 Isaka Y, Fujiwara Y, Ueda N, Kaneda Y, Kamada T, Imai E (1993) Glomerulosclerosis Induced by *in vivo* transfection of transforming growth factor-B or platelet-derived growth factor gene into the rat kidney. *J Clin Invest* 92: 2597–2601

72 Rogy MA, Baumhofer JM, Beinhauer BG, Brandmeier H, Eisenburger P, Losert UM, Philip R (1996) Gene therapy in surgery. Part I: Methods for gene transfer-application to cancer. *Act Chir Austriaca* 28: 358–361

73 Rogy MA, Auffenberg T, Espat NJ, Philip R, Remick D, Wollenberg GK, Copeland EM, Moldawer LL (1995) Human tumor necrosis factor receptor p55 and IL-10 gene transfer in the mouse reduces mortality to lethal endotoxemia and also attenuates local inflammatory responses. *J Exp Med* 181: 2289–2293

74 Baumhofer JM, Beinhauer BG, Wang JE, Brandmeier H, Geissler K, Losert UM, Philip R, Aversa G, Rogy MA (1998) Gene transfer with IL-4 and IL-13 improves survival in lethal endotoxemia in the mouse and ameliorates peritoneal macrophage immune competence. *Eur J Immunol* 28: 610–615

The failure of clinical trials in sepsis: Challenges of pre-clinical models

David Creery and John C. Marshall

Critical Care Medicine Programme, University of Toronto, Department of Critical Care Medicine, Hospital for Sick Children and Toronto Hospital, 200 Elizabeth Street, Toronto, Ontario, Canada M5G 2C4

Introduction

Perhaps no clinical problem lacking effective therapy has been as extensively studied as sepsis. A MEDLINE search under the MESH heading, "sepsis", currently yields more than 35,000 references, including *in vitro* studies, *in vivo* animal studies, and human clinical trials. To date, no effective mediator-directed therapy is available. Promising compounds, with impressive preclinical efficacy and preliminary human benefit in phase II studies, have failed to improve outcome in well-conducted phase III randomized, controlled trials. The potential reasons for these disappointing results are many [1–4]. An important factor has been the applicability of inferences drawn from pre-clinical studies.

In sepsis research, as in biomedical research in general, differing experimental approaches address different scientific objectives. *In vitro* models permit the maximal control over experimental conditions, and therefore are the optimal models for defining biological mechanisms. Pre-clinical studies, usually using an animal model, can show that a biological process produces a physiological effect *in vivo*. Finally, clinical studies in humans are needed to show that a physiological effect observed in an animal model leads to clinical benefit. Although it is relatively easy to design an animal study so that an effect is seen, demonstration of activity in a pre-clinical model does not reliably predict efficacy in humans.

Pre-clinical studies of novel approaches to modulating the host response in sepsis commonly use animals, although endotoxin has been administered to human volunteers to measure the physiological consequences of mediator manipulation. The ideal animal model of sepsis would be one that closely mimics the natural history of the septic response in humans. Given the heterogeneity of patients enrolled in human sepsis trials, such a model clearly does not exist. A novel therapy, therefore, should be subjected to a series of pre-clinical analyses, using different model systems, before human studies are undertaken. The strengths and limitations of each animal model must be considered in extrapolating the experimental results of mediator-directed therapies to human clinical trials. Indeed it can be argued that one of the major conceptual challenges facing sepsis research is not so much finding an animal model that mirrors human disease, but rather identifying and studying homogeneous human diseases that mirror specific animal models.

This chapter will explore the reasons that efficacy in animal models has not been successfully translated into improvements in clinical outcome. Wichterman and colleagues published the first review of animal models of sepsis in 1980 [5]; since then, a number of excellent reviews have appeared [6, 7].

Heterogeneity of outcomes in pre-clinical studies

While it is relatively easy to establish experimental conditions in a pre-clinical model so that an effect – usually a change in mortality – is observed, it is apparent that the direction of that effect can vary with the specific model employed. For example, murine studies evaluating the role of interleukin 10 (IL-10) have generally shown that IL-10 exerts beneficial effects in models of endotoxicosis [8, 9], but detrimental effects when the experimental challenge is a live organism [10–12]. Yet the conclusion that IL-10 is detrimental in the setting of uncontrolled infection is probably simplistic, since administration of IL-10 appears to improve outcome following cecal ligation and puncture [13, 14]. Similarly, the most compelling evidence of benefit for neutralization of tumor necrosis factor (TNF) comes from studies in which the experimental challenge was systemic endotoxin [15]. When the model involves challenge with viable microorganisms in the mouse, blockade of TNF may variously be beneficial [16, 17], detrimental [18, 19], or ineffectual [20]. In a more complex model such as cecal ligation and puncture, blockade of TNF has been shown to result in benefit [21], harm [22], or neither [20].

Although pre-clinical studies can show striking evidence of *in vivo* benefit, the heterogeneity of responses resulting from the experimental model employed makes it difficult to extrapolate the results of animal models to potential benefit in humans. Conversely, however, the heterogeneity of patient populations enrolled in sepsis trials is reproduced by the heterogeneity of responses seen in animal studies. A systematic understanding of the basis for heterogeneity in clinical trials may permit better definition of patient populations likely to benefit from specific therapies. Thus an analysis of the limitations of animal models may shed light on approaches to make the clinical studies better resemble the pre-clinical models.

Sources of variability in pre-clinical models

Species variability in the response to experimental challenge

Although humans share upwards of 98% of our genetic makeup with other mammalian species, the differences between humans and other animals, or even between rodent species, can exert a profound impact on the response to infectious challenge. For example, human dendritic cells are stimulated by lipopolysaccharide (LPS) or TNF to express antigens on their surface, and are unable to process antigens encountered subsequently. Murine dendritic cells, on the other hand, can continue to process subsequently encountered antigens; thus dendritic cell function will be significantly different in humans than in mice when antigen is encountered in an environment that contains TNF or LPS [23]. Mice have lower numbers of circulating neutrophils than do humans, and their neutrophils are functionally different. L-selectin on human neutrophils binds to E-selectin, while mouse L-selectin does not [24]. Mouse neutrophils lack the endotoxin-neutralizing protein, bactericidal/permeability increasing protein (BPI), whereas human neutrophils express it. Mice manifest a more marked TH1/TH2 polarization than do humans; indeed it remains controversial whether this dichotomy is present in human lymphocytes. Finally, TNF inhibits IL-10 production in mice, but stimulates it in humans. Thus there are multiple, often subtle, differences in immune physiology between mice and humans that may have an important bearing on the application of data from murine models to the treatment of human disease.

At the level of the whole organism, there are significant interspecies differences in sensitivity to endotoxin. Murine species vary considerably in the ability of their monocytes to produce TNF in response to endotoxin, and certain strains, notably the C3H HeJ strain, are resistant to large doses of endotoxin [25]. Interestingly, C3H HeJ mice are exquisitely sensitive to lethality induced by infusion of the parent *E. coli* from which the endotoxin was purified [26]. Endotoxin sensitivity in the mouse can be increased through the use of adjuvants such as D-galactosamine [27]. However, although D-galactosamine markedly reduces the lethal dose of endotoxin in mice, it changes the mode of death, inducing fulminant hepatic necrosis. Other adjuvants such as carrageenan, lead acetate, and beryllium phosphate may similarly alter the physiological derangements leading to death.

Endotoxin sensitivity varies significantly between differing animal species [28]. Both rats and dogs are relatively resistant to endotoxin; rabbits, on the other hand, are quite sensitive. Pigs are sensitive to endotoxin, and resemble humans in their physiological responses to an infectious challenge, but are relatively expensive, and difficult to maintain in a chronically instrumented state. Sheep are docile, and exquisitely sensitive to endotoxin, and develop patterns of organ dysfunction that approximate those seen in human sepsis, but are expensive to purchase and maintain. Baboons, although more genetically similar to humans than non-primates, manifest a much greater degree of endotoxin resistance. Moreover, the pedigree of baboons and other primates is often uncertain, and animals may have previously been used in other studies that alter their responsiveness to *de novo* infectious challenge. Rabbits are sensitive to endotoxin, and relatively inexpensive, however their gut flora, unlike that of humans, is dominated by Gram-positive organisms.

335

Genetic variability in the response to challenge

There is an increasing awareness that the response to infectious challenge in humans is strongly influenced by genetic factors [29, 30]. Genetic variability in responsiveness similarly has an important effect on responses in experimental animals. The Balb/c mouse has been a popular strain for experimental purposes, since the animals are docile and have large spleens; of 22 reports on the role of IL-10 in experimental sepsis published through 1997, 14 used Balb/c mice. However Balb/c mice develop a predominantly TH2 type of response to immune stimulation. In contrast, the more aggressive C57bl/6 strain mounts a TH2 type of response [31].

Most commercially available laboratory mice are derived from a limited genetic pool, permitting careful control of their responses to challenge, and minimizing inter-animal variability. However, this homogeneity may limit the extrapolation of findings in one species to animals of different genetic backgrounds. In fact, the availability of rodent strains with characterized genetic defects has proven invaluable in the study of the pathogenesis of a variety of disease processes. The C3H/HeJ mouse differs at a single locus from the C3H/HeN strain, yet this difference in a single gene of as yet undetermined function confers endotoxin resistance on the HeJ animals [32]. Evaluation of differential responses between these two congenic strains has provided important insights into the role of endotoxin in a variety of physiological and pathological processes [33, 34]. Mice of the lpr strain lack the cell surface receptor, Fas, whose engagement triggers apoptosis; gld mice lack Fas ligand expression, and are susceptible to the development of inflammation at normally privileged sites [35]. The SCID mouse can be reconstituted with human bone marrow, and is an attractive model for studying human immune function. However, only 10% of bone marrow cells engraft in the SCID mouse model, and 95% of circulating lymphocytes are CD8+ cells, limiting the applicability of the model for studies in which CD4+ cells play an important role.

The development of techniques to delete specific genes in murine embryonic stem cells has permitted the generation of knockout mouse strains that lack a single gene product [36]. Mice lacking the p55 receptor for TNF, for example, demonstrate resistance to endotoxin challenge, but enhanced susceptibility to infection with pathogens such as *Listeria* [37]. While knockout mice provide insights into the *in vivo* function of a particular protein, these observations must be interpreted with caution, since deletion of a given gene may result in upregulation of another [38]. Refinements of knockout technology permit the study of the role of genes whose deletion during embryological development would otherwise be lethal, or whose function might be compensated for by overexpression of other genes. For example, mice can be generated that have a tetracycline-dependent promotor region for the target gene. Withdrawal of tetracycline results in cessation of expression of the gene of interest. Similarly, tissue-specific gene deletion has become possible [39].

The availability of mouse strains with well-characterized abnormalities in the function of key components of the immune response has contributed significantly to our understanding of the biology of inflammation. On the other hand, the same defects limit the generalizability of these observations to the understanding of a complex process such as human sepsis.

Differential responses to differing challenges

As discussed earlier, the response to mediator manipulation in rodent models is highly dependent on the nature of the experimental challenge, and a single intervention may result in either benefit or harm. Overexpression of the IL-1ra gene, for example, results in protection against endotoxin, but increased susceptibility to Listeria [40].

However, the dichotomy in responsiveness is not simply a consequence of differential responses to live organisms or microbial products. IL-10 improves survival in neonatal mice challenged with group B *Streptococci* [41], but is detrimental in a murine model of pneumococcal pneumonia [42]. Similarly, tumor necrosis factor is beneficial in a murine model of pneumococcal pneumonia [43], whereas neutralization of TNF improves survival following challenge with *Microcystis* [44]. G-CSF is reported to improve survival following *Pseudomonas* challenge in the mouse [45], but to have no effect following lethal challenge with *S. aureus* in the rabbit [46]. Thus, factors such as the state of immune maturation and the locus of infection exert a potent influence on the response to mediator modulation. Moreover, circulating levels of key proinflammatory cytokines such as TNF vary, even within a given animal species, with the specific strain of bacteria employed, and the rate at which the organisms are infused [47].

Pre- versus post-treatment

The vast majority of animal studies have reported the effects of an inflammatory challenge in animals that have first been treated with the experimental agent. These models evaluate the effects of preventing the activation of a mediator response, rather than those of neutralization of a response during its expression. Not surprisingly, the beneficial effects of therapy become less pronounced the longer therapy is delayed. Moreover, the relationship of the timing of therapy to the infectious challenge can alter the response to therapy. IL-10 given 6 h after the onset of peritonitis improves outcome in a cecal ligation and puncture model, but is without effect when given prior to, or simultaneous with, the induction of peritonitis [48].

The impact of supportive therapy

The clinical syndrome of human sepsis is a complex interplay of the effects of the infectious challenge, and those of the many interventions employed to support the patient in the ICU. In contrast, resuscitation and support in animal models is rudimentary. Standard interventions such as fluid resuscitation, antibiotics, and surgical drainage reduce the lethality of animal models [49, 50], and minimize the benefits seen with mediator manipulation. Although physiological support is possible in a rodent model [51], modelling the ICU setting generally requires the use of large animal models, and financial considerations generally preclude the use of a mortality endpoint.

Selection of appropriate endpoints

The syndrome of sepsis in the human is a highly lethal process, with a 28 day mortality of 35 to 40%. For this reason, regulatory agencies such as the American Food and Drug Administration have been unyielding in their expectation that a novel therapy demonstrate mortality benefit prior to attaining licensure [52]. However there is an increasing trend for animal care committees to prohibit the use of experimental designs that require the animal's death as an endpoint, and to request, at a minimum, that animals be euthanized if there is evidence of distress. The shortcomings of surrogate endpoints for mortality in human trials are even greater when applied to unsupported animal models. Hypotension, lethargy, or profound hypothermia, for example, are manifestations of the disorder being treated, rather than outcomes, and their use as an endpoint precludes evaluation of therapy. Mortality endpoints for studies involving non-rodent species or subhuman primates pose even greater problems from the perspective of animal ethics, and become extraordinarily expensive to undertake.

When mortality is used as an endpoint in animal models, the patterns and timing of death may differ from those seen in humans. High dose endotoxin or bacteremia challenges typically result in death within 24 h, or rapid recovery for surviving animals. In human studies, however, 30 to 60% of deaths occur within the first three days, but mortality rates continue to be elevated for as long as 5 years following illness [53]. The cause of death may also differ between models, as well as from that of human sepsis. When endotoxin is given to rodents pre-conditioned with D-galactosamine, death occurs as a result of fulminant hepatic necrosis, a situation not typically encountered in human endotoxemia. Similarly, bile acid injection into the pancreatic duct causes acute pancreatitis with profound hypotension and death within the first 24 h; feeding of a choline-deficient diet also induces acute pancreatitis, but death occurs at 3 to 7 days and results from hypoxemia and renal failure [54].

Finally, it is apparent that the conduct of studies that use animal models has conventionally not been as rigorous as that of human clinical trials with regard to randomization of subjects or blinding of outcome measurement [55]. These inadequacies of study design may introduce bias into reported results.

In summary, then, animal models can provide important insights into the pathogenesis of a disease process, although what is studied is not the disease, but a model of the disease that, while resembling the clinical condition, may or may not reproduce its actual biological abnormalities. In turn, a deeper understanding of the pathogenesis of a disease process permits a more rational approach to therapy, and so the insights from pre-clinical studies can inform the design of clinical trials of novel agents in human diseases. However, it is inappropriate to conclude that an intervention that modulates a biological process in the highly artificial circumstances of an animal model will necessarily bring clinical benefit in the infinitely more complex setting of human illness. Indeed, sepsis is less a disease than an appropriate and adaptive response to an acute threat to life that arises in a host whose genetic background and premorbid state of health is highly variable. The next challenge in the design and interpretation of preclinical studies will be to develop panels or portfolios of models that may be better able to predict when intervention is likely to produce benefit, harm, or neither. In other words, rather than developing animal models of human sepsis, we will need to better understand the human correlates of animal models.

A Hierarchy of pre-clinical models

As a preliminary step towards a systematic understanding of the insights and limitations that derive from information provided by pre-clinical studies, it is instructive to consider the spectrum of models available (Tab. 1). The list is by no means comprehensive, and within each type of model factors such as the selection of species and genetic strain, the use of resuscitative measures, or other co-interventions, and the timing of therapy in relation to experimental challenge can all alter the observed responses.

Systemic endotoxemia or bacteremia

Evaluation of the effects of an intervention on the acute response to an endotoxin challenge is a simple and appealing first step in the assessment of a potential therapeutic approach. Endotoxin is readily characterized and easily stored, and can be administered to each animal in equal doses, minimizing random variability in the observed outcome. Doses can be titrated to mortality rates in untreated controls, and the investigator can therefore select a dose that will be optimal to his or her

Table 1 - Preclinical models of sepsis

Model	Advantages	Uses
Intravenous challenge	Simplicity	To detect a biologic signal, usually mortality
Endotoxin	Low cost	
Live bacteria		
Candida, Listeria	Potential for use of defined animal strains	
Focal infection	Model specific infections	To evaluate effects of an intervention on local antimicrobial defenses
Pneumonia	Model can provide	
Peritonitis	quantitative bacteriology	
	Local	
	Diffuse	
	CLP	
Subcutaneous injection		
Complex, sequential, or combined models (2-hit, immune compromise)	Reflects circumstances of infection in compromised, critically ill patient	To evaluate effects of intervention in a clinically relevant model
Trauma (hemorrhage, burn) followed by infection	Can reproduce both immune suppression and immunological activation	
Malnutrition + infection		
Neutropenia + infection		
Large animals	Permits resuscitation and full clinical support and monitoring	To define physiological consequences of intervention, and model potential clinical use
Pig, dog, sheep, horse, baboon		
Human endotoxemia	Measures effects in species of interest	To detect.a clinically relevant signal and to define therapeutic markers
	Highly defined challenge	

340

needs. Endotoxin can be handled with minimal risk to laboratory personnel, and administered to the experimental animal with relative ease. Its effects are rapid, and, when mortality is used as an endpoint, definitive. However, endotoxemia is an intoxication rather than an infection, and a single bolus injection does not reproduce the clinical circumstances of infection where exposure to the infecting agent occurs over time.

Intravenous challenge with a known inoculum of live organisms produces a clinical picture similar to that of endotoxin challenge and does permit evaluation of the effects of the intervention on antimicrobial defenses. A variety of organisms may be employed including Gram-negative or Gram-positive species, *Candida*, and *Listeria*. As discussed earlier, the response to therapy of an animal challenged with pathogens such as *Candida* or *Listeria* is often the opposite of that which occurs in response to endotoxemia [37]. The use of several different microbial strains permits a more comprehensive assessment of the potential risks and benefits of a given strategy on antimicrobial immunity.

Meningococcemia is probably the closest human correlate of animal models of endotoxemia or systemic bacteremia, although cholangitis or pyelonephritis, as acute infectious processes associated with the sudden release a large inoculum of organisms into the bloodstream, may also show similarities.

Models of local infection

Viable microorganisms or endotoxin can be administered intratracheally to mimic pneumonia or acute lung injury [10]. As with models of intravenous challenge, it is possible to titrate the severity of the model by varying the challenge dose, and to evaluate the response to differing bacterial strains. Pulmonary challenge models allow the use of alternate endpoints to mortality, for example, quantitative lung bacteriology, quantification of neutrophil influx into the lung, or measurement of lung permeability.

There are a great many models of intraperitoneal microbial challenge that reproduce features of bacterial peritonitis [6]. Known concentrations of defined strains of bacteria can be injected intraperitoneally, usually in conjunction with an adjuvant such as barium or hemoglobin to increase the severity of the model. Focal infection can be reproduced by the implantation of bacteria in a gelatin capsule, fibrin clot, or sterile feces.

The cecal ligation and puncture (CLP) model has proven to be a durable model that reproduces many features of complex intraperitoneal infection [5]. A laparotomy is performed in the anaesthetized animal (usually a rat or mouse, although larger animals such as sheep have been used). The cecum is ligated to create a focus of devitalized tissue, and the cecum punctured to permit escape of bacteria; the lethality of the model can be controlled by varying the number of punctures and the size of the needle used to create the puncture hole. CLP is easy to perform, and mimics human peritonitis in inducing a hyperdynamic state with hyperglycemia, followed later by hypoglycemia and lactic acidosis. Blood cultures are positive for a polymicrobial flora within one hour. Cardiac output is increased 2 h following the procedure, but later drops as the model progresses; systemic vascular resistance is reduced. Resuscitation with saline increases survival. Moreover, the necrotic cecum can be excised, antibiotics can be administered and, even in the rat, hemodynamic monitoring and support can be instituted [51]. Thus the model can reproduce many of the features of resuscitated peritonitis in the human.

Models of immunosuppression or priming

Patients enrolled in sepsis trials are typically elderly, with premorbid illnesses that may alter their response to therapy. In addition, the septic insult commonly arises as a consequence of a previous stimulus that may have primed or otherwise changed the baseline defenses of the host. Models in which host defenses have been altered may permit better evaluation of how an approach may affect a critically ill patient.

There are numerous methods of inducing immunosuppression or priming in an animal model. Some involve deleting specific components of innate host defenses. For example, studies of the effect of G-CSF commonly employ animals that have been rendered neutropenic by administration of cytotoxic agents. While such a model reproduces the alterations seen in neutropenia, it cannot be considered a model for a less specific immunological defect, and for studies of agents such a G-CSF or GM-CSF, administration of the agents simply reverses the underlying characteristics of the model. The role of the liver reticuloendothelial system can be studied in models in which Kupffer cell function has been ablated with agents such as gadolinium chloride [56].

A sophisticated model that reproduces some of the more complex abnormalities of critical illness has been reported by Cross and Opal. Rats are rendered neutropenic by cyclophosphamide, and colonized enterally with *Pseudomonas*. The model reproduces the clinical phenomenon of infection with a relevant pathogen occurring continuously across the gut mucosal barrier. In this model, while inhibition of TNF or IL-1 individually are beneficial, their use in combination is detrimental [57].

Models of sequential insults (also known a two-hit models) permit assessment of the effects of mediator manipulation in a system whose function has been altered by a previous insult. Two-hit models include burn injury followed by cecal ligation and puncture or hemorrhage followed by intratracheal challenge with endotoxin or live bacteria.

Large animal models

A better understanding of the physiological effects of a novel agent generally requires the use of large animals that can be instrumented and monitored following infectious challenge. Multiple physiologically and clinically relevant endpoints can be studied [58], although such studies are both costly and time-consuming. The selection of a species whose physiological responses to experimental challenge resemble those of the human is particularly important.

Endotoxin challenge in human volunteers

The evaluation of the consequences of mediator manipulation in human volunteers given an intravenous bolus of endotoxin combines features of pre-clinical and early phase clinical studies. The physiological, hemodynamic, and cytokine response in this model is well-characterized, and thus the biological effects of a given agent can be studied. Responses may vary from those predicted by animal models. For example, although pretreatment with G-CSF confers benefit in a variety of animal studies, in human endotoxemia, G-CSF enhances the release of both pro- and anti-inflammatory cytokines, augments release of neutrophil elastase, and prevents pulmonary leukosequestration [59].

Human endotoxemia models permit characterization of optimal biological markers to monitor the response to therapy; they share many of the shortcomings described above for animal models of endotoxemia.

Conclusions

Pre-clinical studies performed in a variety of mammalian species have provided us with much of our understanding of the pathophysiological changes that occur during the expression of a septic response. However, extrapolation of insights derived from the highly-controlled circumstances of a specific animal model to the complex and highly heterogeneous group of conditions that make up human sepsis is fraught with difficulties. The disappointing results of clinical studies undertaken so far attest to the fact that a more systematic and critical evaluation of the strengths and limitations of pre-clinical models will be a pre-requisite to designing successful studies in the future.

References

1   Abraham E, Raffin T (1994) Sepsis therapy trials. Continued disappointment or reason for hope? *JAMA* 271: 1876–1878

2   Bone RC (1996) Why sepsis trials fail. *JAMA* 276, 7: 565–566

3   Vincent JL (1997) Clinical trials in sepsis: where do we stand? *J Crit Care* 12: 3–6, 1997

4   Marshall JC (1998) The failure of clinical trials in sepsis: Challenges of pre-clinical models. *This volume*

5   Wichterman KA, Baue AE, Chaudry IH (1980) Sepsis and septic shock – a review of laboratory models and a proposal. *J Surg Res* 29: 189–201

6   Fink MP, Heard SO (1990) Laboratory models of sepsis and septic shock. *J Surg Res* 49: 186–196

7   Redl H, Schlag G, Bahrami S, Yao YM (1996) Animal models as the basis of pharmacologic intervention in trauma and sepsis patients. *World J Surg* 20: 487–492

8   Marchant A, Bruyns C, Vandenabeele P, Ducarme M, Gerard C, Delvaux A et al (1994) Interleukin-10 controls interferon-gamma and tumor necrosis factor production during experimental endotoxemia. *Eur J Immunol* 24: 1167–1171

9   Standiford TJ, Strieter RM, Lukacs NW, Kunkel SL (1995) Neutralization of IL-10 increases lethality in endotoxemia. Co-operative effects of macrophage inflammatory protein-2 and tumor necrosis factor. *J Immunol* 155: 2222–2229

10   Greenberger MJ, Strieter RM, Kunkel SL, Danforth JM, Goodman RE, Standford TJ (1995) Neutralization of IL-10 increases survival in a model of *Klebsiella* pneumonia. *J Immunol* 155: 722–729

11   van der Poll T, Marchant A, Keogh CV, Goldman M, Lowry SF (1996) Interleukin-10 impairs host defense in murine pneumococcal pneumonia. *J Infect Dis* 174: 994–100

12   Kelly JP, Bancroft BJ (1996) Administration of interleukin-10 abolishes innate resistance to *Listeria monocytogenes*. *Eur J Immunol* 26: 356–364

13   van der Poll T, Marchant A, Buurman WA, Berman L, Keogh CV, Lazarus et al (1995) Endogenous interleukin-10 protects mice from death during septic peritonitis. *J Immunol* 155: 5397–5401

14   Walley KR, Lukacs NW, Standiford TJ, Strieter RM, Kunkel SL (1996) Balance of inflammatory cytokines related to severity and mortality of murine sepsis. *Infect Immun* 64: 4733–4738

15   Beutler B, Milsark IW, Cerami AC (1985) Passive immunization against cachectin/tumor necrosis factor protects mice from lethal effects of endotoxin. *Science* 229: 869–871

16   Evans TJ, Moyes D, Carpenter A, Martin R, Loetscher H, Lesslauer W et al (1994) Protective effect of 55- but not 75-kD soluble tumor necrosis factor-immunoglobulin G fusion proteins in an animal model of Gram negative sepsis. *J Exp Med* 180: 2173–2179

17   Nakano Y, Shirai M, Mori N, Nakano M (1991) Neutralization of microcystin shock in mice by tumor necrosis factor alpha antiserum. *Appl Env Microbiol* 57: 327–330

18   Cross AS, Sadoff JC, Kelly N, Bernton E, Gemski P (1989) Pretreatment with recombi-

nant murine tumor necrosis factor alpha/cachectin and murine interleukin 1 alpha protects mice from lethal bacterial infection. *J Exp Med* 169: 2021–2027

19   Takashima K, Tateda K, Matsumoto T, Iizawa Y, Nakao M, Yamaguchi K (1997) Role of tumor necrosis factor alpha in pathogenesis of pneumococcal pneumonia in mice. *Infect Immun* 65: 257–260

20   Eskandari MK, Bolgos G, Miller C, Nguyen DT, DeForge LE, Remick DG (1992) Anti-tumor necrosis factor antibody therapy fails to prevent lethality after cecal ligation and puncture or endotoxemia. *J Immunol* 148: 2724–2730

21   Evans GF, Snyder YM, Butler LD, Zuckerman SH (1989) Differential expression of interleukin-1 and tumor necrosis factor in murine septic shock models. *Circ Shock* 29: 279–290

22   Echtenacher B, Falk W, Mannel DN, Krammer PH (1990) Requirement of endogenous tumor necrosis factor/cachectin for recovery from experimental peritonitis. *J Immunol* 145: 3762–3766

23   Watts C (1997) Immunology. Inside the gearbox of the dendritic cell. *Nature* 388: 724–725

24   Zollner O, Lenter MC, Blanks JE, Borges E, Steegmaier M, Zerwes HG et al (1997) L-selectin from human, but not from mouse neutrophils binds directly to E-selectin. *J Cell Biol* 136: 707–716

25   Vas SI, Roy RS, Hobson HG (1973) Endotoxin sensitivity of inbred mouse strains. *Can J Microbiol* 19: 767–769

26   Hagberg L, Hull R, Hull S, McGhee JR, Michalek SM, Svanborg EC (1984) Difference in susceptibility to gram-negative urinary tract infection between C3H/HeJ and C3H/HeN mice. *Infect Immun* 46: 839–844

27   Galanos C, Freudenberg MA, Reutter W (1979) Galactosamine-induced sensitization to the lethal effects of endotoxin. *Proc Natl Acad Sci* 76: 5939–5943

28   Fink MP, Baggs AG (1997) Animal models of sepsis and septic shock. In: Fein AM, Abraham E, Balk R, Bernard GR, Bone R, Dantzker DR, Fink MP (eds): *Sepsis and multiorgan failure*. Williams and Wilkins , Baltimore, 596–613

29   Westendorp RG, Langermans JA, Huizinga TW, Elouali AH, Verwij CL, Boomsma DI, Vandenbrouke JP (1997) Genetic influence on cytokine production and fatal meningococcal disease. *Lancet* 349: 170–173

30   Stuber F, Petersen M, Bokelmann F, Schade U (1996) A genomic polymorphism within the tumor necrosis factor locus influences plasma tumor necrosis factor-alpha concentrations and outcome of paients with severe sepsis. *Crit Care Med* 24: 381–384

31   Fernandes DM, Jiang X, Jung JH, Baldwin CL (1996) Comparison of T cell cytokines in resistant and susceptible mice infected wth virulent *Brucella abortus* strain 2308 FEMS Immunol. Med. Microbiol. 16: 193–203

32   Sultzer BM, Castagna R, Bandekar J, Wong P (1993) Lipopolysaccharide nonresponder cells: the C3H HeJ defect. *Immunobiol* 187: 257–271

33   Amura CR, Chen LC, Hirohashi N, Lei MG, Morrison DC (1997) Two functionally independent pathways for lipopolysaccharide-dependent activation of mouse peritoneal macrophages. *J Immunol* 159: 5079–5083

34   Thieblemont N, Wright SD (1997) Mice genetically hyporesponsive to lipopolysaccha-ride (LPS) exhibit a defect in endocytic uptake of LPS and ceramide. *J Exp Med* 185: 2095–2100

35   Nagata S, Suda T (1995) Fas and Fas ligand: lpr and gld mutations. *Immunol Today* 16: 39–43

36   Kaufmann SH, Ladel CH (1994) Application of knockout mice to the experimental analysis of infections with bacteria and protozoa. *Trends Microbiol* 2: 235–242

37   Pfeffer K, Matsuyama T, Kundig M, Wakeham A, Kishihara K, Shahinian A, Wiegmann K, Ohashi PS, Kronke M, Mak TW (1993) Mice deficient for the 55 kd tumor necrosis factor receptor are resistant to endotoxic shock, yet succumb to *L. Monocytogenes* infection. *Cell* 73: 457–467

38   Shastry BS (1995) Genetic knockouts in mice: an update. *Experientia* 51: 1028–1039

39   Rosenberg MP (1997) Gene knockout and transgenic technologies in risk assessment: the next generation. *Molecular Carcinogenesis* 20: 262–274

40   Hirsch E, Irikura VM, Paul SM, Hirsh D (1996) Functions of interleukin 1 receptor antagonist in gene knockout and overproducing mice. *Proc Natl Acad Sci USA* 93: 11008– 11013

41   Cusumano V, Genovese F, Mancuso G, Carbone M, Fera MT, Teti G (1996) Interleukin-10 protects neonatal mice from lethal group B streptococcal infection. *Infect Immun* 64: 2850–2852

42   van der Poll T, Marchant A, Keogh CV, Goldman M, Lowry SF (1996) Interleukin-10 impairs host defense in murine pneumococcal pneumonia. *J Infect Dis* 174: 994–1000

43   Takashima K, Tateda K, Matsumoto T, Iizawa Y, Nakao M, Yamaguchi K (1997) Role of tumor necrosis factor alpha in pathognesis of pneumococcal pneumonia in mice *Infect Immun* 65: 257–260

44   Nakano Y, Shirai M, Mori N, Nakano M (1991) Neutralization of microcystin shock in mice by tumor necrosis factor alpha antiserum. *Appl Environ Microbiol* 57: 327–330

45   Miura S, Takimoto H, Yoshikai Y, Kumazawa Y, Yamada A, Nomoto K (1992) Protec-tive effect of ren-shen-yang-rong-tang (Ninjin-youei-to) in mice with drug-induced leukopenia against Pseudomonas aeruginosa infection. *Int J Immunopharmacol* 14: 1249–1257

46   Frank U, Chambers HF (1996) Treatment of Staphylococcus aureus catheter-related infection and infective endocarditis with granulocyte colony-stimulating factor in the experimental rabbit model. *Antimicrob Agents Chemother* 40: 1308–1310

47   Cross AS, Opal SM, Sadoff JC, Gemski P (1993) Choice of bacteria in animal models of sepsis. *Infect Immun* 61: 2741–2747

48   Kato T, Murata A, Ishida H, Toda H, Tanaka N, Hayashida H, Monden N, Matsuura n (1995) Interleukin 10 reduces mortality from severe peritonitis in mice. *Antimicrob Agents Chemother* 39: 1336–1340

49   Natanson C, Danner RL, Reilly JM (1990) Antibiotics versus cardiovascular support in a canine model of human septic shock. *Am J Physiol* 259: H1440–H1447

50 Bohnen JM, Matlow AG, Mustard RA, Christie NA, Kavouris B (1988) Antibiotic efficacy in intraabdominal sepsis: a clinically relevant model. *Can J Microbiol* 34: 323–326.

51 Martin CM, Sibbald WJ (1994) Modulation of hemodynamics and organ blood flow by nitric oxide synthase inhibition is not altered in normotensive, septic rats. *Am J Resp Crit Care Med* 150: 1539–1544

52 Schwieterman W, Roberts R (1997) Outcome measures for sepsis trials: The FDA perspective. *Sepsis* 1: 69

53 Quartin AA, Schein RM, Kett DH, Peduzzi PN (1997) Magnitude and duration of the effect of sepsis on survival. *JAMA* 277: 1058–1063

54 Norman J (1998) Pancreatitis as a model of sepsis. *Sepsis; in press*

55 Piper RD, Cook DJ, Bone RC, Sibbald WJ (1996) Introducing critical appraisal to studies of animal models investigating novel therapies in sepsis. *Crit Care Med* 24: 2059–2070

56 Nieuwenhuijzen GAP, Haskel Y, Lu Q, Berg RD, van Rooijen N, Goris RJA, Deitch EA (1993) Macrophage elimination increases bacterial translocation but attenuates symptoms and mortality rate in a model of systemic inflammation. *Arch Surg* 218: 791–799

57 Opal SM, Cross AS, Jhung JW, Young LD, Palardy JE, Parejo NA et al (1996) Potential hazards of combination immunotherapy in the treatment of experimental septic shock. *J Infect Dis* 173: 1415–1421

58 Sevransky JE, Shaked G, Novogrodsky A, Levitzki A, Gazit A, Hoffman A, lin RJ, Quezado ZMN, Freeman BD, Eichacker PQ, Danner RL, Banks SM, Bacher J, Thomas ML, Natanson C (1997) Tyrphostin AG 556 improves survival and reduces multiorgan failure in canine *Escherichia coli* peritonitis. *J Clin Invest* 99: 1966–1973

59 Pajkrt D, Manten A, van der Poll T, Tiel-van Buul MMC, Jansen J, Wouter ten Cate J, van Deventer SJH (1997) Modulation of cytokine release and neutrophil function by granulocyte colony-stimulating factor during endotoxemia in humans. *Blood* 90: 1415–1424

The failure of clinical trials in sepsis: Challenges of clinical trial design

John C. Marshall

Eaton North 9-234, Toronto Hospital, General Division, 200 Elizabeth Street, Toronto, Ontario, Canada M5G 2C4

Introduction

More than two dozen well-designed, randomized, controlled phase II or III clinical trials, published over the past 15 years, have tested the hypothesis that modulating the host inflammatory response can improve clinical outcome for patients with sepsis [1, 2]. Four of these have demonstrated a statistically significant effect on survival- three suggesting clinical benefit [3–5], and one, clinical harm [6]. In excess of one billion U.S. dollars have been expended generating these results, but none of the agents studied has been licensed for clinical use.

From the perspective of the speculator or the cynic, the promise of mediator-targeted therapy has been exposed as a scientific pipe-dream, a notion best discarded and abandoned. Yet for the clinician treating the critically ill, or the scientist studying the intricacies of the host inflammatory response, such nihilism flies in the face of a compelling biological rationale, and an urgent clinical need. Much has been written about the reasons that sepsis trials have failed [7–10]; the potential explanations are many (Tab. 1). A critical review of the many possible explanations for this failure provides a useful insight into the complexities of the biological process and the many pitfalls of clinical research.

Have sepsis trials failed: What is the measure of success?

At the outset, it is important to question the very premise of this review – that sepsis trials have been a failure. While it is true that no new agents have been licensed for use in clinical practice for the treatment of sepsis, it can be argued that published data demonstrate consistent, albeit small evidence of clinical benefit. In a meta-analysis of published studies of mediator-targeted therapy, Zeni and colleagues showed an overall survival benefit of 2–3% for patients enrolled in the experimental arm of sepsis trials [2]. An absolute difference of this magnitude only becomes statistically significant when very large trials are performed. Assuming that the 28

Table 1 - Explanations for the negative results of clinical trials of mediator-directed therapies in sepsis

True negative results

- The mediator has no pathophysiological role in the human population studied.
- The mediator has a pathophysiological role, but the study agent failed to neutralize it because of true biological inactivity, *in vivo* inactivation, *in vivo* competition by other mediators, or a compensatory increase in a separate mediator with similar biological effects

False negative results

- The agent was administered too early or too late in the course of the disease
- The duration of therapy was too short
- The dose was inadequate
- The study population was overly heterogeneous with respect to:
  - the biological expression of the inflammatory response
  - the severity of the physiological derangement
  - the genetic predisposition of the patient
  - premorbid health status
  - the site, bacteriology, or presence of infection
  - the adequacy of surgical source control
  - the adequacy of antimicrobial therapy
  - the adequacy of concomitant ICU supportive care
- The agent produced benefit in some patients, but harm in others
- Combination therapy is required to block redundant and overlapping mediator cascades

day mortality for patients enrolled in the placebo arm of such a study is 40%, we would need to study 8400 patients receiving either placebo or study drug to detect a 3% mortality reduction to 37%, at conventional levels of statistical significance and power. If we wish to detect an absolute difference of 2%, then we must study close to 20, 000 patients. If the placebo mortality is lower, the sample size will be correspondingly larger. Expressed differently, a study of 1000 septic patients (a moderately large trial by current standards) will only achieve statistical significance if mortality is reduced from 40% to 31%, a relative reduction of 23%.

Large trials are the rule in disciplines such as cardiology, where mortality reductions of the same order of magnitude of those actually observed in sepsis trials are anticipated [11]. For logistical and cost reasons, such trials are unrealistic in the area of sepsis. Therefore, a successful sepsis trial will require either an agent with greater efficacy in the populations conventionally studied, a refinement of study entry criteria to enrich the population with patients most likely to benefit, or demonstration of greater benefit using an outcome other than 28 day mortality (and a willingness on the part of regulatory agencies to accept such a demonstration for licensing purposes).

The societal perspective

What comprises success in a clinical trial? In general, a clinician will adopt a new therapy if that therapy can be shown to improve clinical outcome; the health care system, on the other hand, needs evidence not only of clinical benefit, but of an acceptable ratio of cost to benefit. Conversely, an intervention that brought no measurable benefit (and no harm) to a patient, but reduced the costs of providing care would be an attractive therapy from a societal perspective. The more expensive a new therapy, the greater its incremental benefit must be to justify the additional costs to health care providers.

Is a 3% overall reduction in 28 day mortality enough of an effect to justify the introduction of a novel mediator-directed therapy? Recombinant proteins are expensive to produce and the developmental costs in bringing such agents to market is considerable, in excess of $ 100,000,000. If we assume that a course of therapy will cost $ 5000, then, assuming a 3% mortality benefit, 100 patients must be treated to save three lives, and the cost per survivor is approximately $ 170,000. Further, if we make the assumption that survivors of the septic insult, a patient population with significant comorbidity, will gain an additional 4.3 years of life [12], the cost per life year gained is approximately $ 40,000. Based on the assumption, almost certainly erroneous, that 500, 000 patients a year might benefit from treatment, the total cost to the health care system of the agent alone is $ 2.5 billion. The introduction of an effective sepsis therapeutic agent will have a significant impact on health costs. When licensure of the anti-endotoxin monoclonal antibody, HA-1A, appeared imminent, the Pharmacy and Therapeutics committee of at least one large urban hospital was faced with the ethical dilemma of having to contemplate withholding therapy from patients who might benefit because the costs of providing therapy exceeded the money available to purchase the agent [13]. From a societal perspective, therefore, there are strong pressures to contain expenditures by either reducing the cost of the agent or identifying a subpopulation of patients who might achieve the greatest benefit. From an industry perspective, it may not be profitable to expend the necessary developmental costs to produce an agent targeted to a population that is much smaller than the widely quoted estimate of 500,000 cases per year.

It is not the purpose of this chapter to debate the commercial costs of therapy. Rather we will focus on the multiple factors that may serve to reduce the demonstrated benefit of novel therapies for sepsis, and use this approach as a framework for a discussion of the limitations of studies that have been undertaken to date.

Biological challenges

Sepsis has been defined as the host systemic inflammatory response to invasive infection [14]. By definition, then, it is not a disease but a process that has evolved to benefit the host but that can, in certain circumstances, produce harm. It is readily apparent from animal studies that modulation of the septic response can have differing effects on outcome depending on the model studied [15]. It has been shown, for example, that administration of interleukin 10 (IL-10) improves the survival of mice challenged with endotoxin [16] but increases mortality when the challenge is a viable organism such as *Listeria* [17].

Patients meeting the criteria for entry into a sepsis trial represent a highly heterogeneous population with respect to the site, or even presence, of infection, and the infecting organism. Thus it is likely that while some will benefit from a particular intervention, others may not, or may even suffer harm. A phase III trial of HA-1A, a monoclonal antibody against bacterial endotoxin, demonstrated a significant mortality benefit for patients with Gram-negative bacteremia, but the reduction in mortality for the entire population was not statistically significant [18]. More importantly, a followup study with the same agent was terminated when an interim analysis showed a trend towards increased mortality in patients with Gram-positive infections [19].

The redundancy of the inflammatory mediator cascade presents another significant biological challenge to sepsis trials. Activation of a macrophage by bacterial endotoxin, for example, triggers the synthesis and release of a complex cascade of endogenous host mediators that can amplify, modify, or downregulate the expression of inflammation [20]. Each of these mediators, in turn, can trigger host cells to release other pro- and anti-inflammatory molecules, with the result that a single trigger can initiate a self-perpetuating process involving literally hundreds of distinct mediators. Targeting a single mediator, even if that mediator is a key component of the inflammatory cascade such as TNF or IL-1, may not be sufficient to terminate the response once it has been initiated. Animal studies showing dramatic benefits from neutralization of TNF [21] or IL-1 [22] involved administration of the agent prior to the inflammatory challenge. Thus a mediator may be necessary to initiate the response, but may play a relatively minor role once the response has been expressed. Termination of an activated response is likely to require either combination therapy, if the target is a discrete mediator, or downstream blockade of a common signalling or effector pathway.

Finally, a novel therapy may fail to show benefit because it lacks biological activity *in vivo*. Concern has been expressed, for example, that both HA-1A and E5, monoclonal antibodies against Gram-negative endotoxin, have not been reliably shown to neutralize the biological effects of endotoxin, and that the failure of trials with these agents may reflect the use of an inactive agent [23]. More recently, a large multicentre Phase III study of an antibody to TNF (Bayer), enrolling approximately 1900 patients, showed a statistically insignificant 2.5% reduction in all cause mortality. Data on cytokine levels from that trial showed that the antibody only effected a 50% reduction in levels of immunoreactive TNF as measured by ELISA; more significantly, when TNF was measured by bioassay, no evidence of neutralization of its activity could be demonstrated (unpublished data). More subtle antagonism of the effects of a experimental agent could arise because of *in vivo* inactivation, or because of an unmeasured compensatory increase in another mediator with a similar biological effect.

Conceptual limitations

The common hypothesis of studies undertaken so far has been that a particular intervention, applied in a heterogeneous population of patients identified as having the clinical condition of sepsis on the basis of a non-specific constellation of clinical manifestations, will result in a mortality benefit that is significantly robust that it will be evident 28 days after the start of therapy. This assumption is, at best, naive.

The entry criteria for clinical studies of experimental mediator-directed therapy performed to date have been those of sepsis syndrome [24], or systemic inflammation response syndrome (SIRS) [14]. These criteria are arbitrary, non-specific and unvalidated. Sepsis syndrome, for example, was proposed in the early 1980's to identify potential study subjects for a randomized trial of high dose methylprednisolone in septic shock [25]. The intent was to identify clinical parameters that might define a population at high risk of having infection with an activated inflammatory response. Yet neither a retrospective review of the control arm of that study [24], nor a subsequent prospective study of patients meeting criteria for sepsis syndrome [26], provided support for the hypothesis that these patients shared a common pathological process. In the latter study, for example, fewer than half of patients with a clinical suspicion of infection were shown to be infected, and the key proinflammatory cytokines TNF, IL-1, and IL-6 were not consistently present. Although 28 day mortality for patients enrolled in the placebo arm of sepsis trials has been consistently in the range of 35 to 40% [1], a relatively reproducible risk of dying does not imply a common disease. Patients with a ruptured abdominal aortic aneurysm or AIDS with a low CD4 count both have a significant risk of mortality, but common risk clearly does not equate to a common pathophysiological process. Sepsis syndrome criteria can be met by an 86 year old woman with acute congestive heart failure and a concomitant urinary tract infection, or by a 24 year old man with a gunshot wound to the colon, yet it is improbable that both patients would benefit equally from a particular mediator-directed therapy. Conversely, a patient with septic shock from perforated diverticulitis will fail to meet sepsis syndrome criteria if he or she does not have an abnormal temperature.

The criteria for SIRS are equally unsatisfactory [27]. The concept of SIRS was articulated at a consensus conference of the Society of Critical Care Medicine and the American College of Chest Physicians, held in 1991 [14]. The intent had been to underline the emerging concept that a clinical syndrome of acute inflammation could arise in the absence of invasive infection. The specific criteria for SIRS that emerged from that meeting were based on expert opinion, not validated data, and although as a kind of abbreviated SAPS or APACHE score they define an increasing risk of mortality, it remains to be shown that patients with SIRS have a single disease [28]. Indeed it is almost certain that they do not: the criteria for SIRS can be met by patients with severe infection, but are equally common following multiple trauma, or even perfectly healthy physiological stresses such as vigourous exercise, public speaking, or making love.

Similarly, the assumption that patients with suspected, or even microbiologically documented, infection comprise a homogeneous group with respect to their cytokine profiles or response to mediator-targeted therapy has never been formally tested. Is the response of a patient with polymicrobial peritonitis biologically similar to that of a patient with pneumococcal pneumonia or an intravascular catheter infection with coagulase-negative *Staphylococci*? It is apparent from a number of studies that the mortality risk associated with a urinary tract infection is less than that of infections at other sites. Does this differential mortality risk equate to a differing expectation of clinical benefit when the inflammatory response is manipulated?

What is the biological objective of therapy?

Any therapeutic intervention improves survival by altering a biological process. For example, thrombolytic agents increase survival by lysing clots in the coronary arteries, thus restoring blood flow to the myocardium. Insulin improves survival in diabetes by lowering blood sugar levels, and preventing the end organ complications of hyperglycemia. Surgery for a ruptured aneurysm is life-saving because it controls hemorrhage and restores blood flow to vital organs. In each case, a mortality benefit is predicted by an expected influence on a process that can, to a greater or lesser extent, be measured. Changes in the electrocardiogram reflect restoration of oxygenation to the myocardium, a reduction in the blood glucose level reflects the biological activity of insulin, and cessation of bleeding indicates successful repair of the aneurysm. But what is the biologic objective of a novel mediator-targeted therapy? Is it reduction in the circulating levels of the target mediator, or a reduction in some downstream action of that mediator? Is it reversal of the study entry criteria? Is it a more rapid or complete eradication of infection? With few exceptions, sepsis trials have failed to define an acute biological objective of therapy and, as a consequence, have failed to provide any evidence that the agent was biologically active while it was being administered.

At the very least, it would seem reasonable to expect that a novel treatment that can improve 28 day survival in an acute process such as sepsis will cause a more rapid or complete reversal of the study entry criteria. It is implausible, for example, that an antiarrhythmic will improve survival if it does not reduce the frequency or severity of arrhythmias, although, as discussed later, the converse is not necessarily true. Reversal of shock, of sepsis syndrome or SIRS, or of the underlying infection has not been explicitly evaluated in many sepsis trials, and where it has, the results have often been disappointing [29, 30]. Failure to reverse study entry criteria suggests one of two possibilities:

- the experimental therapy is biologically inactive
- the entry criteria do not adequately reflect the potential beneficial action of the drug, and therefore the target population is not one that would necessarily be expected to benefit from the drug.

What are appropriate measures of therapeutic benefit?

Because patients enrolled in sepsis trials have a baseline expected risk of mortality of 35 to 40%, it is reasonable to anticipate that the primary benefit of an effective new therapy will be a reduction in mortality: demonstration of reduced mortality has been required by regulatory agencies before a new agent can be licensed. As discussed above, a recent meta-analysis pooling the results of published trials (albeit combining agents with widely differing modes of action) showed a consistent absolute mortality benefit for the experimental agent of 2 to 3% [2]. Although the hypothesis that effective mediator-targeted therapy might result in the same dramatic survival benefits seen in experimental models is appealing, the degree of mortality benefit in the clinical arena is likely to be much smaller. Despite the fact that mortality is both definitive in its ascertainment, and undeniably important clinically, its shortcomings as a study endpoint are many [31, 32].

A mortality benefit will be maximal if the therapy rapidly and effectively alters a pathological process that is immediately linked to death. Thrombolytic agents, for example, lyse intracoronary clots; acute coronary thrombosis is rapidly lethal by virtue of its effects on cardiac function. Therefore, a thrombolytic agent can be legitimately expected to produce a significant mortality benefit. In sepsis, however, the causal link between a specific mediator and death is much less direct. The particular process or processes responsible for death in clinical sepsis remain largely undefined. It is relatively easy to restore satisfactory hemodynamic homeostasis with fluids, to support tissue oxygenation with ventilatory support and vasoactive agents, to control infection with surgery and antibiotics, and to support other failing organ system function with conventional ICU therapy. Despite this, approximately 40% of patients die, and characteristically because the attending intensivist decides that reversal of organ dysfunction is unlikely and discontinues supportive care. Mortality is, in effect, a surrogate for the clinical process responsible for withdrawal of care- the failure of reversal of organ system dysfunction. Mortality as an endpoint is further confounded by the influence of the patient's premorbid state of health. Patients enrolled in sepsis trials are often elderly and medically compromised. Intercurrent illnesses may contribute to death during the study period, or exert a significant impact on the willingness of the intensivist to continue prolonged supportive care.

Objective measures of organ dysfunction reflecting its severity, course, and extent of resolution are attractive alternatives or complements to mortality as endpoints in sepsis trials [33]. When a disorder carries a significant mortality risk, but minimal morbidity for survivors (acute coronary artery thrombosis for example), mortality is the optimal endpoint for use in clinical trials. Conversely, when a disorder produces significant morbidity, but little mortality (rheumatoid arthritis, for example), measures of morbidity, generally reflecting quality of life, are appropriate. Sepsis, however, is associated with both mortality and morbidity in the form of organ dysfunction and dependence on ICU supportive care. Therefore, clinical trials in sepsis should evaluate the effects of a new therapy on both mortality and morbidity. The formal evaluation of organ dysfunction as an outcome in ICU-based trials is a relatively recent development. Several systems are available, and have been incorporated into trials currently in progress [34–37]. However, regulatory agencies have yet to accept a reduction in organ dysfunction as a primary endpoint for a sepsis trial.

Limitations of drug administration

Partly because sensitive, readily obtained measures of the biological effects of experimental therapies are not yet available, experimental agents in sepsis trials are administered in an arbitrary manner. Optimal doses for agents are not well-defined. Vasoactive drugs used in the ICU are titrated to physiological parameters such as blood pressure, cardiac output, or mixed venous oxygen saturation, and administered across a wide range of concentrations. Yet agents expected to have efficacy in the treatment of septic shock are given in single doses, driven by protocol rather than by patient response. Moreover, the duration of therapy is dictated by protocol, rather than by clinical parameters and, as a rule, although the primary endpoint, mortality, is measured at 28 days, readministration of study drug during this period is not permitted.

It is also unknown when during the clinical syndrome a given agent should be administered. Animal studies, by and large, evaluate outcome when an agent is administered prior to the septic challenge [38]. Obviously this is not possible in human sepsis and there may be a limited window of opportunity for therapy with a given agent. Studies in human volunteers challenged with endotoxin show that a single bolus results in the sequential release of host-derived mediators with an early peak of TNF and a later, sustained release of IL-6 [39]. Whether such sequential activation of the cytokine cascade occurs in clinical sepsis is unknown, however, the temporal pattern of mediator expression is likely an important determinant of response to a particular therapeutic strategy. Variability in the time course of mediator release, and the intrinsic redundancy of overlapping cytokine cascades may mandate the use of combination therapy if clinically relevant benefit is to be achieved. Combination therapy, however, presupposes effective therapy with a single agent, a result that so far has proven elusive. Moreover, both cost considerations and the inherent competitiveness of commercial drug development have precluded serious consideration of trials of combination therapies.

Finally, it is not at all clear that a patient meeting the criteria for sepsis syndrome might benefit equally from the spectrum of agents that have been used in trials conducted to date. Is it feasible, for example, that comparable benefit will result from administration of G-CSF, antagonism of TNF, antagonism of endotoxin, administration of corticosteroids, or antagonism of nitric oxide synthesis? The assumption behind the use of similar entry criteria for trials of each of these agent is that they will.

Challenges resulting from the process of care

Variability in concomitant care can have a striking impact on the results of a multicenter clinical trial. This is particularly true for sepsis trials. Sprung and colleagues showed that deficiencies in the provision of concomitant care were a significant factor in the inability of a trial of a monoclonal antibody to TNF to demonstrate clinical benefit [40]. Pre-clinical studies strongly suggest that the effects of mediator-targeted therapy may be diametrically opposite if infection has not been satisfactorily controlled, however, formal evaluation of surgical source control has not been routinely incorporated into clinical trial design [41].

Similarly it has been observed that both baseline mortality for patients with sepsis, and the apparent response to mediator-directed therapy varies considerably from one country to the next [23]. Possible explanations for the existence of strong centre effects are many and include variability in severity of illness or comorbidity in patient populations, variations in patterns of medical or nursing care, and variability in approaches to concomitant care. Patients enrolled in sepsis trials, by definition, have a life-threatening disorder, and one that is often a consequence of preexisting illness or advanced age. Variability in decisions regarding the appropriateness of sustained life support measures may have a significant impact on trial conduct. A decision was made to forego life-sustaining measures for fully 22% of the 543 patients enrolled in the multicentre trial of HA-1A, an antibody to endotoxin, and one third of these decisions were made within 72 hours of study entry [42]. Unless an experimental therapy has the ability to reverse the physiological abnormalities of sepsis immediately and profoundly, such decisions will inevitably hinder appropriate evaluation of the agent.

Conclusions

The disappointing results of clinical trials of mediator-directed therapy in sepsis completed to date provide an eloquent testimonial to the enormous complexities involved in attempting to improve clinical outcomes by modifying the host inflammatory response. Yet it would be erroneous to conclude that further efforts are futile.

Successful therapy in any medical disorder presupposes that certain conditions be met. We must first be able to define a population of patients who have a disease- a morbid disorder with a single pathological basis. Ideally that pathological derangement must be understood sufficiently well that a rational therapeutic strategy can be articulated and tested. Diabetes, coronary artery disease, or small cell carcinoma of the lung are diseases; sepsis is not a disease but a syndrome. While it can be conceptualized as over expression of an inflammatory response, or even as a state of deranged interactions between pro- and anti-inflammatory states, it cannot yet be definitively characterized as a reproducible alteration in any specific mediator or process that we can treat. Successful mediator-targeted therapy will require the delineation of discrete diseases, and, as has proven so important in oncology, the development of objective systems to stage these diseases.

Secondly, we must employ agents that have appropriate biological activity both *in vitro* and *in vivo*. Efficacy must be evident not only in a panel of preclinical models, but also in humans. Studies evaluating the influence of therapeutic intervention on the subjective and objective response to intravenous endotoxin challenge in human volunteers [43, 44] have the potential to provide important insights into the biological activity of a compound *in vivo*. However, Phase II studies employing intensive clinical and biological surveillance are necessary to confirm that activity occurs in the real life setting of critical illness. Moreover, it is critical that appropriate quality control assays be established to ensure that an agent retains its biological activity over time as production methods change.

We must next ensure that the experimental intervention is administered sufficiently early in the course of the disease that the natural history of the disease process can be altered, and at a sufficient dose and for a sufficient duration of time that an optimal effect can be obtained. Finally, we must employ measures of biological activity and of clinical benefit that are sufficiently specific for the activity of the agent, and sufficiently sensitive to clinically meaningful change so that an effect will be seen if one is truly present.

It is a recurring theme of critiques of the failure of sepsis trials that large and costly Phase III clinical trials are premature, since not enough is known about the preclinical biology of inflammation, or about the epidemiology of human sepsis [7, 38, 45, 46]. A number of avenues are available that may foster the development of a better understanding of the latter (Tab. 2). The development of collaborative, multidisciplinary investigative efforts will clearly be a pre-requisite to realizing the preclinical promise of mediator-directed therapies.

Table 2 - Approaches to an improved understanding of the epidemiology of sepsis

Approach	Advantages and disadvantages
Multi-institutional registries	Comprehensive, with excellent oppportunity for investigator input into design and development. However, costly, difficult to fund, and potential for significant variability in measurement of biological parameters.
Placebo arm of completed studies	Comprehensive and accurate data collection, however, limited by funding, willingness of sponsors to provide access to data, and by initial study entry criteria.
Post-hoc analyses of completed trials	Permit multivariate analyses to define potential reasons for negative results and opportunity to test these if there is more than one treatment arm, or more than one completed trial. However, there is little incentive for a sponsor to expend extra resources on the analysis of a 'negative' study, and analyses are limited by initial trial entry criteria.
Prospective studies in ongoing trials	Optimal approach for data collection, however, run risk that selected study population will prove not to be optimal population for therapy, and thus may jeopardize acceptance of trial for licensing.
Expert consensus meetings	Provide optimal opportunity for scientific interaction and expert articulation of current state of the art, however in the absence of empiric data, cannot answer question.

References

1   Meade MO, Creery D, Marshall JC (1997) Systematic review of outcome measures in randomized trials of mediator-directed therapies in sepsis. *Sepsis* 1: 27–33

2   Zeni F, Freeman B, Natanson C (1997) Anti-inflammatory therapies to treat sepsis and septic shock: A reassessment. *Crit Care Med* 25: 1095–1100

3   Ziegler EJ, McCutchan JA, Fierer J, Glauser MP, Sadoff JC, Douglas H et al (1982) Treatment of gram-negative bacteremia and shock with human antiserum to a mutant *Escherichia coli*. *N Engl J Med* 307: 1225–1230

4   Ziegler EJ, Fisher CJ, Sprung CL, Straube RC, Sadoff JC, Foulke GE et al (1991) Treatment of gram-negative bacteremia and septic shock with HA-1A human monoclonal antibody against endotoxin. *N Engl J Med* 324: 429–436

5   Fisher CJ Jr, Slotman GJ, Opal SM, Pribble JP, Bone RC, Emmanuel G et al (1994) Initial evaluation of human recombinant interleukin-1 receptor antagonist in the treatment of sepsis syndrome: A randomized, open-label, placebo-controlled multicenter trial. *Crit Care Med* 22: 12–21

6   Fisher CJ Jr, Agosti JM, Opal SM, Lowry SF, Balk RA, Sadoff JC, Abraham E, Schein RMH, Benjamin E (1996) Treatment of septic shock with the tumor necrosis factor receptor: Fc fusion protein. *N Engl J Med* 334: 1697–1702

7   Fink MP (1995) Another negative clinical trial of a new agent for the treatment of sepsis: Rethinking the process of developing adjuvant treatments for serious infections. *Crit Care Med* 23: 989–991

8   Bernard GR (1995) Sepsis trials: intersection of investigation, regulation, funding, and practice. *Am J Respir Crit Care Med* 152: 4–10

9   Dellinger RP (1996) Post hoc analyses in sepsis trials: A formula for disappointment? *Crit Care Med* 24: 727–729

10   Bone RC (1995) Sepsis and controlled clinical trials: The odyssey. *Crit Care Med* 23: 1165–1166

11   ISIS-4 (Fourth International Study of Infarct Survival) Collaborative Group (1995) ISIS-4: a randomized factorial trial assessing early oral captopril, oral mononitrate, and intravenous magnesium sulphate in 58 050 patients with suspected acute myocardial infarction. *Lancet* 345: 669–685

12   Schulman KA, Glick HA, Ubin H, Eisenberg JM (1991) Cost-effectiveness of HA-1A monoclonal antibody for Gram-negative sepsis. *JAMA* 266: 3466–3471

13   Luce JM (1993) Introduction of new technology into critical care practice: A history of HA-1A monclonal antibody against endotoxin. *Crit Care Med* 21: 1233–1241

14   Bone RC, Balk RA, Cerra FB, Dellinger RP, Fein AM, Knaus WA et al (1992) Definitions for sepsis and organ failure and guidelines for the use of innovative therapies in sepsis. *Chest* 101: 1644–1655

15   Creery D, Marshall JC (1998) The failure of clinical trials in sepsis. Challenges of preclinical models. *This volume* 333–347

16   Standiford TJ, Strieter RM, Łukacs NW, Kunkel SL (1995) Neutralization of IL-10

increases lethality in endotoxemia. Co-operative effects of macrophage inflammatory protein-2 and tumor necrosis factor. *J Immunol* 155: 2222–2229

17 Kelly JP, Bancroft BJ (1996) Administration of interleukin-10 abolishes innate resistance to Listeria monocytogenes. *Eur J Immunol* 26: 356–364

18 Ziegler EJ, Fisher CJ, Sprung L et al (1991) Treatment of Gram-negative bacteremia and septic shock with HA-1A human monoclonal antibody against endotoxin. *N Engl J Med* 324: 429–436

19 McCloskey RV, Straube RC, Sanders C et al (1994) Treatment of septic shock with human monoclonal antibody HA-1A. A randomized, double-blind, placebo-controlled trial. *Ann Intern Med* 121: 1–5

20 Giroir BP (1993) Mediators of septic shock. New approaches for interrupting the endogenous inflammatory cascade. *Crit Care Med* 21: 780–789

21 Tracey KJ, Fong Y, Hesse DG, Manogue KR, Lee AT, Kuo GC, Lowry SF, Cerami A (1987) Anti-cachectin/TNF monoclonal antibodies prevent septic shock during lethal bacteremia. *Nature* 330: 662–664

22 Wakabayashi G, Gelfand JA, Burke JF, Thompson RC, Dinarelo CA (1991) A specific receptor antagonist for interleukin 1 prevents *Escherichia coli* induced shock in rabbits. *FASEB J* 5: 338–343

23 Warren HS, Danner RL, Munford RS (1992) Anti-endotoxin monoclonal antibodies. *N Engl J Med* 326: 1153–1157

24 Bone RC, Fisher CJ, Clemmer TP, Slotman GJ, Metz CA, Balk RA (1989) Sepsis syndrome: A valid clinical entity. *Crit Care Med* 17: 389–393

25 Bone RC, Fisher CJ, Clemmer TP, Slotman J, Metz CA, Balk RA (1987) A controlled clinical trial of high dose methylprednisolone in the treatment of severe sepsis and septic shock. *N Engl J Med* 317: 654–658

26 Casey LC, Balk RA, Bone RC (1993) Plasma cytokines and endotoxin levels correlate with survival in patients with the sepsis syndrome. *Ann Intern Med* 119: 771–778

27 Vincent JL (1997) Dear SIRS, I'm sorry to say that I don't like you. *Crit Care Med* 25: 372–374

28 Marshall JC (1997) Both the disposition and the means of cure: Severe SIRS, sterile shock, and the ongoing challenge of description. *Crit Care Med* 25: 1765–1766

29 Kett DH, Quartin AA, Sprung CL, Fisher CJ Jr, Pena MA, Heard SO, Zimmerman JL, Albertson TE, Panacek EA, Idelman LA, Schein RMH (1994) An evaluation of the hemodynamic effects of HA-1A human monoclonal antibody. *Crit Care Med* 22: 1227–1234

30 Vincent JL, Slotman G, van Leeuwen PAM, Shelly M, Nasraway SA, Tenaillon A, Bander J, Friedman G, on behalf of the substudy group on acute hemodynamic effects of IL-1ra. IL-1ra administration does not imporve cardiac function in patients with severe sepsis. *submitted*

31 Petros AJ, Marshall JC, Van Saene HKF (1995) Should morbidity replace mortality as an endpoint for clinical trials in intensive care? *Lancet* 345: 369–371

32 Hebert PC (1997) Mortality as an outcome in sepsis trials. *Sepsis* 1: 35–40

33   Marshall JC, Bernard G, Le Gall JR, Vincent JL (1997) The measurement of organ dysfunction/failure as an ICU outcome. *Sepsis* 1: 41–57

34   Marshall JC, Cook DJ, Christou NV, Bernard GR, Sprung CL, Sibbald WJ (1995) Multiple organ dysfunction score: A reliable descriptor of a complex clinical outcome. *Crit Care Med* 23: 1638–1652

35   Vincent JL, Moreno R, Takala J et al (1996) The SOFA (Sepsis-related Organ Failure Assessment) score to describe organ dysfunction/failure. *Intensive Care Med* 22: 707–710

36   Bernard GR, Doig G, Hudson G, et al (1995) Quantification of organ dysfunction for clinical trials in sepsis. *Am J Respir Crit Care Med* 151: A323

37   Le Gall JR, Klar J, Lemeshow S, Saulnier F, Alberti C, Artigas A, Teres D (1996) The Logistic Organ Dysfunction system. A new way to assess organ dysfunction in the intensive care unit. *JAMA* 276: 802–810

38   Dellinger RP for the ACCP, NIAID, NHLBI Workshop (1997) From the bench to the bedside: The future of sepsis research. *Chest* 111: 744–753, 1997

39   Van Deventer SJ, Buller HR, ten Cate JW, Aaarden LA, Hack CE, Sturk A (1990) Exerimental endotoxemia in humans: analysis of cytokine release and coagulation, fibrinolytic, and complement pathways. *Blood* 76: 2520–2526

40   Sprung CL, Finch RG, Thijs LG, Glauser MP (1996) International sepsis trial (INTERSEPT): role and impact of a clinical evaluation committee. *Crit Care Med* 24: 1441–1447

41   Marshall JC, Lowry SF (1995) Evaluation of the adequacy of source control in clinical trials in sepsis. In: Sibbald WJ, Vincent JL (eds): *Clinical trials for the treatment of sepsis*. Springer-Verlag, Heidelberg, 327–344

42   Sprung CL, Eidelman LA, Pizov R, Fisher CJ Jr, Ziegler J, Sadoff JC, Straube RC (1997) Influence of alterations in foregoing life-sustaining treatment practices on a clinical sepsis trial. *Crit Care Med* 25: 383–387

43   Van der Poll T, Coyle SM, Levi M, Jansen PM, Dentener M, Barbosa K, Buurman WA, Hack CE, ten Cate JW, Agosti JM, Lowry SF (1997) Effect of a recombinant dimeic tumor necrosis factor receptor on inflammatory responses to intravenous endotoxin in normal humans. *Blood* 89: 3727–3734

44   Pajrkt D, Doran DE, Koster F, Lerch PG, Arnet B, van der Poll T, ten Cate JW, van Deventer SJ (1996) Antiinflammatory effects of reconstituted high-density lipoprotein during human endotoxemia. *J Exp Med* 184: 1601–1608

45   Cohen J, Heumann D, Glauser MP (1995) Do monoclonal antibodies still have a future in infectious diseases? *Am J Med* 99 (Suppl 6A): 45S–52S

46   Sprung CL, Cohen J, Eidelman LA (1995) A plea for caution in the performance of sepsis trials. *Intensive Care Med* 21: 389–390.

Index

PIR
Progress in Inflammation Research

T Cells in Arthritis

Miossec P.,
Hôpital Edouard Herriot, Lyon, France /
van den Berg W.B.,
University Hospital Nijmegen, Netherlands / **Firestein G.S.,**
UCSD, La Jolla, USA (Ed.)

Rheumatoid arthritis (RA) is the most common and most severe form of inflammatory arthritis. The pathogenesis of RA has been the subject of intense research for several decades. The prevailing hypotheses have changed over the years, and have attempted to incorporate the most recent data. Although T cells represent an important component of the cells which infiltrate the joint synovium, their contribution at a late stage of the disease remains a matter of debate.

The goal of this book is to outline the major arguments and data suggesting that T cells may, or may not, be central players in the pathogenesis of chronic RA. While each of the editors and authors has his/her own bias (as will be clear by reading the respective chapters), our hope is that the readers will enjoy a complete and balanced view of the critical questions and experiments. This is not just an intellectual exercise since the direction of future therapeutic interventions depends heavily on how one interprets the pathogenesis of RA and the contribution of T cells.

Contents

Firestein G.S. and Nguyen K. H.Y.:
T cells as secondary players in rheumatoid arthritis

Fox D. A. and Singer N. G.:
T cell receptor rearrangements in arthritis

Franz J. K., Pap T., Müller-Ladner U., Gay R. E., Burmester G. R., Gay S.:
T cell-independent joint destruction

van den Berg W. B.:
Role of T cells in arthritis: lessons from animal models

Miossec P.
The Th1/ Th2 ccytokine balnce in arthritis

Burger D. and Dayer J.-M.
Interactions between T cell plasma membranes and monocytes

Oppenheimer-Marks N. and Lipsky P. E.
Adhesion molecules in arthritis: Control of T cell migration into the synovium

Bonneville M., Scotet E., Peyrat M.-A., Lim A., David-Ameline J., Houssaint E.:
T cell reactivity to Epstein-Barr virus in rheumatoid arthritis

Sieper J., Braun J.
T cell responses in reactive and lyme arthritis

Breedveld F. C.
T cell directed therapies and biologics

Falta M. T. and Kotzin B. L.
T cells as primary players in rheumatoid arthritis

	PIR – Progress in Inflammation Research
	Miossec P., et al (Ed.)
	T Cells in Arthritis
	1998. 238 pages. Hardcover
	sFr. 168.– / DM 198.– / öS 1446.–
	ISBN 3-7643-5853-X

BioSciences with Birkhäuser

(Prices are subject to change without notice. 9/98)

For orders originating from all over the world except USA and Canada:

Birkhäuser Verlag AG
P.O. Box 133
CH-4010 Basel / Switzerland
Fax: +41 / 61 / 205 07 92
e-mail: orders@birkhauser.ch

For orders originating in the USA and Canada:

Birkhäuser Boston, Inc.
333 Meadowland Parkway
USA-Secaucus, NJ 07094-2491
Fax: +1 / 201 348 4033
e-mail: orders@birkhauser.com

Birkhäuser

PIR
Progress in Inflammation Research

Chemokines and Skin

Kownatzki E. / Norgauer J.,
Albert-Ludwigs-Universität, Freiburg, Germany (Ed.)

http://www.birkhauser.ch

Check our Highlights for new and notable titles selected monthly in each field

The present volume summarizes the state of information on chemokines focussing on skin diseases. The first three chapters deal with the structure and molecular biology of chemokines and their receptors. The following three review information on the interaction of chemokines with lymphocytes, mast cells and eosinophilic granulocytes. One chapter deals with the expression of chemokines in several inflammatory skin diseases. The final chapter reports on in vitro evidence for a growth-promoting activity of chemokines in skin-derived tumor cells.

The volume is of use for the basic scientist interested in practical aspects and for the physician in search for basic mechanisms of skin diseases.

Contents

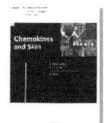

PIR - Progress in Inflammation Research
E. Kownatzki / J. Norgauer (Ed.)
Chemokines and Skin
1998. 140 pages. Hardcover
sFr. 148.– / DM 178.– / öS 1300.–
ISBN 3-7643-5818-1

BioSciences with Birkhäuser

(Prices are subject to change without notice. 9/98)

For orders originating from all over the world except USA and Canada:

For orders originating in the USA and Canada:

Birkhäuser Verlag AG
P.O. Box 133
CH-4010 Basel / Switzerland
Fax: +41 / 61 / 205 07 92
e-mail: orders@birkhauser.ch

Birkhäuser Boston, Inc.
333 Meadowland Parkway
USA-Secaucus, NJ 07094-2491
Fax: +1 / 201 348 4033
e-mail: orders@birkhauser.com

Birkhäuser

PIR
Progress in Inflammtion Research

Medicinal Fatty Acids in Inflammation

Kremer J.M.,
Albany Medical College, Albany, USA (Ed.)

This volume is a unique assembly of contributions focusing on the biochemical, immunological and clinical benefits of n-3 fatty acids in inflammation.

Leading clinical investigators from fields as diverse as rheumatology, dermatology, nephrology, gastroenterology and neurology have authored chapters. The basic scientific underpinnings of their findings are elucidated as well.

The work is a highly accessible, one-of-a-kind source which will well serve lipid researchers, graduate students, dieticians and members of the food industry.

Contents

List of contributors

Preface

Calder P. C.:
n-3 Polyunsaturated fatty acids and mononuclear phagocyte function

Zurier R. B.:
Gammalinolenic acid treatment of rheumatoid arthritis

Ziboh V. A.:
The role of n-3 fatty acids in psoriasis

Horrobin D. F.:
n-6 Fatty acids and nervous system diorders

Fernandes G.:
n-3 Fatty acids on autoimmune disease and apoptosis

Belluzzi A. and Miglio F.:
n-3 Fatty acids in the treatment of Crohn's disease

Rodgers J. B.:
n-3 Fatty acids in the treatment of ulcerative colitis

Geusens P. P.:
n-3 Fatty acids in the treatment of rheumatoid arthritis

Grande J. P. and Donadio J. V.:
n-3 Polyunsaturated fatty acids in the treatment of patients with IgA nephropathy

Subject index

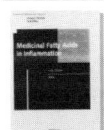

PIR – Progress in Inflammtion Research
Kremer J.M. (Ed.)
Medicinal Fatty Acids in Inflammation
1998. 154 pages. Hardcover
sFr. 148.– / DM 178.– / öS 1300.–
ISBN 3-7643-5854-8

BioSciences with Birkhäuser

(Prices are subject to change without notice. 9/98)

For orders originating from all over the world except USA and Canada:

For orders originating in the USA and Canada:

Birkhäuser Verlag AG
P.O. Box 133
CH-4010 Basel / Switzerland
Fax: +41 / 61 / 205 07 92
e-mail: orders@birkhauser.ch

Birkhäuser Boston, Inc.
333 Meadowland Parkway
USA-Secaucus, NJ 07094-2491
Fax: +1 / 201 348 4033
e-mail: orders@birkhauser.com

Birkhäuser